2012
YEAR BOOK OF
UROLOGY®

The 2012 Year Book Series

Year Book of Anesthesiology and Pain Management™: Drs Chestnut, Abram, Black, Gravlee, Lien, Mathru, and Roizen

Year Book of Cardiology®: Drs Gersh, Cheitlin, Elliott, Gold, Graham, and Thourani

Year Book of Critical Care Medicine®: Drs Dries, Zanotti-Cavazzoni, Latenser, Martinez, Rincon, and Zwank

Year Book of Dermatology and Dermatologic Surgery™: Dr Del Rosso

Year Book of Diagnostic Radiology®: Drs Elster, Abbara, Oestreich, Offiah, Rosado de Christenson, Stephens, and Strickland

Year Book of Emergency Medicine®: Drs Hamilton, Bruno, Handly, Minczak, Mullin, Quintana, and Ramoska

Year Book of Endocrinology®: Drs Schott, Apovian, Clarke, Eugster, Meikle, Oetgen, Ovalle, Schteingart, and Toth

Year Book of Hand and Upper Limb Surgery®: Drs Yao, Adams, Isaacs, Lee, and Rizzo

Year Book of Medicine®: Drs Barker, Garrick, Gersh, Khardori, LeRoith, Panush, Talley, and Thigpen

Year Book of Neonatal and Perinatal Medicine®: Drs Fanaroff, Benitz, Donn, Neu, Papile, and Van Marter

Year Book of Neurology and Neurosurgery®: Drs Klimo, Minagar, Gandhi, House, Kevill, Liu, Mazia, Panagariya, Ragel, Riesenburger, Robottom, Schwendimann, Shafazand, Uhm, and Yang

Year Book of Obstetrics, Gynecology, and Women's Health®: Drs Dungan and Shulman

Year Book of Oncology®: Drs Arceci, Bauer, Chiorean, Gordon, Lawton, Murphy, Thigpen, and Tsao

Year Book of Ophthalmology®: Drs Rapuano, Cohen, Flanders, Hammersmith, Milman, Myers, Nagra, Nelson, Penne, Pyfer, Sergott, Shields, Talekar, and Vander

Year Book of Orthopedics®: Drs Morrey, Huddleston, Rose, Swiontkowski, and Trigg

Year Book of Otolaryngology-Head and Neck Surgery®: Drs Sindwani, Balough, Franco, Gapany, and Mitchell

Year Book of Pathology and Laboratory Medicine®: Drs Raab and Bissell

Year Book of Pediatrics®: Dr Stockman

Year Book of Plastic and Aesthetic Surgery™: Drs Miller, Gosman, Gurtner, Gutowski, Ruberg, Salisbury, and Smith

2012
The Year Book of
UROLOGY®

Editors

Gerald L. Andriole, Jr, MD

Professor and Chief of Urology, Washington University School of Medicine; Chief of Urology, Barnes-Jewish Hospital, St Louis, Missouri

Douglas E. Coplen, MD

Associate Professor of Surgery (Urology), Washington University School of Medicine; Director of Pediatric Urology, St Louis Children's Hospital, St Louis, Missouri

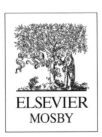

ELSEVIER
MOSBY

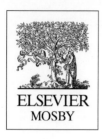

ELSEVIER
MOSBY

Vice President, Continuity: Kimberly Murphy
Editor: Stephanie Donley
Production Supervisor, Electronic Year Books: Donna M. Skelton
Electronic Article Manager: Mike Sheets
Illustrations and Permissions Coordinator: Dawn Vohsen

2012 EDITION

Printed and bound by CPI Group (UK) Ltd, Croydon, CR0 4YY
Composition by TNQ Books and Journals Pvt Ltd, India
Transferred to digital print 2012

Editorial Office:
Elsevier
Suite 1800
1600 John F. Kennedy Blvd
Philadelphia, PA 19103-2899

International Standard Serial Number: 0084-4071
International Standard Book Number: 978-0-323-08896-1

Contributors

Brian M. Benway, MD
Assistant Professor, Division of Urologic Surgery, Department of Surgery, Washington University School of Medicine, St Louis, Missouri

J. Quentin Clemens, MD
Associate Professor of Urology; Director, Division of Neurourology and Pelvic Reconstructive Surgery, University of Michigan, Ann Arbor, Michigan

Adam S. Kibel, MD
Chief of Urologic Surgery, Brigham and Women's Hospital; Professor of Urology, Harvard Medical School, Boston, Massachusetts

Venkatesh Krishnamurthi, MD
Director, Kidney/Pancreas Transplant, Cleveland Clinic Foundation, Cleveland, Ohio

Eric S. Rovner, MD
Professor of Urology, Medical University of South Carolina; Attending Surgeon, Medical University Hospital, Charleston, South Carolina

Alan Shindel, MD
Assistant Professor and Director of Men's Health, UC Davis School of Medicine, Sacramento, California

Table of Contents

Journals Represented

Journals represented in this YEAR BOOK are listed below.

Acta Obstetricia et Gynecologica Scandinavica
AJR American Journal of Roentgenology
American Journal of Infection Control
American Journal of Obstetrics and Gynecology
American Journal of Public Health
American Journal of Surgical Pathology
Archives of Internal Medicine
Archives of Sexual Behavior
British Journal of Medical & Surgical Urology
British Journal of Obstetrics and Gynaecology
British Journal of Urology International
British Medical Journal
Cancer
Circulation
Clinical Pediatrics
Clinical Pharmacology & Therapeutics
Clinical Radiology
European Urology
Fertility and Sterility
Gynecologic Oncology
International Journal of Epidemiology
Journal of Andrology
Journal of Clinical Oncology
Journal of General Internal Medicine
Journal of Orthopaedic Trauma
Journal of Pediatric Surgery
Journal of Pediatrics
Journal of Sexual Medicine
Journal of the American College of Cardiology
Journal of the American Geriatrics Society
Journal of the American Medical Association
Journal of the National Cancer Institute
Journal of Ultrasound in Medicine
Journal of Urology
Lancet
New England Journal of Medicine
Obstetrics & Gynecology
Pediatric Research
Pediatrics
Proceedings of the National Academy of Sciences of the United States of America
Scandinavian Journal of Urology and Nephrology
Seminars in Nuclear Medicine
Spine

Transplantation
Urology

STANDARD ABBREVIATIONS

The following terms are abbreviated in this edition: acquired immunodeficiency syndrome (AIDS), cardiopulmonary resuscitation (CPR), central nervous system (CNS), cerebrospinal fluid (CSF), computed tomography (CT), deoxyribonucleic acid (DNA), electrocardiography (ECG), health maintenance organization (HMO), human immunodeficiency virus (HIV), intensive care unit (ICU), intramuscular (IM), intravenous (IV), magnetic resonance (MR) imaging (MRI), ribonucleic acid (RNA), ultrasound (US), and ultraviolet (UV).

NOTE

The YEAR BOOK OF UROLOGY is a literature survey service providing abstracts of articles published in the professional literature. Every effort is made to assure the accuracy of the information presented in these pages. Neither the editors nor the publisher of the YEAR BOOK OF UROLOGY can be responsible for errors in the original materials. The editors' comments are their own opinions. Mention of specific products within this publication does not constitute endorsement.

To facilitate the use of the YEAR BOOK OF UROLOGY as a reference tool, all illustrations and tables included in this publication are now identified as they appear in the original article. This change is meant to help the reader recognize that any illustration or table appearing in the YEAR BOOK OF UROLOGY may be only one of many in the original article. For this reason, figure and table numbers will often appear to be out of sequence within the YEAR BOOK OF UROLOGY.

1 Clinical Outcomes

Accuracy of a urinary catheter surveillance protocol
Burns AC, Petersen NJ, Garza A, et al (Michael E. DeBakey Veterans Affairs Med Ctr, Houston, TX; et al)
Am J Infect Control 40:55-58, 2012

Background.—Many hospitals are increasing surveillance for catheter-associated urinary tract infections, which requires documentation of urinary catheter device-days. However, device-days are usually obtained by chart review or nursing reports. The aim of this study was to demonstrate that chart review can provide accurate urinary catheter data compared with physical inspection of the urinary catheter at the bedside.

Methods.—We compared 2 methods for collecting urinary catheter data over a 6-month period on 10 wards at our VA hospital. For the chart reviews, we created a daily bed-occupancy roster from the electronic medical record. Catheter data were extracted from the daily progress notes for each patient using a standardized review process. Bedside reviews were conducted by visiting the ward and verifying the presence and type of urinary catheters. Agreement between the 2 methods was calculated.

Results.—We obtained urinary catheter data by both methods in 621 cases. The presence or type of urinary catheter differed between chart and bedside review in only 10 cases (1.6%). Chart review had a sensitivity of 100%, a specificity of 97.7%, raw agreement of 98.4%, and a κ value of 0.96.

Conclusions.—Individual chart review in the electronic medical record provided very accurate data on urinary catheter use.

▶ The Center for Medicaid and Medicare Services (CMS) is focusing on decreasing or eliminating nosocomial infections. There has been a specific focus on catheter-associated urinary tract infection (CAUTI). Hospitals are developing and adopting care pathways aimed at reducing the rate of CAUTI. These guidelines and recommendations include surveillance for catheter use, which is necessary to ensure both appropriate catheter usage and to monitor whether interventions to decrease inappropriate catheter use are effective. Surveillance can be complicated by the fact that the medical record may not accurately reflect the presence of an indwelling urinary catheter or the indications for catheterization. The majority of catheters are generally placed without a physician's order and are maintained without specific documentation in the medical record. At the Houston Veteran's Administration Medical Clinic, catheter monitoring required chart-based and bedside spot checks by a full-time research assistant and the employ of a data coordinator. Although this approach is very accurate, it is also very time intensive and expensive. Use of electronic medial records is a practical way to automate and monitor patients by requiring, for example, nurses to document the presence and indications for all invasive devices on a regular basis. This will hopefully improve care and decrease the incidence of CAUTI.

D. E. Coplen, MD

Use, Costs and Comparative Effectiveness of Robotic Assisted, Laparoscopic and Open Urological Surgery

Yu H-Y, Hevelone ND, Lipsitz SR, et al (Harvard Med School, Boston, MA)
J Urol 187:1392-1398, 2012

Purpose.—Although robotic assisted laparoscopic surgery has been aggressively marketed and rapidly adopted, there are few comparative effectiveness studies that support its purported advantages compared to open and laparoscopic surgery. We used a population based approach to assess use, costs and outcomes of robotic assisted laparoscopic surgery vs laparoscopic surgery and open surgery for common robotic assisted urological procedures.

Materials and Methods.—From the Nationwide Inpatient Sample we identified the most common urological robotic assisted laparoscopic surgery procedures during the last quarter of 2008 as radical prostatectomy, nephrectomy, partial nephrectomy and pyeloplasty. Robotic assisted laparoscopic surgery, laparoscopic surgery and open surgery use, costs and inpatient outcomes were compared using propensity score methods.

Results.—Robotic assisted laparoscopic surgery was performed for 52.7% of radical prostatectomies, 27.3% of pyeloplasties, 11.5% of partial nephrectomies and 2.3% of nephrectomies. For radical prostatectomy robotic assisted laparoscopic surgery was more prevalent than open surgery among white patients in high volume, urban hospitals (all $p \leq 0.015$). Geographic variations were found in the use of robotic assisted laparoscopic surgery vs open surgery. Robotic assisted laparoscopic surgery and laparoscopic surgery vs open surgery were associated with shorter length of stay for all procedures, with robotic assisted laparoscopic surgery being the shortest for radical prostatectomy and partial nephrectomy (all $p < 0.001$). For most procedures robotic assisted laparoscopic surgery and laparoscopic surgery vs open surgery resulted in fewer deaths, complications, transfusions and more routine discharges. However, robotic assisted laparoscopic surgery was more costly than laparoscopic surgery and open surgery for most procedures.

Conclusions.—While robotic assisted and laparoscopic surgery are associated with fewer deaths, complications, transfusions and shorter length of hospital stay compared to open surgery, robotic assisted laparoscopic surgery is more costly than laparoscopic and open surgery. Additional studies are needed to better delineate the comparative and cost-effectiveness of robotic assisted laparoscopic surgery relative to laparoscopic surgery and open surgery.

▶ Robotic-assisted laparoscopy (RAL) has been widely adopted without evidence demonstrating superior outcomes compared with laparoscopic surgery and open surgery. Consumer advertising has resulted in patient demand for RAL. While RAL may be associated with a shorter length of hospital stay, decreased blood loss, and acute complications, it may be associated with a higher incidence of postoperative incontinence and erectile dysfunction.[1] The authors confirm the wide adoption of RAL for 4 different surgeries. The data set does not include disease-specific characteristics and does not allow assessment of long-term outcomes (eg, positive margins, cancer survival, recurrent obstruction requiring repeat pyeloplasty). It is clear that RAL is associated with increased cost when compared with laparoscopic surgery. Because the postprocedure morbidity is likely similar in both groups, it is imperative that future studies evaluate long-term outcomes and not just short-term hospitalization-related data that are not related to survival and quality of life.

D. E. Coplen, MD

Reference

1. Hu JC, Gu X, Lipsitz SR, et al. Comparative effectiveness of minimally invasive vs open radical prostatectomy. *JAMA*. 2009;302:1557-1564.

Repeated Botulinum Toxin Type A Injections for Refractory Overactive Bladder: Medium-Term Outcomes, Safety Profile, and Discontinuation Rates
Dowson C, Watkins J, Khan MS, et al (Guy's Hosp, London, UK; Guy's and St Thomas NHS Foundation Trust & King's College London School of Medicine, London, UK)
Eur Urol 61:834-839, 2012

Background.—Efficacy and safety of botulinum toxin type A (BoNTA) injection is supported by level 1 evidence, but data regarding repeated injections are limited in patients with refractory overactive bladder (OAB) and idiopathic detrusor overactivity (IDO).

Objectives.—Describe medium-term outcomes and discontinuation rates for patients adopting repeated BoNTA as a management strategy for IDO.

Design, Setting, and Participants.—Prospective data from a single centre were collected from the first 100 patients.

Intervention.—Bladder injection of BoNTA (predominantly 200 U onabotulinumtoxinA; Allergan Ltd., Marlow, Buckinghamshire, UK) in an outpatient setting.

Measurements.—OAB symptoms, quality of life, discontinuation rates, interinjection interval, and adverse events were recorded. Data comparisons were performed using a generalised linear model or a chi-square test where appropriate.

Results and Limitations.—Two hundred seven injections were performed in 100 patients. All patients had 1 injection, 53 had a total of 2, 20 had 3, 13 had 4, 10 had 5, 5 had 6, 3 had 7, 1 had 8, 1 had 9, and 1 had 10 injections. Statistics were applied up to five repeated injections. A statistically significant reduction in frequency, urgency, and urge urinary incontinence were seen following the first BoNTA injection compared to baseline. This improvement was maintained after repeated injections and was not statistically different when comparing differences between injections. Thirty-seven patients stopped treatment after the first two injections; thereafter, dropouts were rare. The most common reasons for discontinuing treatment were poor efficacy (13%) and clean intermittent self-catheterisation (CISC)—related issues (11%). The incidence of CISC after the first injection was 35%. Bacteriuria was detected in 21% of patients. The mean interinjection interval was 322 d. Limitations included the concurrent use of antimuscarinic drugs in some patients.

Conclusions.—BoNTA can provide a safe and effective medium-term management option for patients with refractory IDO. The most common reasons cited for stopping treatment were poor efficacy and CISC-related issues.

▶ Botulinum toxin injections are effective in reducing symptoms of both neurogenic overactive bladder (OAB) and idiopathic OAB. OnabotulinumtoxinA (Botox) is Food and Drug Administration (FDA)—approved for the treatment of neurogenic OAB, and a request for FDA approval of this agent for the treatment of idiopathic OAB has been submitted. Limited longitudinal data exist about the outcomes of serial onabotulinumtoxinA injections for idiopathic OAB. This study found that 25% of patients with idiopathic OAB did not proceed beyond the first injection, mostly because of a poor clinical response or development of urinary retention. The typical duration of response was 9 or 10 months, and the efficacy did not appear to decline with serial injections. These longitudinal results are virtually identical to those observed for the treatment of neurogenic OAB. Approximately 35% of patients required intermittent catheterization (IC) because of symptomatic residual urine volumes above 150 cc. As would be expected, those who required IC had a higher rate of urinary tract infection than those who did not. All of those who required IC after a single injection also required IC after subsequent injections with the same dose. It is important to note that the typical onabotulinumtoxinA dose administered in this study was 200 U. Previous studies have suggested that a dose of 100 U of this agent provides a similar effect with reduced incidence of urinary retention. Regardless of the dose administered, any patient considering this therapy must be willing and able to manage urinary retention should it occur.

J. Q. Clemens, MD

2 Clinical Research

Complications of Foley Catheters–Is Infection the Greatest Risk?
Leuck A-M, Wright D, Ellingson L, et al (Univ of Minnesota, Minneapolis)
J Urol 187:1662-1666, 2012

Purpose.—Foley catheters cause a variety of harms, including infection, pain and trauma. Although symptomatic urinary tract infection and asymptomatic bacteriuria are frequently discussed, genitourinary trauma receives comparatively little attention.

Materials and Methods.—A dedicated Foley catheter nurse prospectively reviewed the medical records of inpatients with a Foley catheter at the Minneapolis Veterans Affairs Medical Center from August 21, 2008 to December 31, 2009. Daily surveillance included Foley catheter related bacteriuria and trauma. Data were analyzed as the number of event days per 100 Foley catheter days.

Results.—During 6,513 surveyed Foley catheter days, urinalysis/urine culture was done on 407 (6.3%) days. This testing identified 116 possible urinary tract infection episodes (1.8% of Foley catheter days), of which only 21 (18%) involved clinical manifestations. However, the remaining 95 asymptomatic bacteriuria episodes accounted for 39 (70%) of 56 antimicrobial treated possible urinary tract infection episodes (for proportion of treated episodes with vs without symptomatic urinary tract infection manifestations, $p = 0.005$). Concurrently 100 instances of catheter associated genitourinary trauma (1.5% of Foley catheter days) were recorded, of which 32 (32%) led to interventions such as prolonged catheterization or cystoscopy. Trauma prompting an intervention accounted for as great a proportion of Foley catheter days (0.5%) as did symptomatic urinary tract infection (0.3%) ($p = 0.17$).

Conclusions.—In this prospective surveillance project, intervention triggering Foley catheter related genitourinary trauma was as common as symptomatic urinary tract infection. Moreover, despite recent increased attention to the distinction between asymptomatic bacteriuria and symptomatic urinary tract infection in catheterized patients, asymptomatic bacteriuria accounted for significantly more antimicrobial treatment than did symptomatic urinary tract infection. Elimination of unnecessary Foley catheter use could prevent symptomatic urinary tract infection, unnecessary antimicrobial therapy for asymptomatic bacteriuria and Foley catheter related trauma.

▶ In 2008, Medicare regulations stopped reimbursement for nosocomial catheter-associated urinary tract infections (UTIs). Obviously, there has been increased focus on this adverse outcome. It is concerning that asymptomatic bacteriuria is just as likely to be treated as a symptomatic UTI. This clearly increases the incidence of antimicrobial resistance. The authors evaluate other potential harms of Foley catheterization. They confirm that placement and maintenance of an indwelling catheter is not innocuous. Genitourinary trauma is at least as common a complication as symptomatic UTI. Although much of this trauma is minor, a urologic intervention was required in one-third of patients and long-term sequelae are unknown. The clinical focus should be reduction of unnecessary catheterization and not just UTI. The best way to avoid a complication of an indwelling urethral catheter is to decrease unnecessary catheter placement.

D. E. Coplen, MD

The prevalence of urinary incontinence 20 years after childbirth: a national cohort study in singleton primiparae after vaginal or caesarean delivery
Gyhagen M, Bullarbo M, Nielsen TF, et al (Sahlgrenska Academy at Gothenburg Univ, Sweden)
BJOG 2012 [Epub ahead of print]

Objective.—To investigate the prevalence and risk factors for urinary incontinence (UI) 20 years after one vaginal delivery or one caesarean section.

Design.—Registry-based national cohort study.

Setting.—Women who returned postal questionnaires (response rate 65.2%) in 2008.

Population.—Singleton primiparae who delivered in the period 1985–1988 with no further births ($n = 5236$).

Methods.—The Swedish Pregnancy, Obesity and Pelvic Floor (SWEPOP) study linked Medical Birth Register (MBR) data to a questionnaire about UI.

Main Outcome Measures.—Prevalence of UI and UI for more than 10 years (UI >10 years) were assessed 20 years after childbirth.

Results.—The prevalence of UI (40.3 versus 28.8%; OR 1.67; 95% CI 1.45–1.92) and UI >10 years (10.1 versus 3.9%; OR 2.75; 95% CI 2.02–3.75) was higher in women after vaginal delivery than after caesarean section. There was no difference in the prevalence of UI or UI >10 years after an acute caesarean section or an elective caesarean section. We found an 8% increased risk of UI per current body mass index (BMI) unit, and age at delivery increased the UI risk by 3% annually.

Conclusions.—Two decades after one birth, vaginal delivery was associated with a 67% increased risk of UI, and UI >10 years increased by 275% compared with caesarean section. Our data indicate that it is necessary to perform eight or nine caesarean sections to avoid one case of UI. Weight control is an important prophylactic measure to reduce UI. Current BMI was the most important BMI-determinant for UI, which is important, as BMI is modifiable.

▶ It is common to attribute female urinary incontinence (UI) to previous vaginal delivery, and yet the studies that have examined this association have yielded inconsistent results. This study differs from others in that it was limited to women who had delivered only a single child. This allowed a cleaner assessment of the effect of various methods of delivery on UI. The results make intuitive sense: vaginal delivery was associated with an increased risk of UI, and increased infant birth weight was associated with an increased risk of UI in women who delivered vaginally. Increased body mass index was also associated with increased UI risk. Other studies have demonstrated an increased risk of pelvic prolapse following vaginal delivery.

The authors note that 8 or 9 caesarian sections would need to be performed to prevent 1 case of UI. Prevention of future pelvic floor disorders is one reason women may choose elective caesarean section over vaginal delivery. However, this approach does not come without risks. At my institution, we are seeing more bladder injuries during caesarian section as well as more patients with placentas percreta—both are sequelae of prior caesarian section deliveries.

J. Q. Clemens, MD

3 Endourology and Stone Disease

Shock Wave Lithotripsy vs Ureteroscopy: Variation in Surgical Management of Kidney Stones at Freestanding Children's Hospitals
Wang H-HS, Huang L, Routh JC, et al (Children's Hosp Boston, MA)
J Urol 187:1402-1407, 2012

Purpose.—Although shock wave lithotripsy has long been considered the gold standard for treatment of kidney stones in children, ureteroscopy has become increasingly common. The factors determining procedure choice at individual centers are unclear. We sought to identify patient and hospital factors associated with the choice between shock wave lithotripsy and ureteroscopy.

Materials and Methods.—We searched the Pediatric Health Information System hospital database to identify patients with renal calculi who underwent inpatient or outpatient shock wave lithotripsy or ureteroscopy between 2000 and 2008. We used multivariate regression to evaluate whether procedure type was associated with hospital level factors, including treating hospital, region, size and teaching status, or patient level factors, including age, race, gender and insurance type.

Results.—We identified 3,377 children with renal stones, of whom 538 (16%) underwent surgery (shock wave lithotripsy in 48%, ureteroscopy in 52%). Procedures in 445 patients at hospitals performing both procedures were included. The relative proportion of ureteroscopy increased during the study period (24% from 2000 to 2002 vs 50% from 2006 to 2008, $p = 0.0001$). Procedure choice was not significantly associated with patient age ($p = 0.2$), gender ($p = 0.1$), race ($p = 0.07$), insurance ($p = 0.9$), hospital size ($p = 0.6$) or teaching status ($p = 0.99$). Procedure choice varied significantly by geographical region ($p = 0.05$), regional population ($p = 0.002$) and stone location ($p < 0.0001$). On multivariable analysis controlling for stone location, gender and treatment year the treating hospital was still highly associated with procedure choice.

Conclusions.—There is wide variation in procedure choice for children with kidney stones at freestanding children's hospitals in the United States.

Treatment choice depends significantly on the hospital at which a patient undergoes treatment.

▶ Over the last decade, ureteroscopic stone treatment has become increasingly popular in children secondary to technical advances and instrumentation. This database analysis shows increased utilization of ureteroscopy over an 8-year period. It is important to note that the authors excluded centers performing only ureteroscopy or shock wave lithotripsy (SWL) during this period. Ureteroscopic equipment is always available, but most pediatric centers do not have a dedicated shock wave lithotripsy machine, and this may impact therapeutic decision making in children requiring urgent intervention for symptomatic urolithiasis. Stone position was categorized as ureteral or renal, and the exact position may impact treatment modality. SWL is not utilized for treatment of distal ureteral stones in women and is associated with poorer results in lower pole calculi. There is no information on stone size, and there are no data on clinical outcomes. The authors are concerned about treatment variation. More data are required to ascertain whether clinical factors or institutional preferences drive treatment.

D. E. Coplen, MD

Metabolic Syndrome in Obese Adolescents is Associated with Risk for Nephrolithiasis
Tiwari R, Campfield T, Wittcopp C, et al (Baystate Med Ctr/Tufts Univ School of Medicine and Tufts Univ School of Medicine, Boston, MA)
J Pediatr 160:615-620, 2012

Objectives.—To examine the relationship between urinary pH and metabolic syndrome risk factors along with insulin resistance in obese adolescents, and to evaluate the relationship between other urinary stone-forming and -inhibiting markers and metabolic syndrome.

Study Design.—A total of 46 obese adolescents were enrolled. Twenty-four hour and randomly obtained urine samples were analyzed for urinary pH, promoters of stone formation (ie, uric acid, oxalate, and relative saturation ratio of calcium oxalate [RSR-CaOx]), and inhibitors of stone formation (ie, citrate and osteopontin). Other data collected included height, weight, blood pressure, and fasting lipid, insulin, and glucose levels.

Results.—The subjects had a mean age of 14.6 ± 2.0 years and a mean body mass index of 36 ± 6.3 kg/m^2. Random urine pH and the number of risk factors for metabolic syndrome were negatively correlated ($r = -0.34$; $P = .02$). RSR-CaOx was correlated with both homeostasis model assessment of insulin resistance score ($r = 0.38$; $P < .01$) and number of risk factors for metabolic syndrome ($r = 0.47$; $P = .001$).

Conclusion.—Decreased urinary pH and increased RSR-CaOx are associated with risk factors for metabolic syndrome in obese adolescents.

▶ The incidence of urolithiasis and obesity in children is increasing. It is unclear if there is any relationship between weight gain/diet and stone formation.

Insulin resistance alters renal ammonium production and decreases urinary pH. Urine pH is important in uric acid precipitation, which is important for both uric acid and calcium oxalate stone formation. The authors stratified urinalysis results by the number of metabolic syndrome risk factors (high-density lipoprotein level, triglycerides, blood pressure, abnormal fasting glucose, and type 2 diabetes). There was no correlation between obesity and urine pH or other stone-forming risk factors. The data show a strong relationship between urine pH, calcium oxalate saturation, and the number of risk factors for metabolic syndrome. These are possible mechanisms that increase the risk of stones in obese children, although none of the children in this study had a known history of stone disease. Certainly, if these risks develop in childhood, the lifetime risk of stone formation is higher.

D. E. Coplen, MD

Obstetric Complications of Ureteroscopy During Pregnancy
Johnson EB, Krambeck AE, White WM, et al (Dartmouth-Hitchcock Med Ctr, Lebanon, NH; Mayo Clinic, Rochester, MN; Univ of Tennessee Med Ctr, Knoxville; et al)
J Urol 188:151-154, 2012

Purpose.—During pregnancy a ureteral stone and its management may pose risks for the mother and fetus. Definitive ureteroscopic management of an obstructing stone during pregnancy has been increasingly used without a reported increased incidence of urological complications. However, the rate of obstetric complications of ureteroscopy during pregnancy remains undefined.

Materials and Methods.—Charts of pregnant women who had undergone ureteroscopy at 5 tertiary centers were reviewed. Patient and procedure characteristics were collected. Records were evaluated for the occurrence of obstetric complications in the postoperative period.

Results.—A total of 46 procedures were performed in 45 patients at 5 institutions. There were 2 obstetric complications (4.3%), including 1 preterm labor managed conservatively and 1 preterm labor resulting in preterm delivery. There was no fetal loss. No statistically significant characteristics were identified differentiating those patients having obstetric complications.

Conclusions.—Ureteroscopy performed during pregnancy has been previously reported to be urologically safe and effective for addressing ureteral stones. In our multi-institutional series a 4% rate of obstetric complications was observed. Based on this risk a multidisciplinary approach is prudent for the pregnant patient undergoing ureteroscopy.

▶ When the symptoms of urolithiasis during pregnancy are refractory to analgesics, antiemetics, and hydration, a ureteral stent or percutaneous nephrostomy can be placed. These interventions are definitively indicated when urolithiasis is complicated by infection. The authors evaluate outcomes of therapeutic ureteroscopy performed during the second and third trimester of pregnancy. There was no fetal loss in 45 cases. A stone was not identified in 7 patients. A low-dose computed tomography (CT) scan was falsely positive in 1 patient, but ultrasound can and magnetic resonance imaging were falsely positive in 28% and 20%, respectively. The sensitivity of the preprocedure imaging needs to be considered prior to proceeding with ureteroscopy in pregnant patients. Fluoroscopy time was not reported in these patients. The risk of obtaining low-dose CT and intra-operative radiation exposure to the fetus needs to be considered, although this is in theory safer later in pregnancy. However, given the current concerns regarding radiation exposure in children, the decision to proceed with ureteroscopy during pregnancy should not be taken lightly.

D. E. Coplen, MD

4 Transplantation

A Simplified Donor Risk Index for Predicting Outcome After Deceased Donor Kidney Transplantation

Watson CJE, Johnson RJ, Birch R, et al (Addenbrooke's Hosp, Cambridge, UK; NHS Blood and Transplant, Bristol, UK)
Transplantation 93:314-318, 2012

Background.—We sought to determine the deceased donor factors associated with outcome after kidney transplantation and to develop a clinically applicable Kidney Donor Risk Index.

Methods.—Data from the UK Transplant Registry on 7620 adult recipients of adult deceased donor kidney transplants between 2000 and 2007 inclusive were analyzed. Donor factors potentially influencing transplant outcome were investigated using Cox regression, adjusting for significant recipient and transplant factors. A United Kingdom Kidney Donor Risk Index was derived from the model and validated.

Results.—Donor age was the most significant factor predicting poor transplant outcome (hazard ratio for 18−39 and 60+ years relative to 40−59 years was 0.78 and 1.49, respectively, $P < 0.001$). A history of donor hypertension was also associated with increased risk (hazard ratio 1.30, $P = 0.001$), and increased donor body weight, longer hospital stay before death, and use of adrenaline were also significantly associated with poorer outcomes up to 3 years posttransplant. Other donor factors including donation after circulatory death, history of cardiothoracic disease, diabetes history, and terminal creatinine were not significant. A donor risk index based on the five significant donor factors was derived and confirmed to be prognostic of outcome in a validation cohort (concordance statistic 0.62). An index developed in the United States by Rao et al., Transplantation 2009; 88: 231−236, included 15 factors and gave a concordance statistic of 0.63 in the UK context, suggesting that our much simpler model has equivalent predictive ability.

Conclusions.—A Kidney Donor Risk Index based on five donor variables provides a clinically useful tool that may help with organ allocation and informed consent.

▶ Given the increasing number of kidney transplant candidates and the relatively stable number of organ donors, greater numbers of "marginal" donors are being considered for transplantation. The long-term success of these donor organs is expected to be inferior, but the degree of diminished survival is unclear. Transplant physicians may benefit from a tool that aids in predicting graft survival.

In this study, the authors examined the outcome of 7620 primary deceased donor renal transplants during a contemporary era (January 2000 to December 2007) in the United Kingdom. Using 60% of this population (4570 transplants), they developed a predictive model for kidney transplant survival over 3 prespecified time periods: 0 to 3 months, 3 months to 3 years, and more than 3 years. In the development of the model, the investigators controlled for recipient characteristics known to affect survival, such as age, primary renal disease, gender, human leukocyte antigen match and others. Five donor characteristics were found to be significantly predictive for graft survival at the various time points: age, history of hypertension, weight, days in hospital, and use of epinephrine. Both donor age and history of hypertension were also significantly predictive of overall survival. Based on these 5 characteristics, the authors developed an easily computable donor risk index in which the "reference" donor had a risk index equal to 1. Donor with improved survival had an index less than 1, and donors with diminished survival compared with the reference group had an index greater than 1. The model was then applied to the remaining 40% of the population (3050 transplants) and found to have reasonable predictive ability (concordance statistic $= 0.62$).

The utility of this manuscript lies in the relative simplicity of the risk index calculation. As the authors indicate, only 5 donor characteristics are required. Interestingly, the investigators compared this model with a similar index developed on United States transplant recipients. Although the US index required 15 donor variables, its predictive ability was equal to that of the UK donor risk index.

Transplant professionals should familiarize themselves with this article and develop a comfort level in using the donor risk index. Understandably, variables that are often predictive of donor quality, such as donor cause of death, were not predictive in this model, and the significance of their absence remains to be studied. By using the authors' relatively simple calculation, donor quality can be readily assessed, which can allow a more informed discussion with a potential recipient regarding the short- and long-term graft survival following kidney transplantation.

V. Krishnamurthi, MD

Management of Primary Symptomatic Lymphocele After Kidney Transplantation: A Systematic Review

Lucewicz A, Wong G, Lam VWT, et al (The Univ of Sydney, Australia)
Transplantation 92:663-673, 2011

Background.—Management of lymphoceles after kidney transplantation is highly variable. The aim of this study was to evaluate and compare the different approaches of lymphocele management among kidney transplant recipients.

Methods.—MEDLINE and EMBASE were systematically searched for case studies published between 1954 and 2010. Inclusion criteria were symptomatic lymphoceles developing in recipients of deceased or living donor kidneys with specified intervention and outcome. Primary outcome was the rate of recurrence. Secondary outcomes were the rate of conversion from laparoscopic to open surgery, hospital stay, and complication rates.

Results.—Fifty-two retrospective case series with 1113 cases of primary lymphocele were selected for review. No randomized controlled trials or prospective cohort studies were located. Primary treatment modalities included were as follows: aspiration (n=218), sclerotherapy (n=155), drainage (n=219), laparoscopic surgery (n=333), and open surgery (n=188). Of the 218 cases of lymphocele managed with aspiration alone, 141 recurred with a recurrence rate of 59% (95% confidence interval [CI]: 52—67). Among those who received laparoscopic and open surgery, the recurrence rates were 8% (95% CI: 6—12) and 16% (95% CI: 10—24), respectively. The conversion rate from laparoscopic to open surgery was 12% (95% CI: 8—16).

Conclusions.—Laparoscopic fenestration of a symptomatic lymphocele is associated with the lowest risk of lymphocele recurrence. However, the evidence base to support a recommendation for laparoscopic surgery as first line treatment is weak and highlights the need for a multicenter prospective cohort study to examine the benefits of incorporating initial simple aspiration into the management of lymphocele after kidney transplantation.

▶ Lymphoceles remain relatively common surgical complications following kidney transplantation. Predisposing factors for lymphocele formation, the incidence of symptomatic lymphoceles and the efficacy of the various treatment options are not well known. Perhaps the main reason for this lack of knowledge is the infrequent occurrence of lymphocele and lack of standardized imaging, treatment, and follow-up approaches.

In this meta-analysis, the authors reviewed existing literature between 1954 and 2010 and identified articles analyzing symptomatic lymphoceles. Because there were no prospective, controlled trials, the authors identified 52 retrospective studies yielding 1113 patients. Of note, all of the studies were retrospective, did not always contain a control group, and frequently had variable and incomplete patient follow-up.

The incidence of symptomatic lymphocele was approximately 5%. Five therapeutic options (simple aspiration, sclerotherapy, drain placement, laparoscopic marsupialization, and open surgical marsupialization) were compared for treatment efficacy (recurrence free outcome) and complications.

Laparoscopic marsupialization had the lowest lymphocele recurrence rate at 8%, along with a low complication rate of approximately 7%. Approximately 12% of laparoscopic cases were converted to open procedures. Although the complication rate for percutaneous procedures was low, the lymphocele recurrence rate was approximately 50%.

The strength of this study lies in the fact that it is the first comprehensive review of the literature. The study includes a large patient population and accurately acknowledges the limitations in analyzing small, uncontrolled retrospective studies. Notwithstanding these limitations, this study provides important information about a common problem that many transplant practioners will encounter.

V. Krishnamurthi, MD

5 Female Urology

Diagnostics

Changes in Urodynamic Measures Two Years After Burch Colposuspension or Autologous Sling Surgery

Kraus SR, for the Urinary Incontinence Treatment Network (Univ of Texas Health Sciences Ctr, San Antonio; et al)
Urology 78:1263-1268, 2011

Objective.—To characterize the urodynamic (UDS) changes in subjects 24 months after Burch urethropexy and autologous fascial sling surgery for stress urinary incontinence.

Methods.—In the Stress Incontinence Surgical Treatment Efficacy Trial (SISTEr), 655 women underwent standardized UDSs before and 2 years after Burch or sling surgery. Paired t tests were used to compare the pre- and postoperative UDS measures by treatment group. Analysis of variance models were fit predicting the change in UDS measures, controlling for the treatment group.

Results.—The noninstrumented maximal flow rate decreased 3.6 mL/s in the Burch group and 4.7 mL/s in the sling group ($P = .42$). The average flow rates also decreased (2.4 mL/s in the Burch group and 3.8 mL/s in the sling group, $P = .039$). No difference was found in the increases in first sensation between the Burch and sling groups (23.3 and 29.3 mL, respectively, $P = .61$). Also, no differences were found in the reduction in the pressure flow study maximal flow rates (2.3 mL/s in the Burch group and 4.4 mL/s in the sling group, $P = .11$). An increased detrusor pressure at maximal flow rate (11.4 cm H_2O, $P < .001$) was seen only after the sling procedure. Increases in the bladder outlet obstruction index occurred after both procedures, with greater increases seen after sling surgery (change, Burch +6.27 vs sling +20.12, $P = .001$).

Conclusion.—The Burch colposuspension and autologous fascial sling procedures were associated with similar decreases in noninstrumented flow rates, and the sling was associated with greater increases in the detrusor pressure at maximal flow rate and bladder outlet obstruction index. These changes suggest that both procedures are effective, in part, because of increased outlet resistance. However, the sling procedure might be more obstructive.

▶ In yet another analysis following the Stress Incontinence Surgical Treatment Efficacy Trial (SISTEr), these investigators looked at urodynamic changes

2 years postoperatively. The data suggest that both procedures are, to some degree, obstructive in nature, since there was an increase in the bladder outlet obstruction index in both groups. Additionally, based on urodynamic parameters, the sling appeared to be somewhat more obstructive than the Burch procedure. In the initial publication of this dataset, there was a higher rate of de novo voiding dysfunction in the sling group, which was also suggestive of a greater degree of obstruction in this group.

There are some significant limitations to this urodynamic dataset. The most obvious is that only 180 of the 655 patients had satisfactory pressure flow urodynamic data for analysis. Although the authors note that there was no significant bias in the patients who remained for analysis in both groups, it would seem that patients who would be more likely to follow-up would be those who had some degree of difficulty after their initial procedure. If such a bias did exist, the urodynamic data in this paper may be misleading with respect to its conclusions.

E. S. Rovner, MD

The Impact of OAB on Sexual Health in Men and Women: Results from EpiLUTS

Coyne KS, Sexton CC, Thompson C, et al (United BioSource Corporation, Bethesda, MD; et al)
J Sex Med 8:1603-1615, 2011

Introduction.—Prior research suggests that overactive bladder (OAB) is common and adversely affects sexuality in both men and women. However, more data are needed from population-based studies to evaluate the impact OAB on sexual health.

Aim.—To describe sexual health outcomes in men and women with continent and incontinent OAB (C-OAB, I-OAB) compared to those with no/minimal urinary symptoms (NMS) and to evaluate correlates of decreased sexual activity and enjoyment in men and women, and correlates of erectile dysfunction (ED), ejaculatory dysfunction (EjD), and premature ejaculation (PE) in men.

Methods.—A cross-sectional, population-representative survey was conducted via the Internet in the United Kingdom, Sweden, and United States. OAB was assessed via a questionnaire based on current International Continence Society definitions. Descriptive statistics were used to compare outcomes for those with I-OAB, C-OAB and NMS, and logistic regressions were used to evaluate predictors of sexual functioning.

Main Outcome Measures.—Participants responding to the sexual health portion of the survey were asked questions about sexual activity and satisfaction. Other outcomes included two domains from the Abbreviated Sexual Function Questionnaire, the erectile function domain of the International Index of Erectile Function, and questions assessing EjD and PE.

Results.—Survey response was 59.2%; 6,326 men and 8,085 women participated in the sexual health portion of the survey. Across outcomes,

I-OAB and C-OAB were associated with worse sexual health as compared to those with NMS. Logistic regressions showed that those with I-OAB and C OAB were significantly ($P < 0.0001$) more likely to report diminished sexual activity and enjoyment of sex. I-OAB and C-OAB were also significant predictors of ED and EjD in men, but not PE.

Conclusions.—The impact of OAB is evident across domains of sexual health in both men and women. Sexual health should be assessed in men and women presenting with OAB.

▶ The intimate relationship between the organs of urination and sexual function makes it a foregone conclusion that issues with one organ system will predispose an individual to problems with the other. This has been well established with respect to erectile dysfunction (ED) and benign prostate hyperplasia in men and incontinence and sexual dysfunction in women. This large-scale internet study investigates the coincidence of lower urinary tract symptoms and sexual problems in both men and women. It was determined that symptoms of overactive bladder (OAB), with or without incontinence, portended poorer sexual function, lower sexual frequency, decreased enjoyment of sex, and higher risk of pain in the bladder during sex for both genders. In women, decreased desire and arousal were more prevalent with increasing OAB symptoms. In men, ED and ejaculatory dysfunction (both premature and delayed) were more prevalent. These relationships were maintained even after multivariate adjustment for age, health, and demographic factors.

It is incumbent on providers evaluating patients with complaints of OAB to inquire about sexual perturbations.

A. W. Shindel, MD

Interstitial Cystitis

Randomized Multicenter Clinical Trial of Myofascial Physical Therapy in Women With Interstitial Cystitis/Painful Bladder Syndrome and Pelvic Floor Tenderness

Fitzgerald MP, for the Interstitial Cystitis Collaborative Research Network (Loyola Univ Med Ctr, Maywood, IL; et al)
J Urol 187:2113-2118, 2012

Purpose.—We determined the efficacy and safety of pelvic floor myofascial physical therapy compared to global therapeutic massage in women with newly symptomatic interstitial cystitis/painful bladder syndrome.

Materials and Methods.—A randomized controlled trial of 10 scheduled treatments of myofascial physical therapy vs global therapeutic massage was performed at 11 clinical centers in North America. We recruited women with interstitial cystitis/painful bladder syndrome with demonstrable pelvic floor tenderness on physical examination and a limitation of no more than 3 years' symptom duration. The primary outcome was the proportion of responders defined as moderately improved or markedly improved in overall symptoms compared to baseline on a 7-point global response assessment scale. Secondary outcomes included ratings for pain, urgency and frequency, the O'Leary-Sant IC Symptom and Problem Index, and reports of adverse events. We compared response rates between treatment arms using the exact conditional version of the Mantel-Haenszel test to control for clustering by clinical center. For secondary efficacy outcomes cross-sectional descriptive statistics and changes from baseline were calculated.

Results.—A total of 81 women randomized to the 2 treatment groups had similar symptoms at baseline. The global response assessment response rate was 26% in the global therapeutic massage group and 59% in the myofascial physical therapy group ($p = 0.0012$). Pain, urgency and frequency ratings, and O'Leary-Sant IC Symptom and Problem Index decreased in both groups during followup, and were not significantly different between the groups. Pain was the most common adverse event, occurring at similar rates in both groups. No serious adverse events were reported.

Conclusions.—A significantly higher proportion of women with interstitial cystitis/painful bladder syndrome responded to treatment with myofascial physical therapy than to global therapeutic massage. Myofascial physical therapy may be a beneficial therapy in women with this syndrome.

▶ The AUA Guidelines for Interstitial Cystitis/Bladder Pain Syndrome (IC/BPS) list pelvic floor physical therapy (PFPT) as a second-line therapy, after patient education and behavioral modification. This trial provides level I evidence that PFPT is effective. For study inclusion, the IC/BPS patients had to demonstrate pelvic floor muscle tenderness on examination—identified by transvaginal palpation of the levator muscles, which are located posterolaterally. This is not something that most urologists are trained to evaluate, but it is not difficult to do. It is not known if PFPT is effective in women who do not demonstrate muscle tenderness on examination. The active therapy group received focused pelvic floor therapy, including vaginal tissue manipulation, from highly trained therapists and nurses. The control group received standard massage therapy, similar to what would be offered at a hotel spa. Studies suggest that the majority of women with IC/BPS have pelvic muscle tenderness, and I have found this therapy to be among the most effective that we have to offer. It is important that the therapy is provided by someone with expertise in pelvic floor tissue manipulation. Many therapists are accustomed to treating women who have incontinence, where the goal is to improve pelvic muscle strength (Kegel exercises, etc). In patients with pelvic pain, muscle strengthening exercises like these can worsen their symptoms. In contrast, PFPT in this setting is oriented toward improving range of motion, muscle relaxation, and reducing muscle pain.

J. Q. Clemens, MD

Non-Pharmacologic Therapy

Fluid intake and risk of stress, urgency, and mixed urinary incontinence
Townsend MK, Jura YH, Curhan GC, et al (Brigham and Women's Hosp and Harvard Med School, Boston, MA; Massachusetts General Hosp and Harvard Med School, Boston, MA; et al)
Am J Obstet Gynecol 205:73.e1-73.e6, 2011

Objective.—We investigated the relation between total fluid intake and incident urinary incontinence in the Nurses' Health Study cohorts.

Study Design.—We measured daily fluid intake using food frequency questionnaires among 65,167 women, who were 37-79 years old, without urinary incontinence at study baseline (2000-2001). Women reported incontinence incidence on questionnaires during 4 years of follow-up evaluation. Multivariable-adjusted hazard ratios and 95% confidence intervals were calculated with Cox proportional hazards models.

Results.—We found no association between total fluid intake and risk of incident incontinence (hazard ratio, 1.04; 95% confidence interval, 0.98—1.10; comparing top vs bottom quintile of fluid intake). In analyses of incontinence type, total fluid intake was not associated with risks of incident stress, urgency, or mixed incontinence.

Conclusion.—No significant risk of incident urinary incontinence was found with higher fluid intake in women. These findings suggest that women should not restrict their fluid intake to prevent incontinence development.

▶ This is an interesting secondary analysis from the Nurses' Health Study (NHS) cohorts. These authors looked at a large number of continent women at entry into the NHS I and II datasets and found that there was no association between total fluid intake and development of urinary incontinence during the study. Although a substantial number of the patients developed urinary incontinence over the 4 years of follow-up, there was no relationship between the fluid intake and the development of incontinence. These results should not be extrapolated to mean that fluid intake does not impact either urinary symptoms in continent women or incontinent women or symptoms in those who already are incontinent. There are many studies suggesting that alteration of fluid intake in patients who are incontinent can substantially and favorably impact their symptoms.

E. S. Rovner, MD

Pelvic Prolapse

Reanalysis of a randomized trial of 3 techniques of anterior colporrhaphy using clinically relevant definitions of success

Chmielewski L, Walters MD, Weber AM, et al (Cleveland Clinic, OH)
Am J Obstet Gynecol 205:69.e1-69.e8, 2011

Objective.—The purpose of this study was to reanalyze the results of a previously published trial that compared 3 methods of anterior colporrhaphy according to the clinically relevant definitions of success.

Study Design.—A secondary analysis of a trial of 114 subjects who underwent surgery for anterior pelvic organ prolapse who were assigned randomly to standard anterior colporrhaphy, ultralateral colporrhaphy, or anterior colporrhaphy plus polyglactin 910 mesh from 1996–1999. For the current analysis, success was defined as (1) no prolapse beyond the hymen, (2) the absence of prolapse symptoms (visual analog scale ≤2), and (3) the absence of retreatment.

Results.—Eighty-eight percent of the women met our definition of success at 1 year. One subject (1%) underwent surgery for recurrence 29 months after surgery. No differences among the 3 groups were noted for any outcomes.

Conclusion.—Reanalysis of a trial of 3 methods of anterior colporrhaphy revealed considerably better success with the use of clinically relevant outcome criteria compared with strict anatomic criteria.

▶ A randomized trial that compared 3 different methods of surgical correction of anterior vaginal prolapse was published in 2001.[1] Using an anatomic definition of failure (recurrent descent of the anterior vaginal wall to within 1 cm of the hymenal ring), the authors reported a 2-year success rate of only 30% to 46% depending on the surgical technique used. This study was frequently interpreted to indicate that the success of traditional prolapse repair techniques was unacceptably low and to justify the use of mesh-augmented techniques or alternative techniques (eg, abdominal sacral colpopexy) for the treatment of anterior vaginal wall prolapse. In this study, the authors reanalyzed the data at 1 year (to minimize the impact of missing data) and defined success as (1) no prolapse beyond the hymen, (2) absence of prolapse symptoms, and (3) absence of retreatment for prolapse (surgery or pessary). They found that 88% of the women had a successful outcome at 1 year.

These findings indicate that the outcomes of prolapse repair vary considerably based on the definition used, and that anatomic outcomes do not correlate well with patient-reported outcomes. They also suggest that the outcomes of traditional anterior repair techniques may not be as poor as previously thought. Of course, these results are only at 1 year, and it remains to be seen if patients remain satisfied with longer follow-up.

J. Q. Clemens, MD

Reference

1. Weber AM, Walters MD, Piedmonte MR, Ballard LA. Anterior colporrhaphy: a randomized trial of three surgical techniques. *Am J Obstet Gynecol.* 2001;185: 1299-1306.

Trocar-Guided Mesh Compared With Conventional Vaginal Repair in Recurrent Prolapse: A Randomized Controlled Trial

Withagen MI, Milani AL, den Boon J, et al (Radboud Univ Nijmegen Med Centre, The Netherlands; Reinier de Graaf Group, Delft, The Netherlands; Isala Clinics, Zwolle, The Netherlands; et al)

Obstet Gynecol 117:242-250, 2011

Objective.—To compare efficacy and safety of trocar-guided tension-free vaginal mesh insertion with conventional vaginal prolapse repair in patients with recurrent pelvic organ prolapse.

Methods.—Patients with recurrent pelvic organ prolapse stage II or higher were randomly assigned to either conventional vaginal prolapse surgery or polypropylene mesh insertion. Primary outcome was anatomic failure (pelvic organ prolapse stage II or higher) in the treated vaginal compartments. Secondary outcomes were subjective improvement, effects on bother, quality of life, and adverse events. Questionnaires such as the Incontinence Impact Questionnaire and Urogenital Distress Inventory were administered at baseline, 6 months, and 12 months. Anatomic outcomes were assessed by an unblinded surgeon. Power calculation with $\alpha=0.05$ and $\beta=0.80$ indicated that 194 patients were needed.

Results.—Ninety-seven women underwent conventional repair and 93 mesh repair. The follow-up rate after 12 months was 186 of 190 patients (98%). Twelve months postsurgery, anatomic failure in the treated compartment was observed in 38 of 84 patients (45.2%) in the conventional group and in eight of 83 patients (9.6%) in the mesh group ($P < .001$; odds ratio, 7.7; 95% confidence interval, 3.3—18). Patients in either group reported less bulge and overactive bladder symptoms. Subjective improvement was reported by 64 of 80 patients (80%) in the conventional group compared with 63 of 78 patients (81%) in the mesh group. Mesh exposure was detected in 14 of 83 patients (16.9%).

Conclusion.—At 12 months, the number of anatomic failures observed after tension-free vaginal mesh insertion was less than after conventional vaginal prolapse repair. Symptom decrease and improvement of quality of life were equal in both groups.

Clinical Trial Registration.—ClinicalTrials.gov, www.clinicaltrials.gov, NCT00372190.

Level of Evidence.—I.

▶ The use of vaginal mesh for the treatment of pelvic organ prolapse (POP) has been a subject of considerable debate, given the recent Food and Drug

Administration warning about these techniques (http://www.fda.gov/medical devices/safety/alertsandnotices/publichealthnotifications/ucm061976.htm; http://www.fda.gov/medicaldevices/safety/alertsandnotices/ucm262435.htm). The results from this randomized controlled trial from the Netherlands underscore the primary discussion points in this controversy.

1. In this study, the use of vaginal mesh was associated with better anatomic outcomes at 12 months' follow-up in women with recurrent pelvic prolapse. Similar results have been observed in other clinical trials, and proponents of mesh techniques use these results to suggest that mesh techniques are superior.

2. Despite the observed anatomic differences, symptomatic vaginal bulge symptoms reported by the patients did not differ between the mesh and nonmesh groups. In other words, while the vaginal support appeared better on examination after mesh placement, this difference was not detectable for the patients. This has also been observed in previous clinical trials.

3. At 12 months, vaginal mesh extrusion was observed in 17% of women who had mesh placed. It is clear that the use of mesh for POP repair is associated with unique complications, some of which can be debilitating. Minor vaginal mesh extrusions can be observed expectantly or can be treated with simple office excision under local anesthesia. However, some mesh extrusions involve large areas of the mesh and require 1 or more operative procedures to address. Mesh erosion (into the urethra or bladder) may also occur (although none were observed in this study); these are associated with much greater morbidity and are more difficult to treat.

4. Pelvic pain and dyspareunia were common before and after surgery, whether or not mesh was placed. At baseline, 26% of the women reported pelvic or abdominal pain, and 29% of sexually active women reported dyspareunia. These symptoms resolved in approximately 10% of patients after surgery, while another approximately 10% developed de novo pain after the surgery. In this study, these postoperative pain outcomes were not impacted by the use of mesh. It is clear that vaginal mesh placement can result in persistent pain that necessitates mesh removal. In some patients, the pain symptoms can persist even after the mesh is removed. However, it is important to recognize that postoperative pain can also occur after nonmesh POP surgery.

5. This study assessed outcomes after 12 months, which is typical for trials of surgical treatments for POP. Of course, patients undergo POP surgery with an expectation that the results will last much longer than 12 to 24 months, but at this time we have no long-term data related to vaginal mesh outcomes. It is not clear whether the improved short-term anatomic outcomes seen with mesh techniques will ultimately translate into improved clinical outcomes as well. Similarly, it is unknown whether mesh-related complications such as extrusions and erosions are mostly a short-term phenomenon. Until longer-term studies are available, the debate about mesh will continue to be fueled by inadequate data.

6. The results appeared to differ considerably across treatment sites. For instance, vaginal exposure rates varied from 0% to 100% across the 13

participating treatment centers. This finding suggests that complications associated with vaginal mesh may be attributed to the surgeon rather than to the mesh techniques themselves. However, even if this were true, the specific reasons for poor outcomes are not currently clear. Are there technical differences or errors that result in high extrusion rates? Or is proper patient selection the most important factor? Or both?

J. Q. Clemens, MD

Reconstructions/Outcomes

5-Year Continence Rates, Satisfaction and Adverse Events of Burch Urethropexy and Fascial Sling Surgery for Urinary Incontinence

Brubaker L, for the Urinary Incontinence Treatment Network (Loyola Univ Chicago, IL; et al)
J Urol 187:1324-1330, 2012

Purpose.—We characterized continence, satisfaction and adverse events in women at least 5 years after Burch urethropexy or fascial sling with longitudinal followup of randomized clinical trial participants.

Materials and Methods.—Of 655 women who participated in a randomized surgical trial comparing the efficacy of the Burch and sling treatments 482 (73.6%) enrolled in this long-term observational study. Urinary continence status was assessed yearly for a minimum of 5 years postoperatively. Continence was defined as no urinary leakage on a 3-day voiding diary, and no self-reported stress incontinence symptoms and no stress incontinence surgical re-treatment.

Results.—Incontinent participants were more likely to enroll in the followup study than continent patients (85.5% vs 52.2%) regardless of surgical group ($p < 0.0001$). Overall the continence rates were lower in the Burch urethropexy group than in the fascial sling group ($p = 0.002$). The continence rates at 5 years were 24.1% (95% CI 18.5 to 29.7) vs 30.8% (95% CI 24.7 to 36.9), respectively. Satisfaction at 5 years was related to continence status and was higher in women undergoing sling surgery (83% vs 73%, $p = 0.04$). Satisfaction decreased with time ($p = 0.001$) and remained higher in the sling group ($p = 0.03$). The 2 groups had similar adverse event rates (Burch 10% vs sling 9%) and similar numbers of participants with adverse events (Burch 23 vs sling 22).

Conclusions.—Continence rates in both groups decreased substantially during 5 years, yet most women reported satisfaction with their continence status. Satisfaction was higher in continent women and in those who underwent fascial sling surgery, despite the voiding dysfunction associated with this procedure.

▶ The authors present the 5-year follow-up data from a landmark randomized controlled trial of autologous rectus fascia pubovaginal sling versus Burch urethropexy for the treatment of female stress urinary incontinence (SUI). The previous study found that continence rates at 2 years were superior for the pubovaginal sling, but that more sling patients had experienced voiding dysfunction. These findings persisted at 5 years. Readers should not be discouraged by the low reported continence rates, as the definition of continence used for this study was extremely strict, and the majority of patients (73% in the Burch group, 83% in the sling group) were satisfied with the surgical outcomes. Only 2% of the sling patients had undergone repeat surgery for SUI, compared with 12% of the Burch group. It will be interesting to compare these results with upcoming 5-year data for synthetic midurethral sling surgery from the same group of investigators.

J. Q. Clemens, MD

The clinical relevance of cell-based therapy for the treatment of stress urinary incontinence

Gräs S, Lose G (Copenhagen Univ Hosp, Herlev, Denmark)
Acta Obstet Gynecol Scand 90:815-824, 2011

Stress urinary incontinence is a common disorder affecting the quality of life for millions of women worldwide. Effective surgical procedures involving synthetic permanent meshes exist, but significant short- and long-term complications occur. Cell-based therapy using autologous stem cells or progenitor cells presents an alternative approach, which aims at repairing the anatomical components of the urethral continence mechanism. In vitro expanded progenitor cells isolated from muscle biopsies have been most intensely investigated, and both preclinical trials and a few clinical trials have provided proof of concept for the idea. An initial enthusiasm caused by positive results from early clinical trials has been dampened by the recognition of scientific irregularities. At the same time, the safety issue for cell-based therapy has been highlighted by the appearance of new and comprehensive regulatory demands. The influence on the cost effectiveness, the clinical relevance and the future perspectives of the present clinical approach are discussed.

▶ For those interested in the current state of cell-based therapy for the treatment of stress urinary incontinence, this is an excellent and timely review. The great wave of initial enthusiasm for regenerative medicine as a definitive treatment for stress urinary incontinence has been hampered by a combination of factors, including retraction of some publications as well as political, economic, scientific, and regulatory hurdles. This is a wonderfully concise and accurate review of the current state, promise, and limitations of this therapy. Several clinical trials in humans have been completed and are nicely summarized. In these trials, the efficacy of cell-based therapy appears to be similar to that of periurethral bulking agents with satisfactory safety. Many approaches have been used; however, none have proven to be superior. Overall, although enthusiasm has waned, the promise remains.

E. S. Rovner, MD

Tapes and Slings

Single-Incision Mini-Sling Compared With Tension-Free Vaginal Tape for the Treatment of Stress Urinary Incontinence: A Randomized Controlled Trial
Barber MD, for the Foundation for Female Health Awareness Research Network (Cleveland Clinic, OH; et al)
Obstet Gynecol 119:328-337, 2012

Objective.—To compare the efficacy of a single-incision mini-sling, placed in the "U" position, with tension-free vaginal tape (TVT) in the treatment of stress urinary incontinence.

Methods.—Women with urodynamic stress incontinence with or without genital prolapse were randomized to receive a mini-sling or TVT (N = 263). Those randomized to the mini-sling received two "sham" suprapubic incisions to facilitate blinding. The primary outcome was subjective cure (absence of any urinary incontinence or retreatment) as assessed at 1 year. This trial was a noninferiority study design.

Results.—Participants receiving the mini-sling were less likely to have a bladder injury (0.8% compared with 4.8%; $P = 0.46$), more likely to be discharged without a catheter (78.5% compared with 63%; $P = .008$), and had less pain for postoperative days 1–3. One year after surgery, the rate of cure was similar between treatment groups (mini-sling 55.8% compared with TVT 60.6%; mean difference, 4.8%; 95% confidence interval, −16.7 to +7.2); however, this did not meet our predefined noninferiority criteria of −12%. Incontinence severity at 1 year was greater with the mini-sling than with TVT (mean severity score ± SD: 2.2 ± 2.7 compared with 1.5 ± 1.9; $P = .015$), resulting predominantly from a higher proportion of participants with "severe" incontinence postoperatively (16% compared with 5%; $P = .025$).

Conclusion.—The mini-sling placed in the "U" position results in similar subjective cure rates to TVT 1 year after surgery but postoperative incontinence severity is greater with the mini-sling than with TVT.

Level of Evidence.—I.

▶ This trial was conducted by an experienced group of pelvic floor surgeons. In the article, they comment that mini-slings appear to require more tension to achieve efficacy than typical tension-free midurethral slings placed via the retropubic or transobturator route. They also note that approximately 9% of the mini-sling surgeries encountered technical difficulties that required the use of a second mini-sling device as a replacement or alternate sling. This suggests that mini-slings may not be as simple to place as might be expected. Although the same number of patients in each treatment group were continent at 1 year following surgery, there were clear differences in the failures. In those who were not continent following surgery, the mini-sling patients reported much more severe incontinence. It is not clear if the mini-sling surgery made the incontinence worse in some patients or if it was simply less effective in reducing continence in the noncured patients. Given the relative paucity of data related to single incision mini-slings, the Food and Drug Administration issued a post-market surveillance order on January 3, 2012, requiring manufacturers of these devices to conduct additional studies to better determine their safety and effectiveness.

J. Q. Clemens, MD

Outcomes of Pregnancy Following Surgery for Stress Urinary Incontinence: A Systematic Review
Pollard ME, Morrisroe S, Anger JT (Univ of California-Los Angeles)
J Urol 187:1966-1970, 2012

Purpose.—Although few data have been published on the safety of childbearing after surgery for stress urinary incontinence, a large proportion of physicians recommend that women wait to complete childbearing before pursuing surgical treatment for stress urinary incontinence. We systematically reviewed the available literature to examine the safety of pregnancy after stress urinary incontinence surgery, and to measure the effect of such pregnancy on continence outcomes.

Materials and Methods.—The review was conducted according to the recommendations of the MOOSE (Meta-Analysis of Observational Studies in Epidemiology) group. We performed a systematic review to identify articles published before January 2011 on pregnancy after incontinence surgery. Databases searched include PubMed®, EMBASE® and the Cochrane Review. Our literature search identified 592 titles, of which 20 articles were ultimately included in the review.

Results.—Data were tabulated from case reports, case series and physician surveys. The final analysis in each category included 32, 19 and 67 patients, respectively. Urinary retention developed during pregnancy in 2 women, 1 of whom was treated with a sling takedown and the other with intermittent catheterization. Of these 2 women 1 also had an episode of pyelonephritis during pregnancy, possibly related to the intermittent catheterization. The incidence of postpartum stress urinary incontinence ranged from 5% to 18% after cesarean delivery and from 20% to 30% after vaginal delivery.

Conclusions.—Although the data on outcomes in the literature are limited and further studies need to be performed on the subject, the current data suggests that any increase in risks for pregnancy after surgery for stress incontinence may be small. A low risk of urinary retention during pregnancy may exist. Although some data suggest that cesarean deliveries may result in a lower rate of recurrent stress urinary incontinence than vaginal deliveries, a formal analysis could not be performed with the available data.

▶ Young women with bothersome stress urinary incontinence (SUI) present some unique management considerations. They may be considerably more active than older patients, and long-term surgical outcomes and adverse events may assume more importance in management decisions. In addition, many of these patients may be considering future pregnancy. This review highlights the lack of data currently available to inform discussions about the risks of pregnancy following surgery for SUI. It seems wise to delay SUI surgery until childbearing is complete, but that is not always acceptable to these patients, especially those who do not have concrete plans for conception. In the past, I have often used transurethral collagen injections in these patients due to the known temporary effects and lack of significant complications. With collagen no longer available, I am less willing to inject permanent substances. The increased publicity related to mesh-related complications is often a factor, and most of my young patients who choose to have surgery decide to proceed with autologous fascial slings.

J. Q. Clemens, MD

Adverse events over two years after retropubic or transobturator midurethral sling surgery: findings from the Trial of Midurethral Slings (TOMUS) study

Brubaker L, for the Urinary Incontinence Treatment Network (Loyola Univ Chicago, IL; et al)
Am J Obstet Gynecol 205:498.e1-498.e6, 2011

Objective.—To describe surgical complications in 597 women over a 24-month period after randomization to retropubic or transobturator midurethral slings.

Study Design.—During the Trial of Midurethral Slings study, the Data Safety Monitoring Board regularly reviewed summary reports of all adverse events using the Dindo Surgical Complication Scale. Logistic regression models were created to explore associations between clinicodemographic factors and surgical complications.

Results.—A total of 383 adverse events were observed among 253 of the 597 women (42%). Seventy-five adverse events (20%) were classified as serious (serious adverse events); occurring in 70 women. Intraoperative bladder perforation (15 events) occurred exclusively in the retropubic group. Neurologic adverse events were more common in the transobturator group than in retropubic (32 events vs 20 events, respectively). Twenty-three (4%) women experienced mesh complications, including delayed presentations, in both groups.

Conclusion.—Adverse events vary by procedure, but are common after midurethral sling. Most events resolve without significant sequelae.

▶ This is yet another publication from the Urinary Incontinence Treatment Network group as part of the National Institutes of Health/National Institute of Diabetes and Digestive and Kidney Diseases— sponsored Trial of Midurethral Slings trial originally reported several years ago.[1] That seminal trial reported essentially therapeutic equivalence between the retropubic and transobturator sling approaches for the treatment of female stress urinary incontinence. This article by Brubaker et al describes the adverse events experienced at 2 years from study closure. A near full accounting of adverse events was collected with the only notable exception being dyspareunia. This article suggests that the rate of adverse events is considerably less in the second year following sling compared with the first 12 months postoperatively. For example, of the 17 sling erosions or exposures, only 3 occurred in the second year. Furthermore, of the 53 neurological complications, only 4 remained unresolved at 24 months postoperatively. Unfortunately, the neurological complications are not charac- terized further nor are they attributed to either technique.

E. S. Rovner, MD

Reference

1. Richter HE, Albo ME, Zyczynski HM, et al. Retropubic versus transobturator midurethral slings for stress incontinence. *N Engl J Med.* 2010;362:2066-2076.

Baseline Urodynamic Predictors of Treatment Failure 1 Year After Mid Urethral Sling Surgery

Nager CW, for the Urinary Incontinence Treatment Network (Univ of California San Diego; et al)
J Urol 186:597-603, 2011

Purpose.—We determined whether baseline urodynamic study variables predict failure after mid urethral sling surgery.

Materials and Methods.—Preoperative urodynamic study variables and postoperative continence status were analyzed in women participating in a randomized trial comparing retropubic to transobturator mid urethral sling. Objective failure was defined by positive standardized stress test, 15 ml or greater on 24-hour pad test, or re-treatment for stress urinary incontinence. Subjective failure criteria were self-reported stress symptoms, leakage on 3-day diary or re-treatment for stress urinary incontinence. Logistic regression was used to assess associations between covariates and failure controlling for treatment group and clinical variables. Receiver operator curves were constructed for relationships between objective failure and measures of urethral function.

Results.—Objective continence outcomes were available at 12 months for 565 of 597 (95%) women. Treatment failed in 260 women (245 by subjective criteria, 124 by objective criteria). No urodynamic variable was significantly associated with subjective failure on multivariate analysis. Valsalva leak point pressure, maximum urethral closure pressure and urody- namic stress incontinence were the only urodynamic variables consistently associated with objective failure on multivariate analysis. No specific cut point was determined for predicting failure for Valsalva leak point pressure or maximum urethral closure pressure by ROC. The lowest quartile (Valsalva leak point pressure less than 86 cm H_2O, maximum urethral closure pressure less than 45 cm H_2O) conferred an almost 2-fold increased odds of objective failure regardless of sling route (OR 2.23, 1.20—4.14 for Valsalva leak point pressure and OR 1.88, 1.04—3.41 for maximum urethral closure pressure).

Conclusions.—Women with a Valsalva leak point pressure or maximum urethral closure pressure in the lowest quartile are nearly 2-fold more likely to experience stress urinary incontinence 1 year after transobturator or retropubic mid urethral sling.

▶ This is an analysis of the outcomes data from the Trial of Mid Urethral Slings. This National Institutes of Health/National Institute of Diabetes and Digestive and Kidney Diseases trial was a randomized trial of retropubic midurethral slings versus transobturator midurethral slings. The outcomes and complications data have been published previously. This analysis specifically reviewed whether any urodynamic variables could predict for failure in either group. Although the analysis revealed that there were no definite urodynamic parameters that predicted for failure of transobturator slings versus a retropubic approach, they did find that lower urethral function predicted for failure with both approaches. The authors appropriately note the limitations of this study in evaluating for specific risk factors for one approach versus the other, specifically whether a specific surgical approach should be chosen based on urethral function tests alone. In the only randomized trial looking at failure of retropubic versus transobturator procedures, Schierlitz et al found that poor urethral function predicted for failure with the transobturator approach versus the retropubic approach.[1]

Of note, the preoperative demonstration of detrusor overactivity did not predict for failure collectively or individually in either of the treatment groups. However, only 12% of the total cohort had detrusor overactivity, and overall the patients entered into this study were a highly selected group of patients because the entry criteria included only those with stress-predominant mixed urinary incontinence or pure stress incontinence. Interestingly, it is unclear whether patients with postoperative urinary retention or patients requiring additional procedures for postoperative voiding dysfunction were included in the failure group. If these individuals were included in the failure group, it would be interesting to see whether any voiding parameters preoperatively would have predicted for postoperative voiding dysfunction.

E. S. Rovner, MD

Reference

1. Schierlitz L, Dwyer PL, Rosamilia A, et al. Effectiveness of tension-free vaginal tape compared with transobturator tape in women with stress urinary incontinence and intrinsic sphincter deficiency: a randomized controlled trial. *Obstet Gynecol.* 2008;112:1253-1261.

Single-Incision Mini-Slings Versus Standard Midurethral Slings in Surgical Management of Female Stress Urinary Incontinence: A Meta-Analysis of Effectiveness and Complications

Abdel-Fattah M, Ford JA, Lim CP, et al (Univ of Aberdeen, UK; Grampian NHS, Aberdeen, UK; et al)
Eur Urol 60:468-480, 2011

Context.—Single-incision mini-slings (SIMS) have been introduced for the treatment of female stress urinary incontinence (SUI); however, concerns have been raised regarding their efficacy. No systematic reviews or meta-analyses have previously assessed these relatively new procedures.

Objective.—To assess the current evidence of effectiveness and safety of SIMS compared with standard midurethral slings (SMUS) (retropubic and transobturator tension-free vaginal tapes) in the management of female SUI.

Evidence Acquisition.—We conducted a literature search from 1996 to January 2011. Meta-analysis of all randomised controlled trials (RCTs) comparing SIMS versus SMUS was performed in accordance with the Preferred Reporting Items for Systematic Reviews and Meta-Analyses statement. Data were analysed using Rev-Man 5. Primary outcomes were patient-reported and objective cure rates. Secondary outcomes included perioperative complications, quality of life (QoL) changes, and costs to health services.

Evidence Synthesis.—A total of 758 women in nine RCTs with a mean follow-up of 9.5 mo were included. The mean age (52.3 vs 52.1 yr), body mass index (27.4 vs 27.7), and parity (2.4 and 2.4) were comparable for both groups. SIMS were associated with significantly lower patient-reported and objective cure rates at 6−12 mo compared with SMUS (risk ratio [RR]: 0.83; 95% confidence interval [CI], 0.70−0.99, and RR: 0.85; 95% CI, 0.74−0.97, respectively). SIMS were associated with significantly shorter operative time (weighed mean difference [WMD]: 8.67 min; 95% CI, 17.32 to −0.02), lower day 1 pain scores (WMD: 1.74; 95% CI, −2.58 to −0.09), and less postoperative groin pain (RR: 0.18; 95% CI, 0.04−0.72). Repeat continence surgery (RR: 6.72; 95% CI, 2.39−18.89) and de novo urgency incontinence (RR: 2.08; 95% CI, 1.01−4.28) were significantly higher in the SIMS group. There was no significant difference in the QoL scores between the groups (WMD: 33.46; 95% CI, −20.62 to 87.55). No studies compared cost to health services.

Conclusions.—SIMS are associated with inferior patient-reported and objective cure rates on the short-term follow-up, as well as higher reoperation rates for SUI when compared with SMUS.

▶ The emerging data on single-incision mini-slings are quite variable. Some studies suggest excellent short-term efficacy and safety, whereas others suggest unacceptably poor outcomes. This meta-analysis includes all randomized controlled studies up to and including those published through January 2011. Nine randomized control studies were included, and although data would suggest that inferior outcomes were associated with the single-incision slings, the data are immature and almost certainly biased by the learning curve associated with relatively new single-incision mini-slings. It is important to remember that long-term data (greater than 2 years) is not yet available for the mini-slings. Furthermore, there may be subtle and as yet unrecognized differences between the various types of single-incision mini-slings, all of which were grouped together for purposes of this meta-analysis. Will one type of surgical approach for the treatment of female stress urinary incontinence ultimately emerge as superior to all others, or will each of the various procedures have a niche among a subgroup of patients within the broad spectrum of patients with stress urinary incontinence? Clearly, more, better, and longer-term data are needed before attempting to answer these questions.

E. S. Rovner, MD

Single-Incision Mini-Sling Compared With Tension-Free Vaginal Tape for the Treatment of Stress Urinary Incontinence: A Randomized Controlled Trial

Barber MD, for the Foundation for Female Health Awareness Research Network (Cleveland Clinic, Cleveland OH; et al)

Obstet Gynecol 119:328-337, 2012

Objective.—To compare the efficacy of a single-incision mini-sling, placed in the "U" position, with tension-free vaginal tape (TVT) in the treatment of stress urinary incontinence.

Methods.—Women with urodynamic stress incontinence with or without genital prolapse were randomized to receive a mini-sling or TVT (N = 263). Those randomized to the mini-sling received two "sham" suprapubic incisions to facilitate blinding. The primary outcome was subjective cure (absence of any urinary incontinence or retreatment) as assessed at 1 year. This trial was a noninferiority study design.

Results.—Participants receiving the mini-sling were less likely to have a bladder injury (0.8% compared with 4.8%; $P = .46$), more likely to be discharged without a catheter (78.5% compared with 63%; $P = .008$), and had less pain for postoperative days 1–3. One year after surgery, the rate of cure was similar between treatment groups (mini-sling 55.8% compared with TVT 60.6%; mean difference, 4.8%; 95% confidence interval, -16.7 to $+7.2$); however, this did not meet our predefined noninferiority criteria of -12%. Incontinence severity at 1 year was greater with the mini-sling than with TVT (mean severity score $\pm$ SD: 2.2 ± 2.7 compared with 1.5 ± 1.9; $P = .015$), resulting predominantly from a higher proportion of participants with "severe" incontinence postoperatively (16% compared with 5%; $P = .025$).

Conclusion.—The mini-sling placed in the "U" position results in similar subjective cure rates to TVT 1 year after surgery but postoperative incontinence severity is greater with the mini-sling than with TVT.

Level of Evidence.—I.

▶ This was a well-done randomized controlled trial that demonstrated essentially similar efficacy in the 2 groups at a follow-up of 1 year. There was a trend toward greater improvement in the group that had tension-free vaginal tape, but it was not significant. Complications seemed to be matched evenly in the 2 groups; however, it was surprising that in the mini-sling group, there were ureteral injuries, a bowel injury, and even a bladder injury. They may have been related to concomitant procedures being performed at the same time as the sling procedure.

The Kaplan-Meier survival curve for the development of any urinary incontinence symptoms after surgery seemed to diverge between the 2 procedures with ongoing follow-up but did not reach statistical significance. It will be interesting to see whether these curves continue to diverge as this data set is analyzed in the future with longer follow-up. Which sling is better? These data are unable to answer this question definitively at this time. As with many other types of surgical procedures, clinical outcomes are likely to be more closely related to surgical experience, expertise, and patient selection.

E. S. Rovner, MD

6 Renal Tumors

Cryoablation

National Trends in the Use of Partial Nephrectomy: A Rising Tide That Has Not Lifted All Boats
Patel SG, Penson DF, Pabla B, et al (Vanderbilt Univ Med Ctr, Nashville, TN; Vanderbilt Univ School of Medicine, Nashville, TN)
J Urol 187:816-821, 2012

Purpose.—Treatment of organ confined renal masses with partial nephrectomy has durable oncologic outcomes comparable to radical nephrectomy. Partial nephrectomy is associated with lower risk of chronic kidney disease and in some series with better overall survival. We report a contemporary analysis on national trends of partial nephrectomy use to determine partial nephrectomy use over time, and whether nontumor related factors such as structural attributes of the treating institution or patient characteristics are associated with the underuse of partial nephrectomy.

Materials and Methods.—We performed an analysis of the NIS (National Inpatient Sample), which contains 20% of all United States inpatient hospitalizations. We included patients who underwent radical or partial nephrectomy for a renal mass between 2002 and 2008. Survey weights were applied to obtain national estimates of nephrectomy use and to evaluate nonclinical predictors of partial nephrectomy.

Results.—A total of 46,396 patients were included in the study for a weighted sample of 226,493. There was an increase in partial nephrectomy use from 15.3% in 2002 to 24.7% in 2008 ($p < 0.001$). On multivariate analysis hospital attributes (urban teaching status, nephrectomy volume, geographic region) and patient socioeconomic status (higher income ZIP code and private/HMO payer) were independent predictors of partial nephrectomy use.

Conclusions.—Since 2002 the national use of partial nephrectomy for the management of renal masses has increased. However, the adoption of partial nephrectomy at smaller, rural and nonacademic hospitals lags behind that of larger hospitals, urban/teaching hospitals and higher volume centers. A lower rate of partial nephrectomy use among patients without private insurance and those living in lower income ZIP code areas highlights the underuse of partial nephrectomy as a quality of care concern.

▶ In the most recent American Urological Association guidelines for the management of small renal masses partial nephrectomy (PN) is the preferred management. The bar graph in the article demonstrates the surgical management of renal masses between 2002 and 2008. Given that during this time interval renal masses were smaller (secondary to early detection via cross-sectional imaging), it is surprising that over 60% of tumors are removed via open nephrectomy and that only 24% of tumors are managed with partial nephrectomy. This is indicative of slow adoption of minimally invasive techniques by the urologic community. This delay may be related to technical skills, but the increased operative time and increased chance of postoperative complications may also factor into decision making. To improve the care of patients with renal masses, PN techniques will have to be disseminated or surgical treatment or renal cell cancer will need to be centralized at high-volume centers.

D. E. Coplen, MD

7 Prostate Cancer

Screening

Prostate-Cancer Mortality at 11 Years of Follow-up
Schröder FH, for the ERSPC Investigators (Erasmus Univ Med Ctr, Rotterdam, The Netherlands; et al)
N Engl J Med 366:981-990, 2012

Background.—Several trials evaluating the effect of prostate-specific antigen (PSA) testing on prostate-cancer mortality have shown conflicting results. We updated prostatecancer mortality in the European Randomized Study of Screening for Prostate Cancer with 2 additional years of follow-up.

Methods.—The study involved 182,160 men between the ages of 50 and 74 years at entry, with a predefined core age group of 162,388 men 55 to 69 years of age. The trial was conducted in eight European countries. Men who were randomly assigned to the screening group were offered PSA-based screening, whereas those in the control group were not offered such screening. The primary outcome was mortality from prostate cancer.

Results.—After a median follow-up of 11 years in the core age group, the relative reduction in the risk of death from prostate cancer in the screening group was 21% (rate ratio, 0.79; 95% confidence interval [CI], 0.68 to 0.91; $P = 0.001$), and 29% after adjustment for noncompliance. The absolute reduction in mortality in the screening group was 0.10 deaths per 1000 person-years or 1.07 deaths per 1000 men who underwent randomization. The rate ratio for death from prostate cancer during follow-up years 10 and 11 was 0.62 (95% CI, 0.45 to 0.85; $P = 0.003$). To prevent one death from prostate cancer at 11 years of follow-up, 1055 men would need to be invited for screening and 37 cancers would need to be detected. There was no significant between-group difference in all-cause mortality.

Conclusions.—Analyses after 2 additional years of follow-up consolidated our previous finding that PSA-based screening significantly reduced mortality from prostate cancer but did not affect all-cause mortality. (Current Controlled Trials number, ISRCTN49127736.)

▶ This article shows that with additional follow-up, the approximate 20% relative reduction in the risk of death from prostate cancer is maintained in the screening group of the European Randomised Study of Screening for Prostate

Cancer (ERSPC). A protocol analysis adjusting for noncompliance places the relative risk reduction up to 29%. To prevent 1 death from prostate cancer, 1055 men would need to be invited for screening, and 37 cancers would be detected and potentially treated.

What is of a little concern about the ERSPC is that the results are reported in only a predefined core group of men aged 55 to 69 rather than the entire cohort, and not all of the center's patients have been included in the analysis. There were significant treatment differences between the 2 arms. Finally, elimination of either the Rotterdam or Göteborg section makes the results of the reported group not statistically significant.

Prostate cancer screening probably has a small effect on prostate cancer risk reduction.[1-4]

The US Preventive Services Task Force issued a draft grade D recommendation for prostate-specific antigen (PSA)—based screening. They did this on the basis of their analysis of four key questions:

1. Does PSA-based screening decrease prostate cancer—specific or all-cause mortality?
2. What are the harms of PSA-based screening for prostate cancer?
3. What are the benefits of treatment of early stage or screen-detected prostate cancer?
4. What are the harms of treatment of early stage or screen-detected prostate cancer?

PSA-based screening certainly has no effect on all-cause mortality. It probably has a relatively modest 20% to 40% relative risk reduction for prostate cancer—specific mortality, but it is worthwhile to point out that this has not been demonstrated in all studies. In the ERSPC trial, for example, it was observed only in a core group of participants, and elimination of 2 of the 9 study sites caused the overall ERSPC to be negative. Moreover, there are certain recognized harms of PSA-based screening. These include the data that show that 12% to 15% of screened men will have false-positive results and serious complications occur after 0.5% to 1% of prostate biopsies, and that radical prostatectomy for clinically detected prostate cancer benefited only men less than 65 years of age in the Scandinavian trial. In the US Prostate Cancer Intervention Versus Observation Trial, there was no benefit for most patients with screen-detected prostate cancer. The group considered that treating about 3 men with radical prostatectomy and about 7 men with radiation therapy would result in 1 additional case of erectile dysfunction and 5 men with radical prostatectomy would result in 1 additional case of incontinence.

These editorials collectively raise a few points that are worth considering when evaluating PSA-based screening. First, prostate cancer remains a major public health problem, and this problem will worsen as the population ages. Eliminating screening will return us to the pre-PSA era. Independent models have suggested that about half of the 40% prostate cancer mortality reduction seen since the pre-PSA era is due to screening, with the remainder due to treatment. Furthermore, notwithstanding the morbidity of biopsies and the numbers needed to treat with radical prostatectomy, these numbers are similar for prostate cancer and for many other screened cancers in the United States. Furthermore, the US Preventive Task Force did not consider reduction in the development of clinical metastatic disease as an important endpoint, and all clinicians know that it is. Another important point is that most of the screening trials evaluated by the Task Force used a PSA threshold as a guide for biopsy. We now know that we could use PSA better starting at a younger age and using velocity thresholds to identify which men are at risk for aggressive prostate cancer. Finally, our screening efforts are apt to get better as we can better identify which patients are at highest risk for getting or dying from prostate cancer.

For now I think that we should not embrace mass screening for prostate cancer but rather should take a more nuanced targeted approach toward men who are at increased risk of getting and dying of prostate cancer.

G. L. Andriole, Jr, MD

References

1. Volk RJ, Wolf AMD. Grading the new US preventive services task force prostate cancer screening recommendation. *JAMA.* 2011;306:2715-2716.
2. Kim J, Davis JW. Prostate cancer screening—time to abandon one-size-fits-all approach? *JAMA.* 2011;306:2717-2718.
3. Miller DC, Hollenbeck BK. Missing the mark on prostate-specific antigen screening. *JAMA.* 2011;306:2719-2720.
4. Chou R, LeFevre ML. Prostate cancer screening—the evidence, the recommendations, and the clinical implications. *JAMA.* 2011;306:2721-2722.

Prostate Cancer Screening in the Randomized Prostate, Lung, Colorectal, and Ovarian Cancer Screening Trial: Mortality Results after 13 Years of Follow-up
Andriole GL, for the PLCO Project Team (Washington Univ School of Medicine, St Louis, MO; et al)
J Natl Cancer Inst 104.125-132, 2012

Background.—The prostate component of the Prostate, Lung, Colorectal, and Ovarian (PLCO) Cancer Screening Trial was undertaken to determine whether there is a reduction in prostate cancer mortality from screening using serum prostate-specific antigen (PSA) testing and digital rectal examination (DRE). Mortality after 7—10 years of follow-up has been reported previously. We report extended follow-up to 13 years after the trial.

Methods.—A total of 76 685 men, aged 55—74 years, were enrolled at 10 screening centers between November 1993 and July 2001 and randomly assigned to the intervention (organized screening of annual PSA testing for 6 years and annual DRE for 4 years; 38 340 men) and control (usual care, which sometimes included opportunistic screening; 38 345 men) arms. Screening was completed in October 2006. All incident prostate cancers and deaths from prostate cancer through 13 years of follow-up or through December 31, 2009, were ascertained. Relative risks (RRs) were estimated as the ratio of observed rates in the intervention and control arms, and

95% confidence intervals (CIs) were calculated assuming a Poisson distribution for the number of events. Poisson regression modeling was used to examine the interactions with respect to prostate cancer mortality between trial arm and age, comorbidity status, and pretrial PSA testing. All statistical tests were two-sided.

Results.—Approximately 92% of the study participants were followed to 10 years and 57% to 13 years. At 13 years, 4250 participants had been diagnosed with prostate cancer in the intervention arm compared with 3815 in the control arm. Cumulative incidence rates for prostate cancer in the intervention and control arms were 108.4 and 97.1 per 10 000 person-years, respectively, resulting in a relative increase of 12% in the intervention arm (RR = 1.12, 95% CI = 1.07 to 1.17). After 13 years of follow-up, the cumulative mortality rates from prostate cancer in the intervention and control arms were 3.7 and 3.4 deaths per 10 000 person-years, respectively, resulting in a non-statistically significant difference between the two arms (RR = 1.09, 95% CI = 0.87 to 1.36). No statistically significant interactions with respect to prostate cancer mortality were observed between trial arm and age ($P_{interaction} = .81$), pretrial PSA testing ($P_{interaction} = .52$), and comorbidity ($P_{interaction} = .68$).

Conclusions.—After 13 years of follow-up, there was no evidence of a mortality benefit for organized annual screening in the PLCO trial compared with opportunistic screening, which forms part of usual care, and there was no apparent interaction with age, baseline comorbidity, or pretrial PSA testing.

▶ This article presents an additional 3 years of follow-up, totally 13 years, for 76 000 men randomized to screening in the Prostate, Lung, Colorectal, and Ovarian (PLCO) cancer screening trial. Men in the screened arm did not have a lower prostate cancer-specific survival. This could be because 40% to 50% of patients in the usual care arm also underwent screening. This relatively high contamination suggests that the correct conclusion from PLCO is that organized annual screening with prostate-specific antigen when compared to opportunistic screening does not further increase prostate cancer-specific mortality.

G. L. Andriole, Jr, MD

Prediction of Significant Prostate Cancer Diagnosed 20 to 30 Years Later With a Single Measure of Prostate-Specific Antigen at or Before Age 50
Lilja H, Cronin AM, Dahlin A, et al (Memorial Sloan-Kettering Cancer Ctr, NY; Lund Univ, Malmö, Sweden)
Cancer 117:1210-1219, 2011

Background.—We previously reported that a single prostate-specific antigen (PSA) measured at ages 44-50 was highly predictive of subsequent prostate cancer diagnosis in an unscreened population. Here we report an additional 7 years of follow-up. This provides replication using an independent data set and allows estimates of the association between early

PSA and subsequent advanced cancer (clinical stage ≥T3 or metastases at diagnosis).

Methods.—Blood was collected from 21,277 men in a Swedish city (74% participation rate) during 1974-1986 at ages 33-50. Through 2006, prostate cancer was diagnosed in 1408 participants; we measured PSA in archived plasma for 1312 of these cases (93%) and for 3728 controls.

Results.—At a median follow-up of 23 years, baseline PSA was strongly associated with subsequent prostate cancer (area under the curve, 0.72; 95% CI, 0.70-0.74; for advanced cancer, 0.75; 95% CI, 0.72-0.78). Associations between PSA and prostate cancer were virtually identical for the initial and replication data sets, with 81% of advanced cases (95% CI, 77%-86%) found in men with PSA above the median (0.63 ng/mL at ages 44-50).

Conclusions.—A single PSA at or before age 50 predicts advanced prostate cancer diagnosed up to 30 years later. Use of early PSA to stratify risk would allow a large group of low-risk men to be screened less often but increase frequency of testing on a more limited number of high-risk men. This is likely to improve the ratio of benefit to harm for screening (Fig 2).

▶ As was pointed out by the US Preventive Health Task Force, mass, widespread screening of men with prostate cancer is associated with a very modest, if any, effect on prostate cancer—specific mortality, has no effect on overall mortality, and potentially is in the net harmful because many men undergo unnecessary biopsies or receive unnecessary treatments if prostate cancer is diagnosed. For these reasons, a risk-adjusted strategy has been abdicated. This article identifies

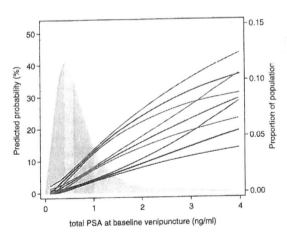

total PSA at baseline venipuncture (ng/ml)

FIGURE 2.—Long-term risk of prostate cancer according to PSA at ages 44-50 is shown (thick blue line, any prostate cancer; thick red line, palpable cancer; thick black line; advanced cancer). Thin lines represent quartiles of the population-based distribution of PSA values (0.42, 0.63, and 0.95 ng/mL). The curves differ from the curves for any cancer, shown in Figure 1, because the analysis was not restricted to men diagnosed at ages 20-25 years after venipuncture. (Reprinted from Lilja H, Cronin AM, Dahlin A, et al. Prediction of Significant Prostate Cancer Diagnosed 20 to 30 Years Later with a Single Measure of Prostate-Specific Antigen at or Before Age 50. *Cancer*. 2011;117:1210–1219, Copyright 2011 American Cancer Society. This material is reproduced with permission of Wiley-Liss, Inc., a subsidiary of John Wiley & Sons, Inc.)

a potentially powerful means to risk stratify men for prostate cancer, that is, serum prostate-specific antigen (PSA) level at or before the age of 50. As is shown in Fig 2, the patient's lifetime risk of any prostate cancer or clinically relevant prostate cancer could be correlated with his PSA level at this relatively young age. For men younger than 50, PSA level may, in fact, be a marker of prostate tumor volume more than of prostate size, as few such men will have significant BPH. In this analysis, which was derived from the Malmo Preventive Project, about half of the metastatic or lethal prostate cancers occurred in men in their 40s who are in the top decile for PSA values. This corresponded to a serum PSA level of greater than 1.3. Moreover, men whose serum PSA level was below the median (< 0.65) had a very low chance of ever developing metastatic or lethal prostate cancer. This may, therefore, represent another tool to risk stratify men to undergo screening and to adjust the intensity of screening.

G. L. Andriole, Jr, MD

An Empirical Evaluation of Guidelines on Prostate-Specific Antigen Velocity in Prostate Cancer Detection
Vickers AJ, Till C, Tangen CM, et al (Memorial Sloan-Kettering Cancer Ctr, NY; Fred Hutchinson Cancer Res Ctr, Seattle, WA; et al)
J Natl Cancer Inst 103:462-469, 2011

Background.—The National Comprehensive Cancer Network and American Urological Association guidelines on early detection of prostate cancer recommend biopsy on the basis of high prostate-specific antigen (PSA) velocity, even in the absence of other indications such as an elevated PSA or a positive digital rectal exam (DRE).

Methods.—To evaluate the current guideline, we compared the area under the curve of a multivariable model for prostate cancer including age, PSA, DRE, family history, and prior biopsy, with and without PSA velocity, in 5519 men undergoing biopsy, regardless of clinical indication, in the control arm of the Prostate Cancer Prevention Trial. We also evaluated the clinical implications of using PSA velocity cut points to determine biopsy in men with low PSA and negative DRE in terms of additional cancers found and unnecessary biopsies conducted. All statistical tests were two-sided.

Results.—Incorporation of PSA velocity led to a very small increase in area under the curve from 0.702 to 0.709. Improvements in predictive accuracy were smaller for the endpoints of high-grade cancer (Gleason score of 7 or greater) and clinically significant cancer (Epstein criteria). Biopsying men with high PSA velocity but no other indication would lead to a large number of additional biopsies, with close to one in seven men being biopsied. PSA cut points with a comparable specificity to PSA velocity cut points had a higher sensitivity (23% vs 19%), particularly for high-grade (41% vs 25%) and clinically significant (32% vs 22%) disease. These findings were robust to the method of calculating PSA velocity.

TABLE 5.—Distribution of Prostate-Specific (PSA) and Prostate-Specific Antigen Velocity (PSAV) Cut Points for Men Without Other Indications for Biopsy with Corresponding Rates of Cancer, High-Grade Cancer, and Clinically Significant Cancer*

PSA and PSAV Cut Points	All Subjects, No. (%)		All Cancers, No. (%)		High-Grade Cancers, No. (%)		Clinically Significant Cancers, No. (%)	
	Below Cut Point	Above Cut Point	Patients Below Cut Point	Patients Above Cut Point	Patients Below Cut Point	Patients Above Cut Point	Patients Below Cut Point[†]	Patients Above Cut Point[†]
PSA <4 ng/mL, negative DRE								
PSAV, ng mL^{-1} y^{-1}								
0.35	3319 (86)	548 (14)	488 (15)	115 (21)	71 (2)	24 (4)	214/3199 (7)	62/521 (12)
0.5	3523 (91)	344 (9)	538 (15)	65 (19)	78 (2)	17 (5)	240/3394 (7)	36/326 (11)
0.75	3720 (96)	147 (4)	575 (15)	28 (19)	88 (2)	7 (5)	259/3578 (7)	17/142 (12)
PSA, ng/mL								
2	2936 (75)	985 (25)	382 (13)	232 (24)	44 (1)	51 (5)	151/2836 (5)	130/934 (14)
2.5	3346 (85)	575 (15)	475 (14)	139 (24)	56 (2)	39 (7)	192/3220 (6)	89/550 (16)
PSA <2.5 ng/mL, negative DRE								
PSAV, ng mL^{-1} y^{-1}								
0.35	2970 (92)	266 (8)	408 (14)	49 (18)	50 (2)	4 (2)	169/2865 (6)	16/252 (6)
0.5	3098 (96)	138 (4)	438 (14)	19 (14)	51 (2)	3 (2)	179/2986 (6)	6/131 (5)
0.75	3193 (99)	43 (1)	448 (14)	9 (21)	52 (2)	2 (5)	182/3076 (6)	3/41 (7)

*DRE = digital rectal exam. High-grade is Gleason 7 or greater; clinically significant cancer is defined as stage greater than T1c or PSA density of at least 0.15 ng mL^{-1} g^{-1} or Gleason score of at least 7, or tumor in 3 or more cores, or at least one core with more than 50% cancer involvement.

†As data are missing for some men, the denominator is listed for this analysis.

Conclusions.—We found no evidence to support the recommendation that men with high PSA velocity should be biopsied in the absence of other indications; this measure should not be included in practice guidelines (Table 5).

► This interesting analysis of about 5000 men in the placebo arm of the Prostate Cancer Prevention Trial suggests that prostate-specific antigen velocity is not an independent predictor of prostate cancer. As shown in Table 5, various velocity cut points could not predict whether cancer was present and, if so, its grade or implied clinical significance.

G. L. Andriole, Jr, MD

Case 9-2012: A 67-Year-Old Man with a Persistently Elevated PSA Level
Kaufman DS, Zietman AL, McDougal WS, et al (Massachusetts General Hosp, Boston, MA)
N Engl J Med 366:1143-1150, 2012

Background.—About 15% to 20% of prostate cancers are found predominantly in the anterior prostate and arise either in the anterior horn of the peripheral zone or the transition zone. Biopsy specimens of these tumors are difficult to obtain using the transrectal approach or transurethral resection. A transperitoneal template-guided mapping biopsy (TTMB) allows surgeons to perform precise needle biopsies and detect cancers in otherwise inaccessible areas.

Case Report.—Man, 67, had persistently elevated serum levels of prostate-specific antigen (PSA) for over 7 years. Five biopsies were done over that time period but only one indicated a tiny focus of low-grade adenocarcinoma. His prostate gland was 45 mL in volume, nontender, and smooth. Bone scan showed uptake in a rib posteriorly on the right side, in the left side of the skull, and in the maxilla on the left side plus questionable lesions in the lumbar spine, but all were indeterminate for cancer. Computed tomography (CT) found hyperdense lesions in the left acetabulum, sacrum, third lumbar vertebral body on the left, and the ninth and tenth ribs on the right posteriorly. Magnetic resonance imaging (MRI) of the brain showed no metastatic disease. The spine lesions and skull abnormality were considered most likely benign. The patient was given bicalutamide for 10 days, then leuprolide acetate parenterally in two 1-month depot doses.

The patient had hot flashes about 2 to 3 times a week and nocturia once a night, but no other genitourinary, gastrointestinal, rectal bleeding, or other symptoms. He had hypertension, hyperlipidemia, and diverticulitis; partial colectomy for a ruptured diverticulum 14 years previously; and an incisional hernia repaired with mesh.

He was taking simvastatin, hydrochlorothiazide, aspirin (325 mg a day), and a multivitamin. His father died of prostate cancer, his mother had breast cancer but died of a stroke, and his sister had breast cancer and died of metastatic disease, but his children and grandchildren were healthy. His vital signs and oxygen saturation were normal, but his body-mass index (BMI) was 32.7. The prostate was slightly enlarged, his platelet count and IgM levels were low, and his blood urea nitrogen levels were high. His PSA levels were too high for active surveillance, but the surgeon thought it was possible that a more aggressive or advanced cancer was in an area not easily accessed by a transrectal biopsy. Therefore the patient was taken off hormone therapy and TTMB was done 3 months after the initial assessment. All three cores taken from the anterior prostate had adenocarcinoma with a Gleason score of 7, and one minute focus of adenocarcinoma was found in a core taken from the left lateral prostate. The patient chose to be treated with laparoscopic prostatectomy. This was complicated by previous abdominal surgeries, but an extraperiotoneal approach, including pelvic lymphadenectomy, allowed the surgeon to perform a successful surgical dissection. Five months after the procedure the patient's PSA level was less than 0.1 ng/mL and remained undetectable at 10-month follow-up.

Conclusions.—TTMB and other biopsy techniques that target the anterior prostate should be considered if the information needed to make an appropriate treatment decision cannot be obtained by transrectal ultrasound-guided biopsies. The morbidity associated with TTMB is greater than with transrectal biopsies, with a higher incidence of acute urinary obstruction. The costs for TTMB are also far greater than with transrectal biopsies. However, biopsies using a template approach are needed in select patients.

▶ This case report and associated discussion is very timely as it exemplifies the controversy surrounding prostate-specific antigen (PSA) screening, how to interpret PSA values, how to biopsy the prostate, and how to select men in whom cancer is diagnosed for treatment. Especially important is the role of template-guided biopsy, as illustrated in Fig 3 in the original article, to optimally diagnose and characterize the cancer.

G. L. Andriole, Jr, MD

Prostate Cancer Screening in the Randomized Prostate, Lung, Colorectal, and Ovarian Cancer Screening Trial: Mortality Results after 13 Years of Follow-up
Andriole GL, for the PLCO Project Team (Washington Univ School of Medicine, St Louis, MO; et al)
J Natl Cancer Inst 104:125-132, 2012

Background.—The prostate component of the Prostate, Lung, Colorectal, and Ovarian (PLCO) Cancer Screening Trial was undertaken to determine whether there is a reduction in prostate cancer mortality from screening using serum prostate-specific antigen (PSA) testing and digital rectal examination (DRE). Mortality after 7–10 years of follow-up has been reported previously. We report extended follow-up to 13 years after the trial.

Methods.—A total of 76 685 men, aged 55–74 years, were enrolled at 10 screening centers between November 1993 and July 2001 and randomly assigned to the intervention (organized screening of annual PSA testing for 6 years and annual DRE for 4 years; 38 340 men) and control (usual care, which sometimes included opportunistic screening; 38 345 men) arms. Screening was completed in October 2006. All incident prostate cancers and deaths from prostate cancer through 13 years of follow-up or through December 31, 2009, were ascertained. Relative risks (RRs) were estimated as the ratio of observed rates in the intervention and control arms, and 95% confidence intervals (CIs) were calculated assuming a Poisson distribution for the number of events. Poisson regression modeling was used to examine the interactions with respect to prostate cancer mortality between trial arm and age, comorbidity status, and pretrial PSA testing. All statistical tests were two-sided.

Results.—Approximately 92% of the study participants were followed to 10 years and 57% to 13 years. At 13 years, 4250 participants had been diagnosed with prostate cancer in the intervention arm compared with 3815 in the control arm. Cumulative incidence rates for prostate cancer in the intervention and control arms were 108.4 and 97.1 per 10 000 person-years, respectively, resulting in a relative increase of 12% in the intervention arm (RR = 1.12, 95% CI = 1.07 to 1.17). After 13 years of follow-up, the cumulative mortality rates from prostate cancer in the intervention and control arms were 3.7 and 3.4 deaths per 10 000 person-years, respectively, resulting in a non-statistically significant difference between the two arms (RR = 1.09, 95% CI = 0.87 to 1.36). No statistically significant interactions with respect to prostate cancer mortality were observed between trial arm and age ($P_{interaction} = .81$), pretrial PSA testing ($P_{interaction} = .52$), and comorbidity ($P_{interaction} = .68$).

Conclusions.—After 13 years of follow-up, there was no evidence of a mortality benefit for organized annual screening in the PLCO trial compared with opportunistic screening, which forms part of usual care, and there was no apparent interaction with age, baseline comorbidity, or pretrial PSA testing.

▶ The key finding in this study is that "there was no evidence of a mortality benefit for organized annual screening in the PLCO trial compared with opportunistic screening." The key phrase is *opportunistic screening.* Unlike the European trial, many men in the control arm obtained a prostate-specific antigen (PSA) level outside of the trial. Estimates have been as high as 85%. Critics of PSA screening have latched onto this trial as proof that it doesn't work. In my opinion, this conclusion is just wrong. Yearly screening may offer no addition benefit or just a marginal benefit, over a PSA every few years. The key word is "may."

How is this going to affect practice? I hope, not much. Removing PSA from our diagnostic armamentarium will result in patients dying of their disease due to delay in diagnosis. I hope we don't go back to 1985 when the majority of men with disease were destined to die of it.

A. S. Kibel, MD

USPSTF Finds Little Evidence to Support Advising PSA Screening in Any Man
Slomski A
JAMA 306:2549-2551, 2011

Background.—In October 2011 the US Preventive Services Task Force (USPSTF) recommended that men no longer receive prostate-specific antigen (PSA)-n-based screening for prostate cancer. Prostate cancer is the most commonly diagnosed non-skin cancer and the second leading cause of cancer deaths in US men. Two studies formed the basis for the new USPSTF recommendation: the European Randomized Study of Screening for Prostate Cancer (ERSPC) and the US Prostate, Lung, Colorectal, and Ovarian Cancer Screening Trial (PLCO). The ERSPC found fewer prostate cancer deaths (6 per 10,000 men screened), but it was not a statistically significant reduction. Men age 55 to 69 years had a slightly greater benefit and statistical significance. The PLCO revealed an increase in the number of prostate deaths of about 3 per 10,000 men. Thus any benefit to PSA screening would appear to be extremely small.

Risks and Benefits.—High-risk groups are a concern. African American men have a substantially higher prostate cancer incidence rate than white men and are more than twice as likely to die of the disease. However, African American men were not adequately represented in the trials on which the recommendations are based. Physicians should consider both race and family history when determining whether a specific man should undergo PSA screening. Men who have immediate relatives who had or have prostate cancer are at higher risk than those without this family history. Informed consent should be sought from all patients.

Urologists also raise questions concerning the data interpretation and the quality of the trials. The PLCO has been criticized because of possible contamination and culling of patients who had prostate cancer, leaving a low-risk population in the control group. It may therefore compare more screening with less screening. In addition, men who receive a positive PSA test result usually receive biopsies, but about 80% of PSA results are false positives. The test exposes men to adverse events such as fever, infection, bleeding, pain, and transient urinary difficulty. If early treatment, radiation, or androgen deprivation is undertaken, up to 5 in 1000 men will die within 1 month of the surgery and 10 to 70 will have serious complications. Between 20% and 30% of every 1000 men treated with radiotherapy or surgery develop urinary incontinence, and bowel dysfunction can occur with radiotherapy. However, men treated immediately with radical prostatectomy have no higher prostate cancer-specific or all-cause mortality than men who are just observed.

Minimizing Harm.—Men in their 40s may be screened to find lethal prostate cancers at a curable stage. PSA changes between ages 40 and 45 years are highly predictive of the risk of developing clinically important cancer and metastatic prostate cancer. Targeted PSA screening can prevent overdiagnosis and unneeded treatment and offer reduced morbidity and mortality. A study of 4383 men followed for 28 years found stepwise increases in PSA levels predict a 3- to 57-fold increased risk of prostate cancer and a 2- to 16-fold increased risk of prostate cancer mortality. Absolute 10-year risk of prostate cancer was 35% to 80% when the PSA level was higher than 10 ng/mL, but 0.6% to 1.5% when the level was less than 1 ng/mL.

Conclusions.—There are benefits and harmful consequences to PSA screening. A reasonable approach may be to obtain a baseline screening in asymptomatic men age 45 to 50 years if they want to be screened. Those with a baseline PSA level of 2 to 4 ng/mL could be rescreened every 2 to 4 years. Men whose PSA level was less than 2 ng/mL could delay screening for 10 years. Values over 4 ng/mL would prompt an examination for prostate cancer.

▶ This is a must read by anyone who screens patients for prostate cancer. In my opinion, the US Preventive Services Task Force got the facts right but the conclusions wrong. Prostate-specific antigen screening is flawed and we need a better test, but to return to the days of no screening will certainly lead to increased mortality from this disease. This article in *JAMA* provides a much more balanced view. It does discuss the task force's concerns but also discussed counter arguments. I will continue to screen my healthy young patients. I already believe that screening should stop for the majority of patients sometime in the early to mid 70s and certainly by age 80. Nothing in the task force's recommendations has changed my mind.

A. S. Kibel, MD

Prostate-Cancer Mortality at 11 Years of Follow-up
Schröder FH, for the ERSPC Investigators (Erasmus Univ Med Ctr, Rotterdam, the Netherlands; et al)
N Engl J Med 366:981-990, 2012

Background.—Several trials evaluating the effect of prostate-specific antigen (PSA) testing on prostate-cancer mortality have shown conflicting results. We updated prostate-cancer mortality in the European Randomized Study of Screening for Prostate Cancer with 2 additional years of follow-up.

Methods.—The study involved 182,160 men between the ages of 50 and 74 years at entry, with a predefined core age group of 162,388 men 55 to 69 years of age. The trial was conducted in eight European countries. Men who were randomly assigned to the screening group were offered PSA-based screening, whereas those in the control group were not offered such screening. The primary outcome was mortality from prostate cancer.

Results.—After a median follow-up of 11 years in the core age group, the relative reduction in the risk of death from prostate cancer in the screening group was 21% (rate ratio, 0.79; 95% confidence interval [CI], 0.68 to 0.91; $P = 0.001$), and 29% after adjustment for noncompliance. The absolute reduction in mortality in the screening group was 0.10 deaths per 1000 person-years or 1.07 deaths per 1000 men who underwent randomization. The rate ratio for death from prostate cancer during follow-up years 10 and 11 was 0.62 (95% CI, 0.45 to 0.85; $P = 0.003$). To prevent one death from prostate cancer at 11 years of follow-up, 1055 men would need to be invited for screening and 37 cancers would need to be detected. There was no significant between-group difference in all-cause mortality.

Conclusions.—Analyses after 2 additional years of follow-up consolidated our previous finding that PSA-based screening significantly reduced mortality from prostate cancer but did not affect all-cause mortality. (Current Controlled Trials number, ISRCTN49127736.)

▶ The European screening study for prostate cancer has clearly demonstrated an improvement in prostate cancer mortality (Fig 2 in the original article). The benefit is not as large as some would have hoped, but I think the results need to be tempered with a little bit of realism. We know that 3% of men die of prostate cancer. That means that 97% don't die of the disease. Therefore, we will have to screen a large number of men to find the few lethal cancers. This should not mean that we dismiss the problems of prostate-specific antigen (PSA) screening, namely, overdiagnosis. PSA is clearly not going to serve as a marker of tumor aggressiveness. Only with new markers will we begin to define who has disease in need of treatment and who can be safely observed.

A. S. Kibel, MD

Artificial Prostate-Specific Antigen Persistence After Radical Prostatectomy
Poyet C, Hof D, Sulser T, et al (Univ Hosp Zürich, Switzerland)
J Clin Oncol 30:e62-e63, 2012

Background.—Serum prostate-specific antigen (PSA) is a highly useful tool for detecting, staging, and monitoring patients with prostate cancer. It has some limitations as a screening test because it is organ specific, not disease specific. After radical prostatectomy (RP), PSA serves as an excellent tumor marker that is highly specific and sensitive for diagnosing recurrent or residual disease. PSA levels become undetectable within 4 to 6 weeks after RP. If they remain at a significant level after this point, the patient usually has disseminated prostate cancer, requiring further treatment. However, heterophilic antibodies (hAs) can complicate the situation, interfering with PSA results.

> *Case Report.*—Man, 62, underwent RP for a clinically localized prostatic adenocarcinoma. Preoperative serum PSA level was 12.2 ng/mL, digital rectal examination was normal, and a Gleason 6 adenocarcinoma was noted in 1 of 12 cores in the transrectal biopsy. Prostate volume was 45 mL. The pathology report identified an organ-contained adenocarcinoma involving both lobes of the prostate and surgical margins negative for tumor cells. At 6-week follow-up, the blood serum levels of PSA were 7.48 ng/mL. A repeat test 1 week later found levels of 7.94 ng/mL. The persistence of such a high level of PSA was improbable given the patient's clinical status, so his serum was analyzed for possible interferences and hAs were detected. After incubating his serum with a blocking reagent for hAs, PSA level fell below detectable limits. Follow-up 3 months later found no PSA after incubation with the hA blocking reagent.

Conclusions.—The high postoperative PSA serum concentrations in this patient were inconsistent with the low-risk features of his disease, so additional investigations were conducted. hAs are human antibodies against animal antibodies and can bind to both solid-phase immunoglobulin G (IgG) and tracer IgG and lead to false positive results on PSA tests. The blocking reagent neutralizes a broad range of hAs, including human anti-mouse antibodies, human antirabbit antibodies, human antigoat antibodies, human antisheep antibodies, and rheumatoid factor. It also reduces interference of hAs in two-site immunoassays such as that used for PSA measurement. Why hAs are in serum remains a mystery in many cases but it is known to occur in persons routinely exposed to animals or animal serum products. The prevalence of hAs in patient serum samples is reported to be 3% to 40%. Because evidence of disease based on a high PSA level after RP leads to further treatment that is potentially harmful, such as radiotherapy or hormone ablation, physicians should be aware of the effects of hAs on PSA tests and perform tests to identify immunologic interference. If serum hAs are detected, future serum samples should be pretreated with hA blocking reagents or tested using a different PSA test. Undiagnosed hA interference may have falsely elevated the initial PSA levels in this patient. He may have been a suitable candidate for active surveillance because his true PSA level was probably well below 10 ng/mL preoperatively.

▶ I almost never choose case reports to review, but this one was just too good. These authors report a patient with a persistent high prostate-specific antigen (PSA) following radical prostatectomy. They found that the elevation was not due to disease persistence but due to heterophilic antibodies that mimic PSA (Fig 2 in the original article). While I've never had a patient of mine with this problem, I have been referred patients like this. The surgeon swears the surgery went well, and the pathology looks fine. I've always attributed it to retained prostate tissue, though I've always wondered how the PSA could be so high in a patient unless a large piece of prostate was left behind. Now I have another possible explanation.

A. S. Kibel, MD

Risk

Germline Mutations in *HOXB13* and Prostate-Cancer Risk

Ewing CM, Ray AM, Lange EM, et al (Johns Hopkins Univ and the James Buchanan Brady Urological Inst, Baltimore, MD; Univ of Michigan Med School and the Univ of Michigan Comprehensive Cancer Ctr, Ann Arbor; Univ of North Carolina and the Univ of North Carolina Lineberger Comprehensive Cancer Ctr, Chapel Hill; et al)
N Engl J Med 366:141-149, 2012

Background.—Family history is a significant risk factor for prostate cancer, although the molecular basis for this association is poorly understood. Linkage studies have implicated chromosome 17q21-22 as a possible location of a prostate-cancer susceptibility gene.

Methods.—We screened more than 200 genes in the 17q21-22 region by sequencing germline DNA from 94 unrelated patients with prostate cancer from families selected for linkage to the candidate region. We tested family members, additional case subjects, and control subjects to characterize the frequency of the identified mutations.

Results.—Probands from four families were discovered to have a rare but recurrent mutation (G84E) in *HOXB13* (rs138213197), a homeobox transcription factor gene that is important in prostate development. All 18 men with prostate cancer and available DNA in these four families carried the mutation. The carrier rate of the G84E mutation was increased by a factor of approximately 20 in 5083 unrelated subjects of European descent who had prostate cancer, with the mutation found in 72 subjects (1.4%), as compared with 1 in 1401 control subjects (0.1%) ($P = 8.5 \times 10^{-7}$). The mutation was significantly more common in men with early-onset, familial prostate cancer (3.1%) than in those with late-onset, nonfamilial prostate cancer (0.6%) ($P = 2.0 \times 10^{-6}$).

Conclusions.—The novel *HOXB13* G84E variant is associated with a significantly increased risk of hereditary prostate cancer. Although the variant accounts for a small fraction of all prostate cancers, this finding has implications for prostate-cancer risk assessment and may provide new mechanistic insights into this common cancer. (Funded by the National Institutes of Health and others.)

▶ This important article examined more than 200 genes in the 17q21-22 region on 94 unrelated patients with prostate cancer from families selected for linkage to the candidate region and compared additional prostate cancer cases on control subjects to characterize the frequency of the identified mutations. The authors identified a novel *HOXB13* (G84E) variant that is associated with a significantly increased risk of hereditary prostate cancer.

Although this variant seems to account for a relatively small fraction of all prostate cancers, it potentially provides significant insight into risk assessment for this disease.

G. L. Andriole, Jr, MD

Dutasteride in localised prostate cancer management: the REDEEM randomised, double-blind, placebo-controlled trial
Fleshner NE, Lucia MS, Egerdie B, et al (Univ of Toronto, Ontario, Canada; Univ of Colorado School of Medicine, Aurora; Urologic Med Res, Kitchener, Ontario, Canada; et al)
Lancet 379:1103-1111, 2012

Background.—We aimed to investigate the safety and efficacy of dutasteride, a 5α-reductase inhibitor, on prostate cancer progression in men with low-risk disease who chose to be followed up with active surveillance.

Methods.—In our 3 year, randomised, double-blind, placebo-controlled study, undertaken at 65 academic medical centres or outpatient clinics in North America, we enrolled men aged 48–82 years who had low-volume, Gleason score 5–6 prostate cancer and had chosen to be followed up with active surveillance. We randomly allocated participants in a one-to-one ratio, stratified by site and in block sizes of four, to receive once-daily dutasteride 0.5 mg or matching placebo. Participants were followed up for 3 years, with 12-core prostate biopsy samples obtained after 18 months and 3 years. The primary endpoint was time to prostate cancer progression, defined as the number of days between the start of study treatment and the earlier of either pathological progression (in patients with ≥1 biopsy assessment after baseline) or therapeutic progression (start of medical therapy). This trial is registered with ClinicalTrials.gov, number NCT00363311.

Findings.—Between Aug 10, 2006, and March 26, 2007, we randomly allocated 302 participants, of whom 289 (96%) had at least one biopsy procedure after baseline and were included in the primary analysis. By 3 years, 54 (38%) of 144 men in the dutasteride group and 70 (48%) of 145 controls had prostate cancer progression (pathological or therapeutic; hazard ratio 0.62, 95% CI 0.43–0.89; $p=0.009$). Incidence of adverse events was much the same between treatment groups. 35 (24%) men in the dutasteride group and 23 (15%) controls had sexual adverse events or breast enlargement or tenderness. Eight (5%) men in the dutasteride group and seven (5%) controls had cardiovascular adverse events, but there were no prostate cancer-related deaths or instances of metastatic disease.

Interpretation.—Dutasteride could provide a beneficial adjunct to active surveillance for men with low-risk prostate cancer (Table 4).

▶ One of the challenges urologists must face in recommending active surveillance for men with low-risk localized prostate cancer is the patient's perception

TABLE 4.—Biopsy Assessment Characteristics at 18 Months and Final Biopsy

	Latest Biopsy Assessment on or Before 18 Months		Final Biopsy Assessment*	
	Dutasteride Group (n=139)	Placebo Group (n=136)	Dutasteride Group (n=140)	Placebo Group (n=136)
Gleason scores				
No cancer detected	39 (28%)	42 (31%)	50 (36%)	31 (23%)
5	0	1 (1%)	0	0
6	92 (66%)	77 (57%)	71 (51%)	83 (61%)
7–8	8 (6%)	16 (12%)	19 (14%)	22 (16%)
3+4	7 (5%)	10 (7%)	13 (9%)	15 (11%)
4+3	1 (1%)	4 (3%)	4 (3%)	4 (3%)
8	0	2 (1%)	2 (1%)	3 (2%)
Pathological characteristics†				
Mean percentage of cancer-positive cores	13.6% (12.41)	17.0% (17.43)	13.9% (13.51)	19.0% (17.23)
Mean cumulative length of tumours, mm	3.4 (5.76)	4.7 (6.49)	3.9 (5.75)	5.4 (6.83)

Data are n (%) or mean (SD).
*Latest biopsy assessment for a participant, irrespective of when that assessment occurred.
†Percentage of cancer-positive cores and tumour length were recorded as zero for biopsy assessments that did not detect cancer.

that his cancer is silently growing. Because 5 alpha-reductase inhibitors, including dutasteride, are known to shrink prostate cancers, the authors of this study randomly assigned men undergoing active surveillance to 3 years of dutasteride or placebo. The most important findings are shown in Table 4, which are that a higher proportion of patients in the dutasteride arm had no cancer on follow-up biopsies and that among the men who did have cancer, there was no difference in the proportion with aggressive histology (Gleason 7 and above).

This may suggest that dutasteride is a useful adjunct to active surveillance for patients with low-risk cancer. Additionally, such patients, if they have an enlarged prostate and symptoms of benign prostatic hyperplasia may benefit symptomatically as well.

G. L. Andriole, Jr, MD

Posttreatment Prostate Specific Antigen Nadir Predicts Prostate Cancer Specific and All Cause Mortality

Tseng YD, Chen M-H, Beard CJ, et al (Dana Farber Cancer Inst and Brigham and Women's Hosp, Boston, MA; et al)
J Urol 187:2068-2073, 2012

Purpose.—We investigated whether the prostate specific antigen nadir predicts prostate cancer specific and all cause mortality in men treated in a randomized trial of radiation with or without 6 months of androgen deprivation therapy.

Materials and Methods.—The study included 204 men with cT1b-T2bN0M0 prostate adenocarcinoma and at least 1 unfavorable factor, including prostate specific antigen less than 10 to 40 ng/ml, Gleason 7 or greater, or T3 on magnetic resonance imaging. We performed Fine and Gray regression, and Cox multivariable analysis to determine whether an increasing prostate specific antigen nadir was associated with prostate cancer specific and all cause mortality, adjusting for treatment, age, Adult Comorbidity Evaluation 27 score and cancer prognostic factors.

Results.—At a 6.9-year median followup median prostate specific antigen nadir was 0.7 ng/ml for radiation alone and 0.1 ng/ml for radiation plus androgen deprivation therapy. The prostate specific antigen nadir (adjusted HR 1.18/ng/ml increase, 95% CI 1.07−1.31, $p = 0.001$) and Gleason 8 or greater (adjusted HR 8.05, 95% CI 1.01−64.05, $p = 0.049$) significantly predicted increased prostate cancer specific mortality. Moderate/severe comorbidity carried a decreased risk (adjusted HR 0.13, 95% CI 0.02−0.96, $p = 0.045$). Higher prostate specific antigen nadir (adjusted HR 1.10/ng/ml increase, 95% CI 1.04−1.17), older age (adjusted HR 1.10/year, 95% CI 1.04−1.15) and interaction between comorbidity score and randomization arm (each $p < 0.001$) increased the all cause mortality risk. Men who achieved a prostate specific antigen nadir of the median value or less had lower estimated prostate cancer specific and all cause mortality at 7 years (3.7% vs 18.3%, $p = 0.0005$ and 31.5% vs 55.0%, $p = 0.002$).

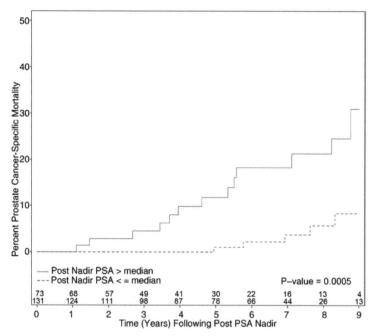

FIGURE 1.—Probability of posttreatment PCSM in men who achieved nPSA of median nPSA or less vs greater than median. (Reprinted from Tseng YD, Chen M-H, Beard CJ, et al. Posttreatment prostate specific antigen nadir predicts prostate cancer specific and all cause mortality. *J Urol.* 2012;187:2068-2073, Copyright 2012, with permission from the American Urological Association.)

Conclusions.—Posttreatment prostate specific antigen nadir is significantly associated with the risk of prostate cancer specific and all cause mortality after radiation with or without androgen deprivation therapy. A suboptimal prostate specific antigen nadir may identify candidates for earlier intervention to prolong survival (Fig 1).

▶ Lower is better, at least in terms of post-radiation therapy prostate-specific antigen levels for men with localized prostate cancer, as illustrated in Fig 1. Hopefully, validation of this finding in other and larger cohorts will allow early identification of men destined to fail after radiation so that additional therapies can be administered before subsequent biochemical or clinical failure. Potentially, that should result in improved outcomes.

G. L. Andriole, Jr, MD

Diagnostics

Short term outcomes of prostate biopsy in men tested for cancer by prostate specific antigen: prospective evaluation within ProtecT study

Rosario DJ, Lane JA, Metcalfe C, et al (Univ of Sheffield, UK; Univ of Bristol, UK; et al)
BMJ 344:d7894, 2012

Objectives.—To measure the effect of the adverse events within 35 days of transrectal ultrasound guided biopsy from the perspective of asymptomatic men having prostate specific antigen (PSA) testing; to assess early attitude to re-biopsy; to estimate healthcare resource use associated with adverse events due to biopsy; and to develop a classification scheme for reporting adverse events after prostate biopsy.

Design.—Prospective cohort study (Prostate Biopsy Effects: ProBE) nested within Prostate Testing for Cancer and Treatment (ProtecT) study.

Participants.—Between 1999 and 2008, 227 000 community dwelling men aged 5069 years were identified at 352 practices and invited to counselling about PSA testing. 111 148 attended a nurse led clinic in the community, and 10 297 with PSA concentrations of 3-20 ng/mL were offered biopsy within ProtecT. Between February 2006 and May 2008, 1147/1753 (65%) eligible men (mean age 62.1 years, mean PSA 5.4 ng/mL) having 10 core transrectal ultrasound guided biopsy under antibiotic cover in the context of ProtecT were recruited to the ProBE study.

Outcome Measures.—Purpose designed questionnaire administered at biopsy and 7 and 35 days after the procedure to measure frequency and effect of symptoms related to pain, infection, and bleeding; patients' attitude to repeat biopsy assessed immediately after biopsy and 7 days later; participants' healthcare resource use within 35 days of biopsy evaluated by questionnaire, telephone follow-up, and medical note review; each man's adverse event profile graded according to symptoms and healthcare use.

Results.—Pain was reported by 429/984 (43.6%), fever by 172/985 (17.5%), haematuria by 642/976 (65.8%), haematochezia by 356/967

(36.8%), and haemoejaculate by 605/653 (92.6%) men during the 35 days after biopsy. Fewer men rated these symptoms as a major/moderate problem—71/977 (7.3%) for pain, 54/981 (5.5%) for fever, 59/958 (6.2%) for haematuria, 24/951 (2.5%) for haematochezia, and 172/646 (26.6%) for haemoejaculate. Immediately after biopsy, 124/1142 (10.9%, 95% confidence interval 9.2 to 12.8) men reported that they would consider further biopsy a major or moderate problem: seven days after biopsy, this proportion had increased to 213/1085 (19.6%, 17.4% to 22.1%). A negative attitude to repeat biopsy was associated with unfavourable experience after the first biopsy, particularly pain at biopsy (odds ratio 8.2, $P < 0.001$) and symptoms related to infection (7.9, $P < 0.001$) and bleeding (4.2, $P < 0.001$); differences were evident between centres ($P < 0.001$). 119/1147 (10.4%, 8.7% to 12.3%) men reported consultation with a healthcare professional (usually their general practitioner), most commonly for infective symptoms. Complete data for all index symptoms at all time points were available in 851 participants. Symptoms and healthcare use could be used to grade these men as follows: grade 0 (no symptoms/contact) 18 (2.1%, 1.3% to 3.3%); grade 1 (minor problem/no contact) 550 (64.6%, 61.4% to 67.8%); grade 2 (moderate/ major problem or contact) 271 (31.8%, 28.8% to 35.1%); grade 3 (hospital admission) 12 (1.4%, 0.8% to 2.4%); and grade 4 (death) 0. Grade of adverse event was associated with an unfavourable attitude to repeat biopsy (Kendall's τ-b ordinal by ordinal 0.29, $P < 0.001$).

Conclusion.—This study with a high response rate of 89% at 35 days in men undergoing biopsy in the context of a randomised controlled trial has shown that although prostate biopsy is well tolerated by most men, it is associated with significant symptoms in a minority and affects attitudes to repeat biopsy and primary care resource use. These findings will inform men who seek PSA testing for detection of prostate cancer and assist their physicians during counselling about the potential risks and effect of biopsy. Variability in the adverse event profile between centres suggests that patients' outcomes could be improved and healthcare use reduced with more effective administration of local anaesthetic and antibiotics.

Trial Registration.—Current Controlled Trials ISRCTN20141297.

▶ This article provides solid data upon which to counsel our patients who are considering an initial or repeat transrectal prostate biopsy. The findings in Box 1 in the original article can be shown to patients, and the associated findings with respect to sepsis and hospital readmission rates (about 1% for each) are eye opening. These findings underscore the need to define a better way of diagnosing prostate cancer (perhaps imaging with subsequent targeted biopsy) and of improving the antibiotic and anesthetic regimens used for prostate biopsy.

G. L. Andriole, Jr, MD

PET in Prostate and Bladder Tumors

Lee ST, Lawrentschuk N, Scott AM (Austin Hosp, Melbourne, Australia; Ludwig Inst for Cancer Res, Melbourne, Australia)
Semin Nucl Med 42:231-246, 2012

^{18}F-fluorodeoxyglucose (FDG) is the most common positron emission tomography (PET) radiotracer used in prostate and bladder cancer evaluation, but its role is hampered by a generally low glucose metabolic rate in primary prostate carcinoma, and physiological excretion of FDG through the urinary system masking FDG uptake in primary bladder and prostate carcinoma. FDG-PET may have a role in selected patients for staging and restaging advanced prostate cancer, particularly in patients with an increasing prostatic-specific antigen (PSA) level. The use of diuresis strategies facilitates the identification of primary bladder cancer, and may be useful in staging extravesical spread of disease. FDG-PET may also be useful in patients with ureteric and urethral cancers. New PET tracers are showing promise in the staging and biological characterization of prostate cancer, which can assist with therapeutic decision making in patients undergoing radiotherapy of primary disease, and in the assessment of metastatic disease (Table 3).

▶ This is an up-to-the-moment summary of the potential role of positron emission tomography (PET) imaging in prostate and bladder cancer. The key areas showing the most promise are the use of PET/computed tomography for staging, choline PET for identification of the site of recurrent disease with a detectable prostate-specific antigen level after radical prostatectomy, and the use of fluoride scans to detect early bone metastases. These are nicely summarized in Table 3.

G. L. Andriole, Jr, MD

TABLE 3.—Summary of Current PET Imaging Applications in Prostate and Bladder Carcinoma

PET/CT Radiotracer	Stage of Disease	Current Status
Prostate Carcinoma ^{18}F-FDG-PET/CT*	Diagnosis, staging and restaging	Potentially useful for visceral and lymph node metastases
PET with other radiotracers eg, ^{11}C-choline, ^{18}F-fluoride†	Diagnosis, staging and restaging	Promising but more clinical data needed
Bladder Carcinoma ^{18}F-FDG-PET/CT‡	Diagnosis, staging and restaging	Potentially useful for visceral, lymph node, and bony metastatic disease
PET with other radiotracers eg, ^{11}C-methionine; ^{18}F-fluoride†	Diagnosis, staging and restaging	Promising but more clinical data needed

*United States Medicare/Medicaid funding does not cover initial treatment strategy for prostate carcinoma and only covers restaging PET for prostate carcinoma for patients who are eligible for entry in the National Oncologic PET Registry.
†^{18}F-fluorine tracer is used widely in the United States for detection of bony metastasis.
‡United States Medicare/Medicaid funding covers initial treatment and subsequent treatment FDG-PET scans in bladder carcinoma, but only in patients eligible for entry into the National Oncologic PET Registry.

Diagnostics/Staging

Impact on the Clinical Outcome of Prostate Cancer by the 2005 International Society of Urological Pathology Modified Gleason Grading System
Dong F, Wang C, Farris AB, et al (Massachusetts General Hosp, Boston)
Am J Surg Pathol 36:838-843, 2012

The 2005 International Society of Urological Pathology (ISUP) Consensus Conference modified the Gleason grading system for prostate cancer. In the modified criteria, ill-defined glands with poorly formed lumina and large cribriform glands with smooth borders, classically described as Gleason pattern 3 adenocarcinoma, were redefined as Gleason pattern 4. To evaluate the clinical outcome of patients upgraded by the ISUP criteria, the histologic slides of 1240 consecutive radical prostatectomy specimens at a single institution were reviewed, and each case of adenocarcinoma was graded on the basis of the original and modified Gleason criteria. A total of 806 patients with prostate cancer of classical Gleason score $3 + 3 = 6$ or $3 + 4 = 7$ and modified Gleason score 6 to 8 were analyzed with a median overall follow-up of 12.6 years. In the study population, 34% of patients with classical Gleason score $3 + 3 = 6$ prostate cancer were upgraded to modified Gleason score 7 or 8 by the ISUP criteria. Compared to patients with modified Gleason score $3 + 3 = 6$ and patients with classical Gleason score $3 + 4 = 7$, the upgraded patients were at intermediate risk for biochemical progression (paired log-rank $P \leq 0.003$) and metastasis (paired log-rank $P \leq 0.04$) after radical prostatectomy. The hazard ratio for upgrading was 1.60 (95% confidence interval, 1.09-2.35, $P = 0.02$) for biochemical recurrence and 5.02 (95% confidence interval, 1.77-14.2, $P = 0.003$) for metastasis. These results validate the prognostic value of the modified Gleason grading system and suggest that the recognition of an intermediate-risk

TABLE 3.—Patient Characteristics

	cGS $3 + 3 = 6$ mGS 6	cGS $3 + 3 = 6$ mGS 7-8	cGS $3 + 4 = 7$ mGS 7-8	P
No. patients	412	210	184	—
Seminal vesicle invasion present (%)	3 (0.7%)	11 (5.2%)	14 (7.6%)	<0.001
Seminal vesicle invasion absent (%)	409 (99.3%)	199 (94.8%)	170 (92.4%)	—
Pathologic stage pT2	383	155	132	
Positive margin (%)	63 (16.4%)	36 (23.2%)	52 (39.4%)	<0.001
Negative margin (%)	320 (83.6%)	119 (76.8%)	80 (60.6%)	—
Pathologic stage pT3	29	55	52	
Positive margin (%)	14 (48.3%)	26 (47.3%)	25 (48.1%)	0.99
Negative margin (%)	15 (51.7%)	29 (52.7%)	27 (51.9%)	—

cGS indicates classic Gleason score; mGS, modified Gleason score.

histological pattern may be useful in the prognosis of patients with prostate cancer (Table 3).

▶ This report supports the use of a modified Gleason score as proposed by International Society of Urological Pathology in 2005 over the classical Gleason score proposed in 1968. As shown in Table 3, upgrading from classical 3 + 3 to modified 7 or above was associated with worse outcome.

G. L. Andriole, Jr, MD

Extent of Cancer of Less Than 50% in Any Prostate Needle Biopsy Core: How Many Millimeters Are There?
Montironi R, Scarpelli M, Mazzucchelli R, et al (Polytechnic Univ of the Marche Region, Ancona, Italy; et al)
Eur Urol 61:751-756, 2012

Background.—Prostate-specific antigen (PSA)-n-based screening has reduced deaths from prostate cancer (PCa) by 20% but also increased PCa overtreatment. Active surveillance (AS) was introduced to help decrease overtreatment. One of the criteria used to select candidates for AS is that there be no more than 50% PCa involved in any needle biopsy core. However, there is no consensus about how to best measure tumor length or percentage on a core, especially foci of PCa are interspersed with benign stroma.

Value of Extent of Involvement.—Needle biopsies permit the diagnosis of PCa but also offer descriptive information such as type of cancer, amount of tumor, and grade. All these characteristics contribute to making accurate decisions about patient management, assessing the potential for local cure, and determining the risk for distant metastasis. Extent of involvement correlates to a degree with the Gleason score, tumor volume, surgical margins, and pathologic stage in radical prostatectomy (RP) specimens. Extent may also predict biochemical recurrence, progression after surgery, and radiation therapy failure. It has been used to predict pathologic stage and seminal vesicle invasion after RP and radiation therapy failure. Combining extent of involvement with the Gleason score, location of the tumor, and serum PSA levels increases prognostic and predictive power.

Reporting Extent of Involvement.—Extent of cancer can be reported as millimeters of cancer per core, total millimeters of cancer among all cores, percentage of cancer per core, total percentage of cancer in the entire specimen, number of positive cores, or fraction of positive cores. The percentage of each core involved with cancer is calculated based on the linear length of the cancer divided by the core length and then multiplied by 100. Visual estimation is an alternative method. The former method is more objective and reproducible than the latter, even if it requires more time.

When cancer and benign prostate tissue are interspersed in a core, one can measure the discontinuous foci of PCa as if they were a single continuous focus or ignore the intervening benign tissue and mentally collapse all separate cancer foci and add up the separate percentages. The same choices can be made if the cancer is measured in millimeters. Few data show which method is best for predicting pathologic outcome at RP. However, one study shows that for PCa in which the needle biopsy grade is representative of the entire tumor in the RP, quantifying cancer extent on biopsy by measuring the tumor from one end to the other rather than subtracting out benign tissue correlates better with organ-confined disease and risk of positive margins.

Factors Influencing Extent of Involvement.—The percentage of core involvement by PCa depends on the final length of the core in the slide, which is influenced by technical factors involved in tissue processing and/ or slide preparation. These include flattening cores between nylon sponges in cassettes, submitting multiple cores in a single cassette, and measuring cancer on fragmented cores. All of these reduce the probability of making the PCa diagnosis because important information is lost.

Conclusions.—The percentage of core involvement can correspond to various millimeters of cancer, so it may be best to actually measure the extent of cancer in millimeters. For a discontinuous sample, measuring the cancer from its beginning to its end gives the minimal diameter of cancer and may better reflect tumor volume.

▶ This article provides a thoughtful assessment of biopsy reporting conventions. As we are entering an era where more men are diagnosed with small prostate cancers and are potentially eligible for active surveillance, an accurate understanding on the part of the patient and physician of the amount of cancer identified on the biopsy is essential. The authors suggest the "total mm of cancer length" is preferable to "% core involvement" for making this assessment.

G. L. Andriole, Jr, MD

Natural History/Outcomes

Cigarette Smoking and Prostate Cancer Recurrence After Prostatectomy
Joshu CE, Mondul AM, Meinhold CL, et al (Johns Hopkins Bloomberg School of Public Health, Baltimore, MD; et al)
J Natl Cancer Inst 103:835-838, 2011

Toward the establishment of evidence-based recommendations for the prevention of prostate cancer recurrence after treatment, we examined the association between smoking and prostate cancer recurrence in a retrospective cohort study of 1416 men who underwent radical prostatectomy. Surgeries were performed by a single surgeon at Johns Hopkins Hospital between January 1, 1993, and March 31, 2006. Smoking status at 5 years before and 1 year after surgery was assessed by survey. Prostate cancer recurrence was defined as confirmed re-elevation of prostate-specific antigen levels, local recurrence, metastasis, or prostate cancer death. The cumulative incidence of recurrence was 34.3% among current smokers, 14.8% among former smokers, and 12.1% among never smokers, with a mean follow-up time of 7.3 years. Men who were current smokers at 1 year after surgery were more likely than never smokers to have disease recurrence after adjusting for pathological characteristics, including stage and grade (hazard ratio for recurrence = 2.31, 95% confidence interval = 1.05 to 5.10). This result suggests an association between cigarette smoking and risk of prostate cancer recurrence.

▶ Patients with newly diagnosed prostate carcinoma always want to know what they can do to prevent recurrences. Recommendations are difficult, because there are no prospective data that any treatment or behavior will decrease risk. In general, I recommend a heart-healthy diet with complex carbohydrates and limited meat and fats. The rationale for this is that there is good epidemiologic evidence that this will decrease risk of disease recurrence. More important, these recommendations are clearly heart-friendly, which is a bigger risk for death. This article provides some evidence that smoking cessation should be added to the recommendations. The authors found that men still smoking 1 year after surgery had more than double the risk of recurrence. Although this sounds impressive, this is only 8 of 51 patients in the entire cohort. In addition, although the authors controlled for multiple confounders, it is entirely possible that men who continue to smoke after a diagnosis of cancer have other characteristics that increase the risk of recurrence. For example, they may be less likely to follow recommendations for adjuvant therapy. However, can one really argue against smoking cessation? Just like the dietary recommendations, it will clearly decrease the risk of cardiovascular disease. If it improves outcomes for prostate cancer as well, that is icing on the cake.

A. S. Kibel, MD

Treatment Comparison

Trends in the treatment of localized prostate cancer using supplemented cancer registry data

Hamilton AS, Albertsen PC, Johnson TK, et al (Univ of Southern California, Los Angeles; Univ of Connecticut Health Ctr, Farmington; Ctr for Devices and Radiological Health, Silver Spring, MD; et al)
BJU Int 107:576-584, 2011

Objective.—To conduct an analysis of localized prostate cancer treatment in the USA between 1998 and 2002.

Patients and Methods.—Results from the National Cancer Institute's Patterns of Care study from 10 regional cancer registries in 1998 and 14 registries in 2002 were compared using univariate and multivariate statistical methods.

Results.—Patients with localized prostate cancer in 2002 were younger, had lower prostate-specific antigen values, and higher Gleason scores compared with those diagnosed in 1998. Little change occurred in age-adjusted percentages of men who were treated with a radical prostatectomy

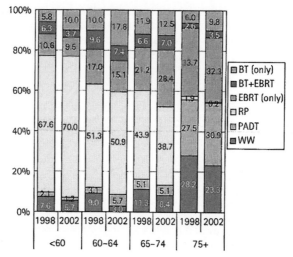

FIGURE 2.—Age-specific percentage distribution of type of initial therapy by diagnosis year. (Reprinted from Hamilton AS, Albertsen PC, Johnson TK, et al. Trends in the treatment of localized prostate cancer using supplemented cancer registry data. *BJU Int.* 2011;107:576-584, with permission from The Authors.)

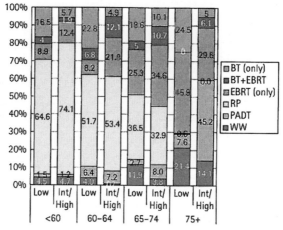

FIGURE 3.—Age-specific percentage distribution of type of initial therapy by risk group (risk group definition: Low = Gleason score <7 and PSA ≤10; Intermediate/High = Gleason score ≥7 or PSA >10) for clinically localized prostate cancer cased diagnosed in 2002. (Reprinted from Hamilton AS, Albertsen PC, Johnson TK, et al. Trends in the treatment of localized prostate cancer using supplemented cancer registry data. *BJU Int.* 2011;107:576-584, with permission from The Authors.)

(45–46%) or by external beam radiation (EBRT) alone (19–20%). The proportion receiving brachytherapy (BT), alone or with EBRT, increased from 14.9 to 17.7%, while the proportion receiving watchful waiting declined from 12.6 to 9.0%. Younger African-American men with intermediate/high-risk disease were less likely to receive any type of aggressive therapy in comparison with Non-Hispanic White men. Over 70% of men who were ≥75 years of age, with low-risk disease, were treated with EBRT or BT.

Conclusions.—Older men with low-risk disease might be overtreated with aggressive therapy, while younger intermediate/high-risk African-American men appear less likely to receive indicated aggressive therapy (Figs 2 and 3).

▶ Men with prostate cancer often seem to get treated irrespective of the patient's age and the tumor-related factors. Fig 2 shows that there has been very little change in distribution of treatments for men of various age strata between 1998 and 2002. Fig 3 shows a very tiny proportion of men are being offered watchful waiting, a recommendation that has been made by the National Institutes of Health's Consensus Conference Panel.

Overtreatment of prostate cancer has been and remains a difficult problem that the medical community should address. Use of dutasteride or focal ablation of tumors as an adjunct of active surveillance may minimize aggressive over-treatment of what is low-risk prostate cancer, which is generally a nonlethal condition.

G. L. Andriole, Jr, MD

Trends in Radical Prostatectomy: Centralization, Robotics, and Access to Urologic Cancer Care
Stitzenberg KB, Wong Y-N, Nielsen ME, et al (Univ of North Carolina, Chapel Hill; Fox Chase Cancer Ctr, Philadelphia, PA)
Cancer 118:54-62, 2012

Background.—Robotic surgery has been widely adopted for radical prostatectomy. We hypothesized that this change is rapidly shifting procedures away from hospitals that do not offer robotics and consequently increasing patient travel.

Methods.—A population-based observational study of all prostatectomies for cancer in New York, New Jersey, and Pennsylvania from 2000 to 2009 was performed using hospital discharge data. Hospital procedure volume was defined as the number of prostatectomies performed for cancer in a given year. Straight-line travel distance to the treating hospital was calculated for each case. Hospitals were contacted to determine the year of acquisition of the first robot.

Results.—From 2000 to 2009, the total number of prostatectomies performed annually increased substantially. The increase occurred almost entirely at the very high-volume centers (≥106 prostatectomies/year). The number of hospitals performing prostatectomy fell 37% from 2000 to 2009. By 2009, the 9% (21/244) of hospitals that had very high volume performed 57% of all prostatectomies, and the 35% (86/244) of hospitals with a robot performed 85% of all prostatectomies. The median travel distance increased 54% from 2000 to 2009 ($P < .001$). The proportion of patients traveling ≥15 miles increased from 24% to 40% ($P < .001$).

Conclusions.—Over the past decade, the number of radical prostatectomies performed has risen substantially. These procedures have been increasingly centralized at high-volume centers, leading to longer patient travel distances. Few prostatectomies are now performed at hospitals that do not offer robotic surgery (Figs 1A and 3).

▶ The introduction of robotic surgery into the management of prostate cancer has profoundly altered the management of the disease on multiple levels. This population-based evaluation of claims data for radical prostatectomy performed in New York, New Jersey, and Pennsylvania from 2000 to 2009 provides some remarkable insights. First and foremost is the tremendous centralization of care. Patients are increasingly managed at a few high-referral base centers (Fig 1A). In addition, patients are traveling farther and farther to seek care (Fig 3).

This is a descriptive study and therefore cannot inform us of the reasons for these shifts; however, one would expect this to be in part due to marketing and in part due to a rational regionalization of complex care. If these changes are due to high-volume centers providing better care, and therefore patients seeking them out, I for one believe this is probably a good thing. If, however, the changes are a result of marketing and are not related to quality of care, I believe that these changes would represent a detriment to care. The biggest impact would be in the Midwest, where robots are fewer. If patients have to travel long distances to get quality care, they may not. The result may (may—by no means certain) result in a decrease in quality of care simply due to access.

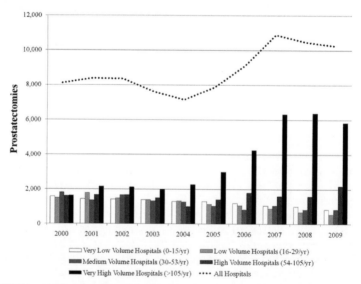

FIGURE 1.—Graph shows the total number of prostatectomies performed annually in New Jersey, New York, and Pennsylvania, 2000-2009. (Reprinted from Stitzenberg KB, Wong Y-N, Nielsen ME, et al. Trends in Radical Prostatectomy: Centralization, Robotics, and Access to Urologic Cancer Care. *Cancer.* 2012;118:54-62, Copyright 2012, American Cancer Society with permission of Wiley-Liss, Inc., a subsidiary of John Wiley & Sons, Inc.)

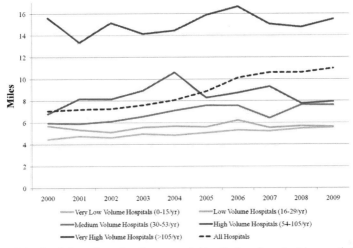

FIGURE 3.—Graph shows the median distance traveled in miles from the patient's home to the hospital where the prostatectomy was performed. (Reprinted from Stitzenberg KB, Wong Y-N, Nielsen ME, et al. Trends in Radical Prostatectomy: Centralization, Robotics, and Access to Urologic Cancer Care. *Cancer.* 2012;118:54-62, Copyright 2012, American Cancer Society with permission of Wiley-Liss, Inc., a subsidiary of John Wiley & Sons, Inc.)

Time will tell if findings in a relative dense part of the country hold true elsewhere.

A. S. Kibel, MD

Watchful Waiting/Outcomes

Active Surveillance for the Management of Prostate Cancer in a Contemporary Cohort
Dall'Era MA, Konety BR, Cowan JE, et al (Univ of California at San Francisco; et al)
Cancer 112:2664-2670, 2008

Background.—Active surveillance followed by selective treatment for men who have evidence of disease progression may be an option for select patients with early-stage prostate cancer. In this article, the authors report their experience in a contemporary cohort of men with prostate cancer who were managed with active surveillance.

Methods.—All men who were managed initially with active surveillance were identified through the authors' institutional database. Selection criteria for active surveillance included: prostate-specific antigen (PSA) <10 ng/mL, biopsy Gleason sum ≤6 with no pattern 4 or 5, cancer involvement of <33% of biopsy cores, and clinical stage T1/T2a tumor. Patients were followed with PSA measurements and digital rectal examination every 3 to 6 months and with transrectal ultrasound at 6- to 12-month intervals. Beginning in 2003, patients also underwent repeat prostate biopsy at

12 to 24 months. The primary outcome measured was active treatment. Evidence of disease progression, defined as an increase in rebiopsy Gleason sum or significant PSA velocity changes (>0.75 ng/mL per year), was a secondary outcome. Chi-square and log-rank tests were used to compare groups. The association between clinical characteristics and receipt of active treatment was analyzed by using Cox proportional hazards regression.

Results.—Three hundred twenty-one men (mean age [± standard deviation]: 63.4 ± 8.5 years) selected active surveillance as their initial management. The overall median follow-up was 3.6 years (range, 1−17 years). The initial mean PSA level was 6.5 ± 3.9 ng/mL. One hundred twenty men (37%) met at least 1 criterion for progression. Overall, 38% of men had higher grade on repeat biopsy, and 26% of men had a PSA velocity >0.75 ng/mL per year. Seventy-eight men (24%) received secondary treatment at a median 3 years (range, 1−17 years) after diagnosis. Approximately 13% of patients with no disease progression elected to obtain treatment. PSA density at diagnosis and rise in Gleason score on repeat biopsy were associated significantly with receipt of secondary treatment. The disease-specific survival rate was 100%.

Conclusions.—Selected individuals with early-stage prostate cancer may be candidates for active surveillance. Specific criteria can be and need to be developed to select the most appropriate individuals for this form of management and to monitor disease progression. A small attrition rate can be expected because of men who are unable or unwilling to tolerate surveillance.

▶ This important article demonstrates that by carefully selecting prostate cancer patients, and by consistently evaluating them over time with prostate-specific antigen (PSA) and a standardized biopsy approach, there is a low transition to definitive therapy for men on an active surveillance regimen. Avoiding aggressive treatment is particularly beneficial as we are learning that overdiagnosis and overtreatment of localized prostate cancer occurs for many men undergoing PSA-based screening.

G. L. Andriole, Jr, MD

Radical Prostatectomy Outcomes

A Clinicopathologic Study of Preoperative and Postoperative Findings with Minute Gleason 3 + 3 = 6 Cancer at Radical Prostatectomy
Osunkoya AO, Carter HB, Epstein JI (The Johns Hopkins Hosp, Baltimore, MD)
Urology 72:638-640, 2008

Objectives.—One would expect cases with small foci of cancer at radical prostatectomy to be associated with correspondingly favorable (Gleason score ≤6, <3 positive cores, no core with greater than 50% cancer) biopsy and preoperative clinical findings.

Methods.—Radical prostatectomies from The Johns Hopkins Hospital (July 2004 to July 2006) with only 1 to 3 slides involved by 3 + 3 = 6 adenocarcinoma of the prostate with no focus of cancer measuring greater than 2 mm in dimension were identified.

Results.—One hundred fifty-one radical prostatectomy specimens were obtained with cancer involving 1 slide in 69 cases (45.7%), 2 slides in 61 cases (40.4%), and 3 slides in 21 cases (13.9%). Predominantly transition zone cancer was present in 1 patient (0.66%). Mean patient age was 57.1 years (41 to 73 years). Twenty-two patients (14.6%) had a suspicious digital rectal examination. Mean serum prostate-specific antigen (PSA) and percentage free PSA were 5.2 ng/dL (0.3 to 16.7 ng/dL) and 15.5% (8% to 36%), respectively. Of 146, 127 (87%) men with available information had PSA density of less than 0.15. Mean number of cores obtained was 12 (4 to 27 cores) and all were Gleason $3 + 3 = 6$ cancers on biopsy. One hundred fourteen cases (75.5%) had 1 core positive, 28 cases (18.5%) 2 cores, and 9 cases (6%) had 3 or more cores positive. One hundred forty-eight cases (98%) had cancer involving 50% or less of 1 core; 2 of these cases with greater than 50% cancer were discontinuous foci.

Conclusions.—Although, typically, biopsy and clinical preoperative findings associated with very limited cancer at radical prostatectomy are correspondingly favorable, exceptions occur in terms of biopsy cancer extent, serum PSA measurements, and digital rectal examination findings.

▶ This study confirms the broadly suspected observation that our current techniques of prostate biopsy often yield misleading results. Sometimes the biopsy misses cancer, undergrades and understages it, or, as in this study, overestimates the tumor size. Clearly, these findings place physicians and patients in a difficult situation when trying to determine the best approach for a given man's cancer. Until imaging techniques improve, I think we should work on developing systematic, template-guided approaches to better identify and classify tumors.

G. L. Andriole, Jr, MD

Adverse Effects of Robotic-Assisted Laparoscopic Versus Open Retropubic Radical Prostatectomy Among a Nationwide Random Sample of Medicare-Age Men

Barry MJ, Gallagher PM, Skinner JS, et al (Massachusetts General Hosp, Boston; Univ of Massachusetts, Boston; The Dartmouth Inst for Health Policy & Clinical Practice, Hanover, NH)
J Clin Oncol 30:513-518, 2012

Purpose.—Robotic-assisted laparoscopic radical prostatectomy is eclipsing open radical prostatectomy among men with clinically localized prostate cancer. The objective of this study was to compare the risks of problems with continence and sexual function following these procedures among Medicare-age men.

Patients and Methods.—A population-based random sample was drawn from the 20% Medicare claims files for August 1, 2008, through December

31, 2008. Participants had hospital and physician claims for radical prostatectomy and diagnostic codes for prostate cancer and reported undergoing
either a robotic or open surgery. They received a mail survey that included
self-ratings of problems with continence and sexual function a median of
14 months postoperatively.

Results.—Completed surveys were obtained from 685 (86%) of 797
eligible participants, and 406 and 220 patients reported having had
robotic or open surgery, respectively. Overall, 189 (31.1%; 95% CI,
27.5% to 34.8%) of 607 men reported having a moderate or big problem
with continence, and 522 (88.0%; 95% CI, 85.4% to 90.6%) of 593 men
reported having a moderate or big problem with sexual function. In
logistic regression models predicting the log odds of a moderate or big
problem with postoperative continence and adjusting for age and educational level, robotic prostatectomy was associated with a nonsignificant
trend toward greater problems with continence (odds ratio [OR] 1.41;
95% CI, 0.97 to 2.05). Robotic prostatectomy was not associated with
greater problems with sexual function (OR, 0.87; 95% CI, 0.51 to 1.49).

Conclusion.—Risks of problems with continence and sexual function
are high after both procedures. Medicare-age men should not expect
fewer adverse effects following robotic prostatectomy.

▶ This interesting study was very eye-opening in that risks of continence and
sexual functions were high for men undergoing open or robotic prostatectomy
and similar among men undergoing open and robotic prostatectomy. Popular
press summarized this article by saying "don't believe the hype about robotic
prostatectomy." Notwithstanding, this lack of data in support of better outcomes,
many individuals continue to doubt advantages to robotic prostatectomy that
have not actually been demonstrated in a comprehensive study.

G. L. Andriole, Jr, MD

**Positive Surgical Margin and Perioperative Complication Rates of Primary
Surgical Treatments for Prostate Cancer: A Systematic Review and Meta-
Analysis Comparing Retropubic, Laparoscopic, and Robotic Prostatectomy**
Tewari A, Sooriakumaran P, Bloch DA, et al (Weill Cornell Med College—New
York Presbyterian Hosp; Stanford Univ School of Medicine, CA; et al)
Eur Urol 62:1-15, 2012

Context.—Radical prostatectomy (RP) approaches have rarely been
compared adequately with regard to margin and perioperative complication rates.

Objective.—Review the literature from 2002 to 2010 and compare
margin and perioperative complication rates for open retropubic RP
(ORP), laparoscopic RP (LRP), and robot-assisted LRP (RALP).

Evidence Acquisition.—Summary data were abstracted from 400 original research articles representing 167 184 ORP, 57 303 LRP, and 62 389

RALP patients (total: 286 876). Articles were found through PubMed and Scopus searches and met a priori inclusion criteria (eg, surgery after 1990, reporting margin rates and/or perioperative complications, study size >25 cases). The primary outcomes were positive surgical margin (PSM) rates, as well as total intra- and perioperative complication rates. Secondary outcomes included blood loss, transfusions, conversions, length of hospital stay, and rates for specific individual complications. Weighted averages were compared for each outcome using propensity adjustment.

Evidence Synthesis.—After propensity adjustment, the LRP group had higher positive surgical margin rates than the RALP group but similar rates to the ORP group. LRP and RALP showed significantly lower blood loss and transfusions, and a shorter length of hospital stay than the ORP group. Total perioperative complication rates were higher for ORP and LRP than for RALP. Total intraoperative complication rates were low for all modalities but lowest for RALP. Rates for readmission, reoperation, nerve, ureteral, and rectal injury, deep vein thrombosis, pneumonia, hematoma, lymphocele, anastomotic leak, fistula, and wound infection showed significant differences between groups, generally favoring RALP. The lack of randomized controlled trials, use of margin status as an indicator of oncologic control, and inability to perform cost comparisons are limitations of this study.

Conclusions.—This meta-analysis demonstrates that RALP is at least equivalent to ORP or LRP in terms of margin rates and suggests that RALP provides certain advantages, especially regarding decreased adverse events.

▶ This is a long run for a short slide: an impressive analysis that shows no substantial outcome differences among open, robotic, and laparoscopic prostatectomy. This seems to validate earlier reports.[1,2]

G. L. Andriole, Jr, MD

References

1. Leff B, Finucane TE. Gizmo idolatry. *JAMA.* 2008;299:1830-1832.
2. Barry MJ, Gallagher PM, Skinner JS, Fowler FJ Jr. Adverse effects of robotic-assisted laparoscopic versus open retropubic radical prostatectomy among a nationwide random sample of Medicare-age men. *J Clin Oncol.* 2012;30:513-518.

Orgasm-Associated Urinary Incontinence and Sexual Life after Radical Prostatectomy

Nilsson AE, Carlsson S, Johansson E, et al (Karolinska Institutet, Stockholm, Sweden; Akademiska Sjukhuset, Uppsala, Sweden)
J Sex Med 8:2632-2639, 2011

Introduction.—Involuntary release of urine during sexual climax, orgasm-associated urinary incontinence, occurs frequently after radical prostatectomy. We know little about its prevalence and its effect on sexual satisfaction.

Aim.—To determine the prevalence of orgasm-associated incontinence after radical prostatectomy and its effect on sexual satisfaction.

Methods.—Consecutive series, follow-up at one point in calendar time of men having undergone radical prostatectomy (open surgery or robot-assisted laparoscopic surgery) at Karolinska University Hospital, Stockholm, Sweden, 2002—2006. Of the 1,411 eligible men, 1,288 (91%) men completed a study-specific questionnaire.

Main Outcome Measure.—Prevalence rate of orgasm-associated incontinence.

Results.—Of the 1,288 men providing information, 691 were sexually active. Altogether, 268 men reported orgasm-associated urinary incontinence, of whom 230 (86%) were otherwise continent. When comparing them with the 422 not reporting the symptom but being sexually active, we found a prevalence ratio (with 95% confidence interval) of 1.5 (1.2—1.8) for not being able to satisfy the partner, 2.1 (1.1—3.5) for avoiding sexual activity because of fear of failing, 1.5 (1.1—2.1) for low orgasmic satisfaction, and 1.4 (1.2—1.7) for having sexual intercourse infrequently. Prevalence ratios increase in prostate-cancer survivors with a higher frequency of orgasm-associated urinary incontinence.

Conclusion.—We found orgasm-associated urinary incontinence to occur among a fifth of prostate cancer survivors having undergone radical prostatectomy, most of whom are continent when not engaged in sexual activity. The symptom was associated with several aspects of sexual life.

▶ This manuscript reports on orgasm-associated urine loss (climacturia) in a cohort of men having undergone radical prostatectomy. Of 691 sexually active men, 268 reported loss of urine with sexual climax. Tellingly, loss of urine occurred only at the time of climax in the vast majority of these men. Men with climaturia appeared to fare worse on a number of metrics pertaining to sexual satisfaction. Interestingly, men who had undergone prior transurethral resection of the prostate and those with persistent erectile dysfunction were at higher risk of climacturia.

Risk of ED and persistent urinary incontinence is routinely discussed with patients undergoing radical prostatectomy, although realistic expectations and outcomes may not always be adequately conveyed. These are critical issues, but of only slightly lesser importance to patients are more subtle issues pertaining to what sex will be like after prostate surgery. Penile length loss and/or new onset curvature is not uncommon[1]; furthermore, leakage of urine at sexual climax may persist for long periods of time, as this article makes clear. To best serve our patients, it is important that the litany of common possible long-term effects of radical pelvic surgery be discussed with patients beforehand; this will help set realistic expectations and goals and hopefully diminish the number of patients who are angered about things "no one ever told me about ..."

A. W. Shindel, MD

Reference

1. Mulhall JP. Penile length changes after radical prostatectomy. *BJU Int.* 2005;96:472-474.

Adverse Effects of Robotic-Assisted Laparoscopic Versus Open Retropubic Radical Prostatectomy Among a Nationwide Random Sample of Medicare-Age Men

Barry MJ, Gallagher PM, Skinner JS, et al (Massachusetts General Hosp, Boston; Univ of Massachusetts, Boston; Dartmouth College and Dartmouth Inst for Health Policy and Clinical Practice, Hanover, NH)
J Clin Oncol 30:513-518, 2012

Purpose.—Robotic-assisted laparoscopic radical prostatectomy is eclipsing open radical prostatectomy among men with clinically localized prostate cancer. The objective of this study was to compare the risks of problems with continence and sexual function following these procedures among Medicare-age men.

Patients and Methods.—A population-based random sample was drawn from the 20% Medicare claims files for August 1, 2008, through December 31, 2008. Participants had hospital and physician claims for radical prostatectomy and diagnostic codes for prostate cancer and reported undergoing either a robotic or open surgery. They received a mail survey that included self-ratings of problems with continence and sexual function a median of 14 months postoperatively.

Results.—Completed surveys were obtained from 685 (86%) of 797 eligible participants, and 406 and 220 patients reported having had robotic or open surgery, respectively. Overall, 189 (31.1%; 95% CI, 27.5% to 34.8%) of 607 men reported having a moderate or big problem with continence, and 522 (88.0%; 95% CI, 85.4% to 90.6%) of 593 men reported having a moderate or big problem with sexual function. In logistic regression models predicting the log odds of a moderate or big problem with postoperative continence and adjusting for age and educational level, robotic prostatectomy was associated with a nonsignificant trend toward greater problems with continence (odds ratio [OR] 1.41; 95% CI, 0.97 to 2.05). Robotic prostatectomy was not associated with greater problems with sexual function (OR, 0.87; 95% CI, 0.51 to 1.49).

Conclusion.—Risks of problems with continence and sexual function are high after both procedures. Medicare-age men should not expect fewer adverse effects following robotic prostatectomy.

▶ This article assessed a sample of men who underwent radical prostatectomy (via open or robotic approach) late in 2008. Participants completed a self-administered survey on bother from urinary and sexual complaints at a median of 14 months after their treatment. It was determined that the odds of moderate to big problems with sexual function did not differ based on surgical modality; however, there was a nonsignificant trend (95% CI, 0.97−2.05) toward greater frequency of urinary bother in men who had undergone a robotic procedure.

The authors made an assumption in their methodology that men who did not report having had a laparoscopic prostatectomy had an open prostatectomy by default. They took some steps to control for this by comparing this to claims' databases, which seems an innocent enough assumption, but it does cast some concern on the eventual conclusions.

Other variables to consider include specific medical comorbidities, relationship issues, and partner status; these factors exert a profound influence on sexual function and sexual function recovery, and they were not assessed. Finally, the great heterogeneity that is always present in random population samples from claims' databases make interpretation difficult.

Nevertheless, in the absence of any compelling data to the contrary, it can be concluded that claims that robotic surgery promises better sexual and urinary outcomes compared to open surgery have likely been overstated. Responsible surgeons should take this to heart and be very forthright with their patients that "robotic surgery" is not *necessarily* "better surgery."

A. W. Shindel, MD

Preoperative Erectile Function Represents a Significant Predictor of Postoperative Urinary Continence Recovery in Patients Treated With Bilateral Nerve Sparing Radical Prostatectomy
Gandaglia G, Suardi N, Gallina A, et al (Univ Vita-Salute San Raffaele, Milan, Italy)
J Urol 187:569-574, 2012

Purpose.—The association between baseline functional status and urinary continence recovery after radical prostatectomy remains controversial. We tested the hypothesis that baseline erectile and urinary function predicts urinary continence recovery after bilateral nerve sparing radical prostatectomy.

Materials and Methods.—The study included 752 patients with prostate cancer treated with bilateral nerve sparing radical prostatectomy between 2003 and 2009. All patients had preoperative functional and oncological data available, including age at surgery, body mass index, prostate specific antigen, and erectile and urinary function. Preoperatively erectile and urinary function was assessed by the erectile function domain of the International Index of Erectile Function and the International Prostatic Symptoms Score. Urinary continence was defined as wearing no pads. Univariate and multivariate Cox regression models were used to test the association between predictors and urinary continence recovery after surgery.

Results.—At a mean postoperative followup of 30.7 months (median 29, range 1 to 80) 611 patients (81.3%) had recovered urinary continence. Overall the urinary continence recovery rate at 1 and 3 years was 73.9% and 82.2%, respectively. On univariate Cox regression analysis patient age and the preoperative score on the erectile function domain of the International Index of Erectile Function were significantly associated with urinary continence recovery (each $p \leq 0.04$). On multivariate analysis age at surgery and the preoperative erectile function domain of the International Index of Erectile Function were the only independent predictors of urinary continence recovery after bilateral nerve sparing radical prostatectomy (each $p \leq 0.04$).

Conclusions.—Age and preoperative erectile function should be considered for urinary continence predictions after bilateral nerve sparing radical prostatectomy and for accurate patient counseling before surgery. Preoperative erectile function might be a marker of pelvic vascular disease, which may affect the status of the external urinary sphincter.

▶ This interesting retrospective, single institution study reports that normal preoperative erectile function (as defined by an International Index of Erectile Function and the International Prostatic Symptoms domain score greater than 26) and younger age were the only independent predictors of postoperative urinary control on multivariable analysis. The authors postulate that this may relate to superior vascular health in the potent men, although it may also be the case that healthier pelvic nerves in men without erectile dysfunction might also play a role.

In this study, continence is defined as wearing no pads; it seems safe to assume from this that leakage is absent or very minimal in those patients categorized as continent. Still, a more specific outcome measure might have changed these results. It is also possible that confounding factors related to postoperative care or psychological adaptations influenced these results. Fundamentally, the mechanistic extrapolations of these authors are logical but not proven by this study, and it remains to be determined how these data can be used in clinical practice.

A. W. Shindel, MD

Adverse Effects of Robotic-Assisted Laparoscopic Versus Open Retropubic Radical Prostatectomy Among a Nationwide Random Sample of Medicare-Age Men

Barry MJ, Gallagher PM, Skinner JS, et al (Massachusetts General Hosp, Boston; Univ of Massachusetts, Boston; Dartmouth College and The Dartmouth Inst for Health Policy & Clinical Practice, Hanover, NH)
J Clin Oncol 30:513-518, 2012

Purpose.—Robotic-assisted laparoscopic radical prostatectomy is eclipsing open radical prostatectomy among men with clinically localized prostate cancer. The objective of this study was to compare the risks of problems with continence and sexual function following these procedures among Medicare-age men.

Patients and Methods.—A population-based random sample was drawn from the 20% Medicare claims files for August 1, 2008, through December 31, 2008. Participants had hospital and physician claims for radical prostatectomy and diagnostic codes for prostate cancer and reported undergoing either a robotic or open surgery. They received a mail survey that included self-ratings of problems with continence and sexual function a median of 14 months postoperatively.

Results.—Completed surveys were obtained from 685 (86%) of 797 eligible participants, and 406 and 220 patients reported having had robotic or open surgery, respectively. Overall, 189 (31.1%; 95% CI, 27.5% to 34.8%) of 607 men reported having a moderate or big problem with continence, and 522 (88.0%; 95% CI, 85.4% to 90.6%) of 593 men reported having a moderate or big problem with sexual function. In logistic regression models predicting the log odds of a moderate or big problem with postoperative continence and adjusting for age and educational level, robotic prostatectomy was associated with a nonsignificant trend toward greater problems with continence (odds ratio [OR] 1.41; 95% CI, 0.97 to 2.05). Robotic prostatectomy was not associated with greater problems with sexual function (OR, 0.87; 95% CI, 0.51 to 1.49).

Conclusion.—Risks of problems with continence and sexual function are high after both procedures. Medicare-age men should not expect fewer adverse effects following robotic prostatectomy.

▶ Surgery for the management of prostate cancer clearly has side effects. The robot is often touted as producing fewer side effects, particularly improved sexual function. There has been a backlash against these claims, which have demonstrated that there are actually more side effects with robot use. Whom do you believe? I personally believe too much of the credit (and blame) is placed on the robot instead of on the surgeon or the patient.

Surgical experience matters. This has been shown over and over again. In this study, how many robotic prostatectomies has each surgeon done—1, 10, 100, or a 1000? The point is we don't know. Patient age and body habitus matter. These are clearly older patients with over 50% being over the age of 70 and 15% over the age of 75. It should come as no surprise that an older patient population is going to have more erectile dysfunction and incontinence. In addition, other patient factors matter—obesity and physical activity, for example. How healthy were the patients in this study? We don't know.

Until we have a randomized trial, we will not know if robotic surgery is better than open. My conclusions from this study are that complications occur, and that patients should seek experienced surgeons—either open or robotic—to remove their prostates.

A. S. Kibel, MD

Chemoprevention/Neoadjuvant Therapy

Denosumab and bone-metastasis-free survival in men with castration-resistant prostate cancer: results of a phase 3, randomised, placebo-controlled trial

Smith MR, Saad F, Coleman R, et al (Massachusetts General Hosp Cancer Ctr, Boston; Univ of Montreal Hosp Ctr, Quebec, Canada; Weston Park Hosp, Sheffield, UK; et al)
Lancet 379:39-46, 2012

Background.—Bone metastases are a major cause of morbidity and mortality in men with prostate cancer. Preclinical studies suggest that osteoclast inhibition might prevent bone metastases. We assessed denosumab, a fully human anti-RANKL monoclonal antibody, for prevention of bone metastasis or death in non-metastatic castration-resistant prostate cancer.

Methods.—In this phase 3, double-blind, randomised, placebo-controlled study, men with non-metastatic castration-resistant prostate cancer at high risk of bone metastasis (prostate-specific antigen [PSA] ≥8·0 µg/L or PSA doubling time ≤10·0 months, or both) were enrolled at 319 centres from 30 countries. Patients were randomly assigned (1:1) via an interactive voice response system to receive subcutaneous denosumab 120 mg or subcutaneous placebo every 4 weeks. Randomisation was stratified by PSA eligibility criteria and previous or ongoing chemotherapy for prostate cancer. Patients, investigators, and all people involved in study conduct were masked to treatment allocation. The primary endpoint was bone-metastasis-free survival, a composite endpoint determined by time to first occurrence of bone metastasis (symptomatic or asymptomatic) or death from any cause. Efficacy analysis was by intention to treat. The masked treatment phase of the trial has been completed. This trial was registered at ClinicalTrials.gov, number NCT00286091.

Findings.—1432 patients were randomly assigned to treatment groups (716 denosumab, 716 placebo). Denosumab significantly increased bone-metastasis-free survival by a median of 4·2 months compared with placebo (median 29·5 [95% CI 25·4–33·3] *vs* 25·2 [22·2–29·5] months; hazard ratio [HR] 0·85, 95% CI 0·73–0·98, $p = 0·028$). Denosumab also significantly delayed time to first bone metastasis (33·2 [95% CI 29·5–38·0] *vs* 29·5 [22·4–33·1] months; HR 0·84, 95% CI 0·71–0·98, $p = 0·032$). Overall survival did not differ between groups (denosumab, 43·9 [95% CI 40·1–not estimable] months *vs* placebo, 44·8 [40·1–not estimable] months; HR 1·01, 95% CI 0·85–1·20, $p = 0·91$). Rates of adverse events and serious adverse events were similar in both groups, except for osteonecrosis of the jaw and hypocalcaemia. 33 (5%) patients on denosumab developed osteonecrosis of the jaw versus none on placebo. Hypocalcaemia occurred in 12 (2%) patients on denosumab and two (<1%) on placebo.

Interpretation.—This large randomised study shows that targeting of the bone microenvironment can delay bone metastasis in men with prostate cancer.

▶ Bone metastases are a major cause for morbidity and mortality in men with prostate cancer. Receptor activator of nuclear factor kappa B ligand (RANKL) inhibitors are known to decrease the frequency of skeletal-related events in men who already have bone metastases. This trial evaluated men who were at high risk for the development of prostate cancer to receive the RANKL inhibitor denosumab or placebo. Men receiving denosumab had increased bone metastases—free survival by a median of 4.2 months compared to placebo (29.5 vs 25.2 months). Overall survival did not differ between the groups, possibly because of crossover to other treatments while on the trial.

Denosumab is useful to prevent androgen deprivation therapy—mediated bone loss and to decrease the rate of skeletal-related adverse events in men who have bone metastasis. This study shows it may have an additional role in delaying the onset of bone metastases.

G. L. Andriole, Jr, MD

Chemotherapy/Immunotherapy

Interdisciplinary Critique of Sipuleucel-T as Immunotherapy in Castration-Resistant Prostate Cancer

Huber ML, Haynes L, Parker C, et al (Trudeau Inst, Saranac Lake, NY; The Royal Marsden NHS Foundation Trust, UK)
J Natl Cancer Inst 104:273-279, 2012

Sipuleucel-T was approved by the US Food and Drug Administration on April 29, 2010, as an immunotherapy for late-stage prostate cancer. To manufacture sipuleucel-T, mononuclear cells harvested from the patient are incubated with a recombinant prostatic acid phosphatase (PAP) antigen and reinfused. The manufacturer proposes that antigen-presenting cells exogenously activated by PAP induce endogenous T-cells to attack PAP-bearing prostate cancer cells. However, the lack of demonstrable tumor responses has prompted calls for scrutiny of the design of the trials in which sipuleucel-T demonstrated a 4-month survival benefit. Previously unpublished data from the sipuleucel-T trials show worse overall survival in older vs younger patients in the placebo groups, which have not been shown previously to be prognostic for survival in castration-resistant prostate cancer patients receiving chemotherapy. Because two-thirds of the cells harvested from placebo patients, but not from the sipuleucel-T arm, were frozen and not reinfused, a detrimental effect of this large repeated cell loss provides a potential alternative explanation for the survival "benefit." Patient safety depends on adequately addressing this alternative explanation for the trial results (Table 2).

▶ Very few treatments for advanced prostate cancer have created as much controversy as sipuleucel-T. The original studies, while not showing any significant objective responses, nonetheless were associated with improved overall survival. This was confirmed in a second study, and, as a result, it was approved in April 2010 by the US Food and Drug Administration for the treatment of

TABLE 2.—Subgroup Analysis by Age Overall Survival of Patients in the Phase III Trials of Sipuleucel-T for Castration-Resistant Prostate Cancer (6)*

| Patient Age, y | Sipuleucel-T | | Placebo | |
	No. of Patients	Median Survival (95% CI), mo	No. of Patients	Median Survival (95% CI), mo
<65	106	29.0 (22.8 to 34.2)	66	28.2 (23.4 to 32.5)
≥65	382	23.4 (22.0 to 27.1)	183	17.3 (13.5 to 21.4)

*CI = confidence interval.

patients with minimally symptomatic castration-resistant prostate cancer. Many members of the urologic and prostate cancer community have been concerned that this treatment may not be as good as the 4.1-month survival benefit, particularly at a cost of more than $90 000. This article reanalyzes the data and suggests that, as shown in Table 2, all of the survival benefits occurred in treated patients over the age of 65. Moreover, the placebo-treated patients had a significantly worse survival than one might have expected. The authors raise a few hypotheses to explain this less-than-expected survival in the placebo group as owing to the inability of these elderly patients to reconstitute the white cells that were removed as part of their placebo therapy. Also, there could have been potentially some effects in patients who received the frozen cells subsequently. In any event, Provenge treatment remains controversial. It has been off putting to many prostate cancer specialists because of the high cost and lack of objective responses. Moreover, in an era of oral therapies (Zytiga and potentially MDB3000), this treatment may not be widely used.

G. L. Andriole, Jr, MD

Advanced Disease

Prostate cancer incidence in patients on 5α-reductase inhibitors for lower urinary tract symptoms: A 14-year retrospective study

Ahmad I, Small DR, Krishna NS, et al (The Beatson Inst for Cancer Res, Glasgow, UK; Southern General Hosp, Glasgow, UK)
Br J Med Surg Urol 5:179-183, 2012

There is still much debate regarding the long-term effect of 5α- reductase inhibitors (5-ARI) on the development of prostate cancer (PC). We tested the incidence of prostate cancer and the tumour Gleason grading in a non-screened population who were prescribed 5-ARIs for lower urinary tract symptoms (LUTS). Data from a prostatic biopsy database were analysed in a retrospective study, and included a period of 14 years (01/01/1997 to 01/01/2011). Those patients who were on 5-ARIs with either finasteride or dutasteride for less than 1 year were excluded. Patients who presented with LUTS and underwent diagnostic prostatic biopsies were included in this study. This patient cohort was further categorised according to their history of 5-ARIs medication.

The incidence of PC in the 5-ARI treated group was 15.4% ($n = 22/143$), comparable to that of the untreated group (16.7%, $n = 332/1990$) ($p = 0.7318$). Mean Gleason sum score and respective grade was the same ($7 = 3 + 4$) (median sum score 7 (range $6-10$)). Average age at the time of PC diagnosis was similar regardless of 5-ARIs treatment: 72 (range $50-84$) and 73 ($45-84$) years for treated and untreated groups, respectively.

In this retrospective study, patients treated with 5-ARIs for LUTS had similar risk in developing PC when compared to those who did not receive

5-ARIs. The Gleason sum scores for the cancers were similar in the two groups.

▶ The association of the higher incidence of higher Gleason score prostate cancer in men receiving 5-alpha-reductase inhibitors was first noted in 2003 for men receiving finasteride as part of the Prostate Cancer Prevention Trial (PCPT). This observational study with a 14-year follow-up does not show any excess high-grade cancer for men with benign prostatic hyperplasia (BPH) who received finasteride as part of therapy for BPH. These data may support the idea that the excess high Gleason score cancers occurring with 5-alpha-reductase inhibitors in randomized trials such as the PCPT may be caused by biases in the study design rather than clinically meaningful endpoints.

G. L. Andriole, Jr, MD

Abiraterone and Increased Survival in Metastatic Prostate Cancer
de Bono JS, for the COU-AA-301 Investigators (Inst of Cancer Res and Royal Marsden Hosp, Sutton, Surrey, UK; et al)
N Engl J Med 364:1995-2005, 2011

Background.—Biosynthesis of extragonadal androgen may contribute to the progression of castration-resistant prostate cancer. We evaluated whether abiraterone acetate, an inhibitor of androgen biosynthesis, prolongs overall survival among patients with metastatic castration-resistant prostate cancer who have received chemotherapy.

Methods.—We randomly assigned, in a 2:1 ratio, 1195 patients who had previously received docetaxel to receive 5 mg of prednisone twice daily with either 1000 mg of abiraterone acetate (797 patients) or placebo (398 patients). The primary end point was overall survival. The secondary end points included time to prostate-specific antigen (PSA) progression (elevation in the PSA level according to prespecified criteria), progression-free survival according to radiologic findings based on prespecified criteria, and the PSA response rate.

Results.—After a median follow-up of 12.8 months, overall survival was longer in the abiraterone acetate—prednisone group than in the placebo—prednisone group (14.8 months vs. 10.9 months; hazard ratio, 0.65; 95% confidence interval, 0.54 to 0.77; $P < 0.001$). Data were unblinded at the interim analysis, since these results exceeded the preplanned criteria for study termination. All secondary end points, including time to PSA progression (10.2 vs. 6.6 months; $P < 0.001$), progression-free survival (5.6 months vs. 3.6 months; $P < 0.001$), and PSA response rate (29% vs. 6%, $P < 0.001$), favored the treatment group. Mineralocorticoid-related adverse events, including fluid retention, hypertension, and hypokalemia, were more frequently reported in the abiraterone acetate—prednisone group than in the placebo—prednisone group.

Conclusions.—The inhibition of androgen biosynthesis by abiraterone acetate prolonged overall survival among patients with metastatic castration-resistant prostate cancer who previously received chemotherapy. (Funded by Cougar Biotechnology; COU-AA-301 ClinicalTrials.gov number, NCT00638690.)

▶ This much-anticipated study shows that inhibition of androgen biosynthesis by abiraterone acetate, which blocks cytochrome P450 c17 (CYP17), a critical enzyme in testosterone synthesis, improves survival of men with metastatic castrate-resistant prostate cancer who previously received docetaxel chemo-therapy. The difference in survival between the placebo and treated groups was 14.8 months versus 10 months. Both treatment arms received prednisone because of abiraterone's potential effect on inhibition of mineralocorticoid synthesis. As can be seen in Fig 2 in the original article, this effect was noted in virtually every subgroup.

This will add to the armamentarium of the treatment for men with advanced prostate cancer.[1] Hopefully, soon there will be other agents (alpha particles and selective androgen receptor inhibitors) that can also be applied to men with metastatic castrate-resistant prostate cancer.

G. L. Andriole, Jr, MD

Reference

1. Antonarakis ES, Eisenberger MA. Expanding treatment options for metastatic prostate cancer. *N Engl J Med.* 2011;364:2055-2058.

Safety and Immunological Efficacy of a DNA Vaccine Encoding Prostatic Acid Phosphatase in Patients With Stage D0 Prostate Cancer
McNeel DG, Dunphy EJ, Davies JG, et al (Univ of Wisconsin Paul P. Carbone Comprehensive Cancer Center, Madison; Univ of Wisconsin, Madison)
J Clin Oncol 27:4047-4054, 2009

Purpose.—Prostatic acid phosphatase (PAP) is a prostate tumor antigen. We have previously demonstrated that a DNA vaccine encoding PAP can elicit antigen-specific CD8+ T cells in rodents. We report here the results of a phase I/IIa trial conducted with a DNA vaccine encoding human PAP in patients with stage D0 prostate cancer.

Patients and Methods.—Twenty-two patients were treated in a dose-escalation trial with 100 μg, 500 μg, or 1,500 μg plasmid DNA, coadminis-tered intradermally with 200 μg granulocyte-macrophage colony-stimulating factor as a vaccine adjuvant, six times at 14-day intervals. All patients were observed for 1 year after treatment.

Results.—No significant adverse events were observed. Three (14%) of 22 patients developed PAP-specific IFNγ-secreting CD8+ T-cells immedi-ately after the treatment course, as determined by enzyme-linked immuno-spot. Nine (41%) of 22 patients developed PAP-specific CD4+ and/or CD8+ T-cell proliferation. Antibody responses to PAP were not detected. Overall, the prostate-specific antigen (PSA) doubling time was observed to increase from a median 6.5 months pretreatment to 8.5 months on-treatment ($P = .033$), and 9.3 months in the 1-year post-treatment period ($P = .054$).

Conclusion.—The demonstration that a DNA vaccine encoding PAP is safe, elicits an antigen-specific T-cell response, and may be associated with an increased PSA doubling time suggests that a multi-institutional phase II trial designed to evaluate clinical efficacy is warranted.

▶ This article by McNeel et al explores the potential utility of a prostatic acid phosphatase (PAP) DNA—based vaccine in treating patients who have biochemical failure following definitive local therapy with either radiation or surgery. This is a high-risk patient population with an average prostate-specific antigen (PSA) doubling time of 6.5 months (range 2.5-30.3 months). The authors report a vigorous immune response to the vaccine, and the vaccine was well tolerated. Seven of 22 patients had a decline in PSA, and there was an increase in the median PSA double time by 1.0 months. However, there were no complete responses and no PSA declines of greater than 50%.

Although these disease-specific endpoints clearly are not overwhelming, this study was not designed to prove the treatment is efficacious; such studies will hopefully be performed later. The study was designed to prove that the vaccine was well tolerated and the immune system could recognize the antigen. Both goals were met. Studies such as this demonstrate that vaccine-based approaches remain promising. Who potentially could benefit the most from an approach such as this? Exactly the patient population this group studied: high enough risk to justify aggressive management, an intact immune system to mount a response, and a disease state in which an immune response could eradicate low-volume disease.

A. S. Kibel, MD

Intensity-Modulated Radiation Therapy, Proton Therapy, or Conformal Radiation Therapy and Morbidity and Disease Control in Localized Prostate Cancer
Sheets NC, Goldin GH, Meyer A-M, et al (Univ of North Carolina at Chapel Hill)
JAMA 307:1611-1620, 2012

Context.—There has been rapid adoption of newer radiation treatments such as intensity-modulated radiation therapy (IMRT) and proton therapy despite greater cost and limited demonstrated benefit compared with previous technologies.

Objective.—To determine the comparative morbidity and disease control of IMRT, proton therapy, and conformal radiation therapy for primary prostate cancer treatment.

Design, Setting, and Patients.—Population-based study using Surveillance, Epidemiology, and End Results—Medicare-linked data from 2000 through 2009 for patients with nonmetastatic prostate cancer.

Main Outcome Measures.—Rates of gastrointestinal and urinary morbidity, erectile dysfunction, hip fractures, and additional cancer therapy.

Results.—Use of IMRT vs conformal radiation therapy increased from 0.15% in 2000 to 95.9% in 2008. In propensity score—adjusted analyses (N = 12 976), men who received IMRT vs conformal radiation therapy were less likely to receive a diagnosis of gastrointestinal morbidities (absolute risk, 13.4 vs 14.7 per 100 person-years; relative risk [RR], 0.91; 95% CI, 0.86-0.96) and hip fractures (absolute risk, 0.8 vs 1.0 per 100 person-years; RR, 0.78; 95% CI, 0.65-0.93) but more likely to receive a diagnosis of erectile dysfunction (absolute risk, 5.9 vs 5.3 per 100 person-years; RR, 1.12; 95% CI, 1.03-1.20). Intensity-modulated radiation therapy patients were less likely to receive additional cancer therapy (absolute risk, 2.5 vs 3.1 per 100 person-years; RR, 0.81; 95% CI, 0.73-0.89). In a propensity score—matched comparison between IMRT and proton therapy (n = 1368), IMRT patients had a lower rate of gastrointestinal morbidity (absolute risk, 12.2 vs 17.8 per 100 person-years; RR, 0.66; 95% CI, 0.55-0.79). There were no significant differences in rates of other morbidities or additional therapies between IMRT and proton therapy.

Conclusions.—Among patients with nonmetastatic prostate cancer, the use of IMRT compared with conformal radiation therapy was associated with less gastrointestinal morbidity and fewer hip fractures but more erectile dysfunction; IMRT compared with proton therapy was associated with less gastrointestinal morbidity.

▶ Is new better? We live in a society that rapidly adopts the latest and greatest without much thought as to whether it is actually better. This well-done study from the University of North Carolina—Chapel Hill explores the changes in radiation therapy treatments from 2000 to 2008. I think the most incredible statistic is that intensity-modulated radiation therapy (IMRT) utilization increased from 0.15% in 2000 to 95.9% in 2008. This is with few data that show it is any better than previous treatments. The authors found that IMRT was associated with lower gastrointestinal (GI) toxicity and hip fractures but at the cost of more impotence. Proton-beam therapy, on the other hand, was found to have more GI toxicity than IMRT. There was not a long enough follow-up to look at cure rates, but there was a trend for patients receiving conformal-beam radiation therapy to need additional therapies, implying that they had failed primary therapy.

What is missing from this discussion is the increased cost of IMRT and proton-beam therapy. Do the results justify the increased cost? I am not an economist, but as money gets tighter, we are going to have to take a hard look at new technology and not simply embrace the latest and greatest!

A. S. Kibel, MD

Other

Appropriate Patient Selection in the Focal Treatment of Prostate Cancer: The Role of Transperineal 3-Dimensional Pathologic Mapping of the Prostate—A 4-Year Experience

Barzell WE, Melamed MR (Urology Treatment Ctr, Sarasota, FL; New York Med College, Valhalla)
Urology 70:27-35, 2007

This study was undertaken to evaluate the usefulness of transperineal mapping biopsy of the prostate as a staging procedure in the appropriate selection of patients for treatment with focal cryoablation. Between October 2001 and January 2006, a total of 80 patients underwent extensive template-guided transperineal pathologic mapping of the prostate (3-DPM), in conjunction with repeat transrectal ultrasound (TRUS)-guided biopsies. Before 3-DPM was performed, the following clinical variables were recorded: age, prostate-specific antigen (PSA), percent free PSA, total prostate volume, transition zone volume, Gleason score, TNM stage, number of positive cores, and maximum percent of positive cores. Results of 3-DPM were compared with those of TRUS-guided biopsies to determine patient suitability for focal cryoablation; this served as the study end point. Of 80 study patients, 43 (54%) were deemed unsuitable for focal cryoablation. When compared with 3-DPM in assessing patient suitability for focal cryoablation repeat TRUS-guided biopsies yielded a false-negative rate of 47%, a sensitivity of 54%, and a negative predictive value of 49%. None of the pre–3-DPM variables correlated significantly with patient suitability for focal ablation. Treatment selected by the 80 study patients included total gland cryoablation (30%), expectant management (23%), radical prostatectomy (18%), focal cryoablation (11%), external irradiation (10%), brachytherapy (6%), and combined external irradiation and brachytherapy (1%); 1% were undecided about treatment selection. In this study, we demonstrated that 3-DPM (1) effectively excluded patients with clinically significant unsuspected cancer outside the area destined to be ablated, (2) appeared to do so more effectively than repeat TRUS-guided biopsies, and (3) was able to precisely locate the site of the cancer to be selectively ablated.

▶ This form of template-guided biopsy, although more cumbersome for the patient and urologist than transrectal biopsy,[1] is nonetheless useful to identify appropriate patients for focal therapy. It stands a good chance of identifying men who appear, on conventional transrectal ultrasound biopsy, to harbor low-risk, unifocal tumors, that actually have larger, multifocal tumors not appropriate for focal ablation. Most urologists who perform brachytherapy can readily perform the steps outlined in the figure.

What we need is a reliable transrectal, template-guided biopsy that accomplishes the same things. The TargetScan approach may be the way to accomplish this in the office setting.

G. L. Andriole, Jr, MD

Reference

1. Andriole GL, Bullock TL, Belani JS, et al. Is there a better way to biopsy the prostate? Prospects for a novel transrectal systematic biopsy approach. *Urology.* 2007; 70:22-26.

8 Testicular Cancer

Laparoscopic Retroperitoneal Lymph Node Dissection for Clinical Stage I Nonseminomatous Germ Cell Tumor: A Large Single Institution Experience

Hyams ES, Pierorazio P, Proteek O, et al (Johns Hopkins Univ, Baltimore, MD; Long Island Jewish Hosp, New Hyde Park, NY)

J Urol 187:487-492, 2012

Purpose.—Primary laparoscopic retroperitoneal lymph node dissection is done at our institution with therapeutic intent and it technically duplicates the open approach. Controversies associated with the procedure include the thoroughness of dissection, the high rate of chemotherapy exposure and the potential deleterious effects of pneumoperitoneum. We present our experience with laparoscopic retroperitoneal lymph node dissection for clinical stage I nonseminomatous germ cell tumors.

Materials and Methods.—We queried the Johns Hopkins minimally invasive surgery database from 1995 to 2010 for patients with a clinical stage I nonseminomatous germ cell tumor undergoing laparoscopic retroperitoneal lymph node dissection. Demographic, perioperative, pathological and followup information was collected and analyzed.

Results.—Of the 91 patients who underwent extended template laparoscopic retroperitoneal lymph node dissection during the study period 60 (66%) had lymphovascular invasion and 55 (60%) had greater than 40% embryonal carcinoma. Median estimated blood loss was 200 cc and mean length of stay was 2.1 days (range 1 to 4). Four patients (4.3%) experienced intraoperative complications and there were 4 open conversions (4.3%). Nine patients (9.8%) experienced postoperative complications. The mean lymph node count was 26.1 (range 7 to 72) and 28 patients (31%) had retroperitoneal metastasis. Followup was available for 55 patients at a median 38.0 months (range 12 to 168). No pN0 case recurred in the retroperitoneum but there were 5 systemic relapses in pN0 cases. Of the 21 patients with pN1 disease 14 elected chemotherapy and 7 elected surveillance. There was no relapse in either group.

Conclusions.—Laparoscopic retroperitoneal lymph node dissection appears to be safe, viable and effective for stage I nonseminomatous germ cell tumors. The lack of retroperitoneal recurrence in pN0—N1 cases supports the oncological efficacy of this approach. Its low morbidity and rapid convalescence compare favorably with those in open series.

▶ The historical standard for retroperitoneal lymph node dissection (RPLND) is open surgery with nearly 100% long-term cure in pN0 and pN1 cases. The cure rate is also high for those requiring chemotherapy for relapse. Patients with lymph-vascular invasion or high-volume embryonal cell carcinoma are at high risk for metastasis; RPLND is a reasonable choice even when cross sectional imaging is normal. Open RPLND is associated with significant potential morbidity, so as long as laparoscopic RPLND has oncologic equivalency, then use should be considered. The authors do show a low operative morbidity and perioperative complications. In most centers, chemotherapy is not routinely administered after open RPLND revealing pN1 disease. In this and other series, several patients receive chemotherapy, and that does not allow a pure evaluation of the completeness of the surgical dissection. Given the decreased morbidity, continued exploration of this technique at centers with skilled laparoscopic surgeons is warranted.

D. E. Coplen, MD

Testicular Adrenal Rest Tumors in Patients With Congenital Adrenal Hyperplasia: Prevalence and Sonographic, Hormonal, and Seminal Characteristics
Delfino M, Elia J, Imbrogno N, et al (Univ of Rome "Sapienza," Italy)
J Ultrasound Med 31:383-388, 2012

Objective.—Testicular adrenal rest tumors have been described in patients with congenital adrenal hyperplasia (CAH). The aim of this work was to (1) evaluate the prevalence of testicular adrenal rest tumors in patients with CAH; (2) study the hormonal profile; (3) define the sonographic features; (4) assess the seminal profile; and (5) initiate a longitudinal study on the possible role of corticotropin (ACTH) plasma levels in the induction and persistence of testicular adrenal rest tumors.

Methods.—Eighteen patients affected by CAH, aged 21 to 41 years, were studied. These were all patients referred to our endocrinology unit for the first time to undergo a clinical evaluation. All of the patients were taking long-term cortisone acetate and fludrocortisone replacement therapy. The study included (1) a physical examination, (2) testis sonography, (3) a hormonal profile, (4) semen analysis.

Results.—Sonography showed testicular adrenal rest tumors in 11 patients (61.1%); of these, 9 cases (50.0%) were bilateral, and 2 (11.1%) were unilateral. The diameter ranged from 4 to 38 mm. In 9 patients, the lesions were hypoechoic, whereas in 2, they were hyperechoic. High plasma ACTH levels were detected in all of the patients with tumors despite long-term therapy. Semen analysis found 2 cases of azoospermia and 6 cases of oligoasthenoteratozoospermia; the 3 remaining patients were normospermic. The preliminary longitudinal study has shown 3 patients with a disappearance or reduction of the tumors after 6 months of modified treatment.

Conclusions.—This study confirms the high prevalence of testicular adrenal rest tumors in patients with CAH and the major role played in its pathogenesis by high plasma ACTH levels.

▶ Ectopic adrenal tissue can be present in the cord and the testicle. Tumors were identified in a majority of asymptomatic men with congenital adrenal hyperplasia (CAH). These are usually clinically insignificant, but the adrenal rests can enlarge and become symptomatic when men with CAH are suboptimally suppressed (glucocorticoids mineralocorticoids) or are noncompliant with therapy. A testicular mass in a man with CAH is a hyperplastic rest until proven otherwise. The images in the article show the variable ultrasound characteristics. Testicular tumor markers (alpha-fetoprotein and β—human chorionic gonadotropin) are normal. Serum 17-OH progesterone will be markedly elevated. Medical treatment and not surgical intervention (radical inguinal orchiectomy) is the cornerstone of management. The tumors regress and symptoms resolve with steroid replacement and normalization of the 17-OH progesterone. There was a relationship between abnormal seminal parameters and the presence of a tumor on ultrasound scan. On that basis, one could argue that orchiectomy would not alter fertility. However, it would be interesting to see if the semen analysis improved after steroid suppression.

D. E. Coplen, MD

9 Sexual Function

Improvement in Sexual Quality of Life of the Female Partner Following Vardenafil Treatment of Men with Erectile Dysfunction: A Randomized, Double-Blind, Placebo-Controlled Study

Martín-Morales A, Graziottin A, Jaoudé GB, et al (Hosp Carlos Haya, Malaga, Spain; H. San Raffaele Resnati, Milan, Italy; Centre d'Etude et de Traitement de la Pathologie de l'Appareil Reproducteur et de la Psychosomatique (CETPARP), Lille, France; et al)
J Sex Med [Epub ahead of print] 2011

Introduction.—Erectile dysfunction (ED) impacts on both members of the couple. Female partners of men with ED are more likely to report reduced sexual quality of life than women whose partners do not have ED.

Aim.—To assess vardenafil efficacy in men with ED and determine the effects of treatment on their female partner's sexual quality of life.

Methods.—Study participants comprised men aged 18–64 years with ED and their female partners. Eligible men had ED of ≥6 months' duration and a female partner who was motivated to support their ED treatment. Eligible women had a total Female Sexual Function Index score >23.55, indicating absence of significant sexual dysfunction. Following a 4-week screening period, men were randomized to treatment with vardenafil 10 mg or placebo, which could be titrated to 20 or 5 mg after 4 weeks.

Main Outcomes Measures.—Primary efficacy variables were question 3 of the Sexual Encounter Profile questionnaire (SEP3) and the quality-of-life domain of the modified Sexual Life Quality Questionnaire (mSLQQ-QOL).

Results.—The intent-to-treat population included 343 couples, with 168 and 175 men receiving vardenafil or placebo, respectively. Vardenafil treatment significantly improved both erection maintenance and the female partners' sexual quality of life. Least squares (LS) mean SEP3 overall success rates after 12 weeks of treatment were 9.5 (baseline) vs. 67.2 (week 12) and 12.4 (baseline) vs. 24.2 (week 12) in the vardenafil and placebo groups, respectively ($P < 0.0001$). In female partners, LS mean mSLQQ-QOL scores were 28.8 (baseline) vs. 68.2 (last observation carried forward [LOCF]) in the vardenafil group and 24.6 (baseline) vs. 40.5 (LOCF) in the placebo group ($P < 0.0001$).

Conclusions.—Vardenafil treatment of men with ED improved both their erectile function and the sexual quality of life of their female partners.

▶ In this 12-week double-blind placebo-controlled study of 343 heterosexual couples (277 of whom completed the entire study), it was demonstrated that treatment with vardenafil significantly improved sexual quality of life and ability to maintain erection to completion of intercourse in men with erectile dysfunction. This is not a novel finding; however, the female partners of these men were also queried and it was determined that the partners of vardenafil-treated men experienced substantial and statistically significant improvements in sexual quality of life as assessed by the modified sexual quality of life questionnaire. Women in this study were required to have no or only mild physical problems at baseline as determined by a Female Sexual Function Index (FSFI) total score of 23.55 or greater; of note, an FSFI-total score of greater than 26.55 is the most frequently used cut-point for "lower risk" of female sexual dysfunction.

The findings of this study with respect to female partners are hardly surprising. Be that as it may, this provides compelling evidence that men and women who are struggling with sexual problems should talk to their significant other about the situation and seek out appropriate treatment; this may be good for both the patient and his or her partner. It is incumbent on health care providers to help initiate this conversation with both their male and female patients and to facilitate appropriate treatment or referral for both members of the couple.

A. W. Shindel, MD

Recreational Use of Erectile Dysfunction Medications in Undergraduate Men in the United States: Characteristics and Associated Risk Factors

Harte CB, Meston CM (Univ of Texas at Austin)
Arch Sex Behav 40:597-606, 2011

Mounting evidence indicates that erectile dysfunction medications (EDMs) have become increasingly used as a sexual enhancement aid among men without a medical indication. Recreational EDM use has been associated with increased sexual risk behaviors, an increased risk for STIs, including incident HIV infection, and high rates of concomitant illicit drug use. The aim of the present study was to investigate the characteristics and associated risk factors for recreational EDM use among young, healthy, undergraduate men. A cross-sectional sample of 1,944 men were recruited from 497 undergraduate institutions within the Unites States between January 2006 and May 2007. The survey assessed patterns of EDM use, as well as demographic, substance use, and sexual behavior characteristics. Four percent of participants had recreationally used an EDM at some point in their lives, with 1.4% reporting current use. The majority of recreational EDM users reported mixing EDMs with illicit drugs and particularly during risky sexual behaviors. Recreational EDM use was independently associated with increased age, gay, or bisexual sexual orientation, drug abuse, lifetime number of sex partners, and lifetime number of "one-night stands." Recreational EDM users also reported a 2.5-fold rate of erectile difficulties compared to nonusers. Overall, recreational use of EDMs was associated with sexual risk behaviors and substance abuse; however, a relatively small proportion of undergraduates reported using EDMs. Results also suggest that a sizable portion of recreational EDM users are heterosexual men, and that use does not solely occur within the environments of venues that cater to men having sex with men.

▶ This survey of undergraduate men in the United States reported an approximately 5% prevalence of erectile dysfunction (ED) medication use in this population. Erectile difficulties were much more likely in the group that had used medications, and in 1% of the overall cohort the medication was dispensed for the management of erectile difficulties. Four percent of this study cohort used ED medications for enhancement of sexual performance, ie, recreational use. Interestingly, one-quarter of the cohort of recreational ED medication users had International Index of Erectile Function scores consistent with at least mild ED, suggesting that the prevalence of clinically relevant erectile difficulty in the ED medication—using cohort was higher than self-report would indicate.

Recreational use of erectogenic medications has been associated with higher risk sexual activity and abuse of other drugs; indeed, the use of these medications for countering of anti-erectogenic effects of illicit drugs was reported by 29% of the medication-using cohort. This has been extensively characterized in men who have sex with men (MSM), but this study makes it clear that recreational PDE5I use is not strictly a public health problem of the MSM population. It is also germane that a substantial proportion of young men endorse International Index of Erectile Function scores consistent with some degree of ED but do not characterize themselves as having the disorder. Increased public awareness about the ubiquity of sexual concerns in men of all ages may help younger men who are struggling with erection problems (organic or psychological) seek out professional advice and treatment rather than relying on black market erectogenic medications.

A. W. Shindel, MD

Low serum testosterone levels are poor predictors of sexual dysfunction
Marberger M, Wilson TH, Rittmaster RS (Univ of Vienna, Austria; Res Triangle Park, NC)
BJU Int 108:256-262, 2011

Objective.—• To identify predictors of sexual dysfunction using baseline data from the reduction by dutasteride of prostate cancer events (REDUCE) study.

Patients and Methods.—• REDUCE was a 4-year randomized, double-blind, placebo-controlled study evaluating the efficacy and safety of once-daily dutasteride 0.5 mg in over 8000 men aged 50–75 years with a prostate-specific antigen (PSA) level of 2.5–10 ng/mL (50–60 years) or 3.0–10 ng/mL (>60 years) and a negative prostate biopsy within 6 months of enrolment.

• Baseline values (mean serum testosterone, age, International Prostate Symptom Score [IPSS], total prostate volume [TPV], body mass index [BMI], and presence of diabetes/ glucose intolerance) were compared in subjects with and without sexual dysfunction (sexual inactivity, impotence, decreased libido or a Problem Assessment Scale of the Sexual Function Index [PAS-SFI] score <9).

Results.—• Multivariate logistic regression showed that baseline age and IPSS were significant predictors of all four sexual function criteria examined ($P < 0.0001$).

• BMI was a significant predictor of decreased libido, impotence and a PAS-SFI score <9, while diabetes/glucose intolerance was a significant predictor of sexual inactivity, impotence and a PAS-SFI score <9.

• Testosterone and TPV were not significant predictors of any sexual function criterion examined.

Conclusions.—• Age, IPSS, BMI and diabetes/glucose intolerance, but not serum testosterone or TPV, were significant independent predictors of sexual dysfunction in the REDUCE study population.

• The lack of association between sexual dysfunction and serum testosterone questions the value of modestly reduced or low normal testosterone levels as criteria for choosing testosterone replacement in older men with sexual dysfunction.

▶ Testosterone is widely touted as a potential cure for all manner of age-associated ills. It is clear that there is a gradual decline in serum testosterone as men age, but correlation does not imply causation and it is less certain that testosterone replacement therapy is the panacea many men and their providers might wish. Be that as it may, it is undeniable that there are men who benefit from replacement therapy; the clinical challenge is selection of the right patient.

This substudy from the REDUCE trial of dutasteride for the prevention of prostate cancer examines the relationship between serum testosterone level and sexual concerns in a large population of men. Serum testosterone was determined based on a single draw at baseline; it does not appear that adjustment was made for potential confounders such as elevated sex hormone binding globulin, which may reduce the free bioavailable fraction.

There was no significant predictive utility of serum testosterone with respect to prevalence of sexual problems. The predictable associations were noted between sexual problems and comorbid conditions including vascular disease, age, and obesity. Although odds ratios were small, it appears that most predictors were examined as continuous variables, so this is not unexpected.

Although compelling, existing evidence has supported a relationship between lower serum testosterone levels and increased risk of both decreased libido and erectile dysfunction[1]; specifically, Wu suggested cutoffs of less than 230 ng/dL and 250 ng/dL for increased risk of decline in sexual thoughts and erectile difficulty, respectively.

Testosterone should still be considered as an option in men with low serum levels and sexual concerns. It is worth consideration, however, that testosterone may be an overstated potential cause of sexual problems in men in the borderline ($\sim$250-300 ng/dL) range.

A. W. Shindel, MD

Reference

1. Wu FC, Tajar A, Beynon JM, et al; EMAS Group. Identification of late-onset hypogonadism in middle-aged and elderly men. *N Engl J Med*. 2010;363:123-135.

Hydrodissection of Neurovascular Bundles During Open Radical Prostatectomy Improves Postoperative Potency

Patel MI, Spernat D, Lopez-Corona E (Westmead Hosp, New South Wales, Australia; Univ of Sydney, New South Wales, Australia; Dodge City Med Ctr and Western Plains Med Complex, KS)
J Urol 186:233-237, 2011

Purpose.—Preservation of the neurovascular bundle during radical prostatectomy is important for postoperative erectile function. We determined whether hydrodissection of the neurovascular bundle during radical prostatectomy would result in improved erectile function postoperatively.

Materials and Methods.—Included in the study were 253 consecutive men who underwent nerve sparing radical prostatectomy, as done by 1 high volume surgeon (MIP). The first 117 and the next 136 men underwent standard dissection and hydrodissection, respectively, of the neurovascular bundle. In all men erectile function was evaluated by Sexual Health Inventory for Men score preoperatively, and 6 weeks and 6 months postoperatively. Time needed to achieve successful intercourse was also determined.

Results.—In men with bilateral neurovascular bundle preservation mean Sexual Health Inventory for Men scores in the hydrodissection group were higher than in the standard dissection group by 2.8 at 6 weeks and by 3.5 at 6 months ($p < 0.05$). In men with unilateral partial neurovascular bundle resection there was also significant improvement between the hydrodissection and standard dissection groups at 6 weeks and 6 months ($p < 0.05$). Men with bilateral neurovascular bundle preservation who underwent hydrodissection and standard dissection required a median of 3 and 6 months, respectively, to achieve successful sexual intercourse with or without a phosphodiesterase-5 inhibitor ($p < 0.05$). A difference was also observed in men who underwent partial neurovascular bundle resection. Hydrodissection was an independent predictor of time to successful intercourse on multivariate Cox regression analysis.

Conclusions.—Hydrodissection of the neurovascular bundle during open radical prostatectomy improves postoperative Sexual Health Inventory for Men scores and the time needed to achieve successful intercourse.

▶ This interesting study suggests that the use of hydrodissection (injection of lidocaine with epinephrine) in the vicinity of the neurovascular bundles during radical prostatectomy accelerates recovery of erectile function postoperatively. Mean postoperative Sexual Health Inventory for Men scores were higher in the hydrodissection group.

Studies such as this are limited in their absence of blinding and randomization. Furthermore, the authors did not use the widely accepted and validated Sexual Encounter Profile questions 2 and 3 to characterize the ability of subjects to attain an erection sufficient for intercourse and maintain the erection until climax, respectively. Although the substance of these questions is contained in the query asked of the patients by these authors, it is not clear that the "recovery" of erectile function experienced by these men was a return to their baseline level of function or simply the ability to accomplish penetration with a markedly less rigid penis.

None of these comments are intended to question the potential utility of this modality in improving recovery of erectile function after prostatectomy; this is a simple and inexpensive intervention that may be of great utility in the future. Replication of these findings by other centers and with more precisely defined and clinically meaningful endpoints is required to verify these results.

A. W. Shindel, MD

Gepirone-ER Treatment of Low Sexual Desire Associated with Depression in Women as Measured by the DeRogatis Inventory of Sexual Function (DISF) Fantasy/Cognition (Desire) Domain—A Post Hoc Analysis
Fabre LF, Smith LC, Derogatis LR (Fabre-Kramer Pharmaceuticals, Houston, TX; Sheppard Pratt Hosp, Baltimore, MD)
J Sex Med 2011 [Epub ahead of print]

Introduction.—Gepirone-extended release (ER) is effective in treating hypoactive sexual desire disorder (HSDD), as measured by the percent of females with HSDD that no longer met criteria for HSDD treatment. Another approach is to determine treatment effect on sexual desire using a recognized rating scale for sexual function. Because gepirone-ER has antidepressant and anxiolytic effects, investigation of these effects on sexual desire is appropriate.

Aim.—The aim of this study was to determine whether gepirone-ER has positive effects on sexual desire as measured by the DeRogatis Inventory of Sexual Function (DISF) in a post hoc analysis of 8- and 24-week studies and if this gepirone effect is independent of its antidepressant or anxiolytic activity.

Main Outcome Measures.—The main outcome measures used for this study were the Hamilton Depression Rating Scale (HAMD-25), change from baseline (CFB), and DISF CFB.

Methods.—Three hundred thirty-four women selected for depressive symptoms, not sexual dysfunction, received gepirone-ER (40–80 mg/day) in a controlled study of atypical depression using the HAMD-25 to measure antidepressant efficacy and a DISF subscale (domain I) to measure sexual cognition/fantasy (desire). After treatment, a 50% reduction from baseline HAMD-25 score identified antidepressant responders. Item 12 of HAMD scale (psychic anxiety) was used to define anxiolytic response scores of 0, 1 as responders, and scores of 2, 3, and 4 as nonresponders.

Results.—Gepirone-ER had no significant antidepressant or an anxiolytic effect in study 134006; however, DISF results demonstrate that gepirone-ER improves sexual desire in short term ($P = 0.043$) and long term ($P = 0.006$). Both gepirone-ER antidepressant and anxiolytic responders have statistically significant improved sexual desire. Gepirone-ER antidepressant and anxiolytic nonresponders also show statistically significant improvement.

Conclusions.—In depressed women, gepirone-ER has three mechanisms of action affecting sexual desire: an antidepressant effect, an anxiolytic effect, and a pro-sexual effect. Gepirone-ER improves sexual desire from the 24th to the 50th percentile according to population norms for the DISF.

▶ Gepirone extended release (ER) is a novel antidepressant that has been touted as an alternative to psychotropic medicines associated with sexual side effects. In this post hoc study, women treated with gepirone for atypical depression were assessed with validated instruments for the depression and anxiety as well as an inventory of sexual thoughts and fantasies. It was determined that gepirone-treated women had increases in sexual thoughts and fantasies irrespective of their response to the medication as an anxiolytic or antidepressant. It is implied that the drug enhances sexual thoughts independent of its efficacy as a psychotropic drug.

This article is a post hoc analysis; it is important to keep in mind that results gleaned from secondary analyses of a study not intended to answer the clinical question of whether gepirone-ER enhances sexual desire must be interpreted with caution. However, given the complete absence of any drug approved for the management of sexual health concerns in women in the United States, new data such as these provide hope that research and development will continue.

A. W. Shindel, MD

Efficacy and Safety of Once-Daily Dosing of Udenafil in the Treatment of Erectile Dysfunction: Results of a Multicenter, Randomized, Double-Blind, Placebo-Controlled Trial
Zhao C, Kim SW, Yang DY, et al (Chonbuk Natl Univ, Jeonju, Korea; Catholic Univ, Seoul, Korea; Hallym Univ, Seoul, Korea; et al)
Eur Urol 60:380-387, 2011

Background.—A once-daily dosing regimen with a phosphodiesterase type 5 inhibitor is needed for the treatment of erectile dysfunction (ED), in part because of the behavioral complexities associated with sexual intimacy. Many patients prefer spontaneous rather than scheduled sexual activities or they anticipate frequent sexual encounters. The pharmacokinetic profiles of udenafil with a time of maximal concentration of $1.0-1.5$ h and a terminal half-life of $11-13$ h make udenafil a good candidate for once-daily dosing.

Objective.—To evaluate the efficacy and safety of once-daily dosing of udenafil in the treatment of ED.

Design, Setting, and Participants.—This multicenter randomized double-blind, placebo-controlled, fix-dosed clinical trial involved 237 patients with ED. The subjects, who were treated with placebo or udenafil (25 mg, 50 mg, or 75 mg) once daily for 12 wk, were asked to complete the International Index of Erectile Function (IIEF), the Sexual Encounter Profile (SEP) diary, and the Global Assessment Questionnaire (GAQ) during the study.

Measurements.—The primary outcome parameter was the change from baseline for the IIEF erectile function domain (EFD) score. The secondary outcome parameters were SEP questions 2 and 3, the shift to normal rate (EFD ≥ 26), and the response to the GAQ.

Results and Limitations.—Compared with placebo, patients who took 50 mg or 75 mg of udenafil had a significantly improved IIEF-EFD score. Similar results were observed in comparing questions 2 and 3 in the SEP diary and the GAQ. Flushing was the most common treatment-related adverse event, which was transient and mild to moderate in severity.

Conclusions.—Udenafil significantly improved erectile function among ED patients when administered in doses of 50 mg or 75 mg once daily for 12 wk. Daily administration of udenafil (50 mg) may be another treatment option for ED.

▶ Udenafil is a phosphodiesterase type 5 inhibitor (PDE5I) that has been approved for management of erectile dysfunction (ED) in South Korea. It has a half-life of 12 hours, a duration that is in between the half-lives of the PDE5Is currently available in the United States. In this study, men with ED who were PDE5I naïve were randomly assigned to treatment with a daily dose of placebo or udenafil at 25-, 50-, and 75-mg doses. Men in the 2 higher dosage schedules had significantly greater improvement in outcome measures compared with those in the placebo and low-dose groups.

This study is lacking in that pharmacokinetic data on udenafil are not included. The higher dosing of daily-dose udenafil compared with that of tadalafil is consistent with this drug's shorter half-life. It will be interesting to acquire additional data on this dosing regimen and determine how often it is preferred compared with on-demand therapy; certainly, daily dosing might permit greater sexual spontaneity and potentially fewer side effects, but this must be balanced against potentially higher costs.

A. W. Shindel, MD

Male circumcision and sexual function in men and women: a survey-based, cross-sectional study in Denmark
Frisch M, Lindholm M, Grønbæk M (Statens Serum Institut, Copenhagen S, Denmark; Natl Inst of Public Health, Copenhagen K, Denmark)
Int J Epidemiol 1-15, 2011

Background.—One-third of the world's men are circumcised, but little is known about possible sexual consequences of male circumcision. In

Denmark ($\sim$ 5% circumcised), we examined associations of male circumcision with a range of sexual measures in both sexes.

Methods.—Participants in a national health survey (n=5552) provided information about their own (men) or their spouse's (women) circumcision status and details about their sex lives. Logistic regression-derived odds ratios (ORs) measured associations of circumcision status with sexual experiences and current difficulties with sexual desire, sexual needs fulfilment and sexual functioning.

Results.—Age at first intercourse, perceived importance of a good sex life and current sexual activity differed little between circumcised and uncircumcised men or between women with circumcised and uncircumcised spouses. However, circumcised men reported more partners and were more likely to report frequent orgasm difficulties after adjustment for potential confounding factors [11 vs 4%, OR_{adj}=3.26; 95% confidence interval (CI) 1.42–7.47], and women with circumcised spouses more often reported incomplete sexual needs fulfilment (38 vs 28%, OR_{adj}=2.09; 95% CI 1.05–4.16) and frequent sexual function difficulties overall (31 vs 22%, OR_{adj}=3.26; 95% CI 1.15–9.27), notably orgasm difficulties (19 vs 14%, OR_{adj}=2.66; 95% CI 1.07–6.66) and dyspareunia (12 vs 3%, OR_{adj}=8.45; 95% CI 3.01–23.74). Findings were stable in several robustness analyses, including one restricted to non-Jews and non-Moslems.

Conclusions.—Circumcision was associated with frequent orgasm difficulties in Danish men and with a range of frequent sexual difficulties in women, notably orgasm difficulties, dyspareunia and a sense of incomplete sexual needs fulfilment. Thorough examination of these matters in areas where male circumcision is more common is warranted.

▶ This report examines sexual satisfaction and quality of life in a population of presumably heterosexual circumcised and uncircumcised Danish men and their female partners. It was determined that circumcised men typically had more part ners as well as greater odds of difficulty reaching orgasm; there was no significant difference in prevalence of erectile dysfunction, premature ejaculation, or pain with intercourse. Female partners of circumcised men reported greater odds of sexual difficulties as well. Of note, just 15% of the 103 circumcised men reported neonatal (6 month) circumcisions; 20 of 71 male partners of female subjects in the study were circumcised at less than 6 months.

This study is novel in that it enrolled many subjects, and great efforts were made to control, as best as possible, for potential confounders of the relationship between sexual function and circumcision status (eg, religion, age, socioeconomics). Validated instruments were not used, and causality cannot be inferred in a cross-sectional survey such as this. Nevertheless, this is as well-designed a study as possible given the nature of the question at hand.

Whether the results can be generalized to parts of the world where circumcision is more prevalent is uncertain. Given the relatively small number of participants who were circumcised or had a circumcised partner, random error might lead to overestimation of difference. This is of particular concern, as an even smaller fraction of the circumcised men had undergone neonatal circumcision, so these data must be interpreted cautiously for this population of men. To their credit, the authors did perform analyses to ascertain whether age at circumcision was an independent association of sexual difficulties. Finally, these data indicate association but cannot prove causation; indeed, studies of sexual satisfaction outcomes after circumcision for human immunodeficiency virus prophylaxis in Africa have generally not indicated a trend toward worsening of sexual function after the procedure.

The author's personal feelings are readily apparent in the first paragraph of the manuscript in which the purported benefits of circumcision are roundly criticized. The authors also make certain to include references stating that decreased orgasm frequency may be predictive of increased mortality. It is quite a stretch to imply an association between circumcision and mortality. Be that as it may, this compelling study does suggest that circumcision should not be applied indiscriminately to male infants. At a minimum, there should be a strong cultural or medical reason to perform circumcision or any other operation in either pediatric or adult male patients.

A. W. Shindel, MD

Effect of Niacin on Erectile Function in Men Suffering Erectile Dysfunction and Dyslipidemia

Ng C-F, Lee C-P, Ho AL, et al (The Chinese Univ of Hong Kong, China)
J Sex Med 2011 [Epub ahead of print]

Introduction.—Dyslipidemia is closely related to erectile dysfunction (ED). Evidence has shown that the lipidlowering agent, 3-hydroxy-3-methylglutaryl-coenzyme A reductase inhibitor (statins), can improve erectile function. However, information about the potential role of another class of lipid-lowering agent, niacin, is unknown.

Aim.—To assess the effect of niacin alone on erectile function in patients suffering from both ED and dyslipidemia.

Methods.—A single center prospective randomized placebo-controlled parallel-group trial was conducted. One hundred sixty male patients with ED and dyslipidemia were randomized in a one-to-one ratio to receive up to 1,500 mg oral niacin daily or placebo for 12 weeks.

Main Outcome Measures.—The primary outcome measure was the improvement in erectile function as assessed by question 3 and question 4 of the International Index of Erectile Function (IIEF Q3 and Q4). Secondary outcome measurements included the total IIEF score, IIEF-erectile function domain, and Sexual Health Inventory for Men (SHIM) score.

Results.—From the overall analysis, the niacin group showed a significant increase in both IIEF-Q3 scores (0.53 ± 1.18, $P < 0.001$) and IIEF-Q4 scores (0.35 ± 1.17, $P = 0.013$) compared with baseline values. The placebo group also showed a significant increase in IIEF-Q3 scores (0.30 ± 1.16, $P = 0.040$) but not IIEF-Q4 scores (0.24 ± 1.13, $P = 0.084$). However, when patients were stratified according to the baseline severity of ED, the patients with moderate and severe ED who received niacin showed a significant improvement in IIEF-Q3 scores (0.56 ± 0.96 [$P = 0.037$] and 1.03 ± 1.20 [$P < 0.001$], respectively) and IIEF-Q4 scores (0.56 ± 1.03 [$P = 0.048$] and 0.84 ± 1.05 [$P < 0.001$], respectively) compared with baseline values, but not for the placebo group. The improvement in IIEF-EF domain score for severe and moderate ED patients in the niacin group were 5.28 ± 5.94 ($P < 0.001$) and 3.31 ± 4.54 ($P = 0.014$) and in the placebo group were 2.65 ± 5.63 ($P < 0.041$) and 2.74 ± 5.59 ($P = 0.027$), respectively. There was no significant improvement in erectile function for patients with mild and mild-to-moderate ED for both groups. For patients not receiving statins treatment, there was a significant improvement in IIEF-Q3 scores (0.47 ± 1.16 [$P = 0.004$]) for the niacin group, but not for the placebo group.

Conclusions.—Niacin alone can improve the erectile function in patients suffering from moderate to severe ED and dyslipidemia.

▶ Treatment of erectile dysfunction (ED) can be prohibitively expensive. Even patients with insurance coverage for erectogenic medications may wish to have intercourse more frequently than their prescription would tend to allow; many others are forced to pay out of pocket, a situation that for many is simply not financially feasible.

Niacin (vitamin B3) is a tried and true treatment for hyperlipidemia that has, in the modern era, been supplanted by the easier-to-tolerate statin drugs. It remains a useful and very affordable therapeutic option for hyperlipidemia. This randomized, placebo-controlled trial in men with dyslipidemia and ED reported significant improvement in response to 2 items from the International Index of Erectile Function (IIEF; relating to ability to attain an erection sufficient for penetration and maintain the erection until climax, respectively) in the niacin-treated arm. This effect was significant only in men with the most severe ED at baseline. Whether the change in IIEF scores was clinically relevant is a separate issue; such small changes may not be of great import to the patient. Furthermore, the change in IIEF in the treatment group compared with the placebo group was relatively modest. Lastly, the niacin-treated group had a higher rate of side effects, particularly flushing and pruritis.

Niacin will certainly not serve as a stand-alone treatment for ED. But it may have a role to play as a low-cost part of an overall lifestyle management protocol designed to improve vascular parameters and boost erectile functioning.

A. W. Shindel, MD

Patient, Resident Physician, and Visit Factors Associated with Documentation of Sexual History in the Outpatient Setting
Loeb DF, Lee RS, Binswanger IA, et al (Univ of Colorado, Aurora; et al)
J Gen Intern Med 26:887-893, 2011

Background.—Providers need an accurate sexual history for appropriate screening and counseling, but data on the patient, visit, and physician factors associated with sexual history-taking are limited.

Objectives.—To assess patient, resident physician, and visit factors associated with documentation of a sexual history at health care maintenance (HCM) visits.

Design.—Retrospective cross-sectional chart review.

Participants.—Review of all HCM clinic notes ($n = 360$) by 26 internal medicine residents from February to August of 2007 at two university-based outpatient clinics.

Measurements.—Documentation of sexual history and patient, resident, and visit factors were abstracted using structured tools. We employed a generalized estimating equations method to control for correlation between patients within residents. We performed multivariate analysis of the factors significantly associated with the outcome of documentation of at least one component of a sexual history.

Key Results.—Among 360 charts reviewed, 25% documented at least one component of a sexual history with a mean percent by resident of 23% (SD = 18%). Factors positively associated with documentation were: concern about sexually transmitted infection (referent: no concern; OR = 4.2 [95% CI = 1.3–13.2]); genitourinary or abdominal complaint (referent: no complaint; OR = 4.3 [2.2–8.5]); performance of other HCM (referent: no HCM performed; OR = 3.2 [1.5–7.0]), and birth control use (referent: no birth control; OR = 3.0 [1.1, 7.8]). Factors negatively associated with documentation were: age groups 46–55, 56–65, and >65 (referent: 18–25; ORs = 0.1, 0.1, and 0.2 [0.0–0.6, 0.0–0.4, and 0.1–0.6]), and no specified marital status (referent: married; OR = 0.5 [0.3–0.8]).

Conclusions.—Our findings highlight the need for an emphasis on documentation of a sexual history by internal medicine residents during routine HCM visits, especially in older and asymptomatic patients, to ensure adequate screening and counseling.

▶ With the expanded role urologists have come to play in managing sexual concerns in men and increasingly in women, inquiry on sexual history in primary care practice is an important step in securing referrals to urologic practices. It was determined in this study of 360 outpatient charts (created by 29 internal medicine residents at 2 clinics) that documentation of sexual history was relatively infrequent and was significantly more common only in cases in which there was a genitourinary or contraceptive presenting concern. Documentation was markedly less frequent in unmarried subjects and subjects older than 45 years. This finding is of particular importance in that older adults are more likely to report sexual problems; from the public health standpoint, older adults also appear to be at greater risk for acquisition of sexually transmitted infections, as educational efforts on barrier usage have largely ignored this segment of the population.

It is common knowledge as well as a published finding that patients are often hesitant to talk about sexual issues to their providers. This article is focused primarily on the need for sexually transmitted infection screening and other health maintenance, although to their credit the authors do invoke the importance of screening for sexual dysfunction and problems. Emphasis on this important quality-of-life indicator is important, as sex is not simply a vector for disease or unplanned pregnancy.

A. W. Shindel, MD

Vasoactive intestinal polypeptide, an erectile neurotransmitter, improves erectile function more significantly in castrated rats than in normal rats
Zhang M-G, Shen Z-J, Zhang C-M, et al (Shanghai Jiaotong Univ School of Medicine, PR China; et al)
BJU Int 108:440-446, 2011

Objective.—• To investigate the regulatory role of androgen in VIP-mediated erectile effect. Androgen is essential for physiological erection. Vasoactive intestinal polypeptide (VIP) is an important erectile neurotransmitter. While previous studies demonstrated that VIP expression in the penis was androgen-independent, it remains controversial whether androgen has any effect on VIP-mediated erection.

Materials and Methods.—• Male SD rats were divided into a control group, a castration group, and a castration-with-testosterone-replacement group. Four weeks later, each group was subdivided into low and high-dose VIP subgroups and subjected to intracavernous injection of 0.5 and 2 μg VIP, respectively.

• Erectile function was tested by recording intracavernosal pressure (ICP) and mean arterial blood pressure (MAP) before and after VIP injection.

• The expressions of the VIP-receptor (VPAC2), G-protein stimulatory and inhibitory alpha subunits (Gs-α, Gi-α), and PDE3A in rat corpus cavernosum (CC) was qualified by real-time PCR and Western blot analysis.

Results.—• Castration reduced erectile function while testosterone restored it. VIP improved erectile function in a dose-dependent manner.

• High-dose VIP significantly enhanced erectile function in castrated rats and there was no difference of ICP/MAP among three groups after injection of high-dose VIP.

• Low-dose VIP also resulted in a higher improvement of erectile function in castrated rats, although the ICP/MAP was lower in these rats than in the other two groups. VPAC2 and Gs-α were up-regulated while Gi-α and PDE3A were down-regulated in CC of castrated rats.

Conclusion.—• VIP improves erectile function much more significantly in hypogonadal condition, mainly due to the higher expression of VPAC2, Gs-α, and lower expression of Gi-α and PDE3A in CC of castrated rats. Androgen may negatively regulate the erectile effect of VIP.

▶ This article investigates the activity of vasoactive intestinal polypeptide (VIP) in erectile physiology of castrated rats with or without androgen replacement compared with intact rats. These authors had previously presented data that VIP receptor is expressed in an androgen-independent fashion.

The study is hampered by lack of a placebo-treated control group; this is an important limitation and makes these findings harder to interpret. Be that as it may, novel targets for erectile dysfunction (ED) pharmacotherapy are always intriguing. Phosphodiesterase type 5 inhibitors have revolutionized the way erectile dysfunction is managed, and while a similar revolution is not to be expected with the next new pharmacotherapy, new options are always welcome in the ED armamentarium. The androgen independence of this VIP effect on erectile function is of particular interest. This may be a more appealing target for the large population of men who are hypogonadal because of either decreased intrinsic production or androgen ablation for prostate cancer.

A. W. Shindel, MD

Comparing Effects of a Low-energy Diet and a High-protein Low-fat Diet on Sexual and Endothelial Function, Urinary Tract Symptoms, and Inflammation in Obese Diabetic Men
Khoo J, Piantadosi C, Duncan R, et al (Changi General Hosp, Singapore; Univ of Adelaide, South Australia, Australia; et al)
J Sex Med 2011 [Epub ahead of print]

Introduction.—Abdominal obesity and type 2 diabetes mellitus are associated with sexual and endothelial dysfunction, lower urinary tract symptoms (LUTS), and chronic systemic inflammation.

Aim.—To determine the effects of diet-induced weight loss and maintenance on sexual and endothelial function, LUTS, and inflammatory markers in obese diabetic men.

Main Outcome Measures.—Weight, waist circumference (WC), International Index of Erectile Function (IIEF-5) score, Sexual Desire Inventory (SDI) score, International Prostate Symptom Scale (IPSS) score, plasma fasting glucose and lipids, testosterone, sex hormone binding globulin (SHBG), inflammatory markers (high-sensitivity C-reactive protein [CRP] and interleukin-6 [IL-6]) and soluble E-selectin, and brachial artery flow-mediated dilatation (FMD) were measured at baseline, 8 weeks, and 52 weeks.

Methods.—Over 8 weeks, 31 abdominally obese (body mass index $\geq$ 30 kg/m^2, WC $\geq$ 102 cm), type 2 diabetic men (mean age 59.7 years) received either a meal replacement-based low-calorie diet (LCD) ~1,000 kcal/day (N = 19) or low-fat, high-protein, reduced-carbohydrate (HP) diet (N = 12) prescribed to decrease intake by ~600 kcal/day. Subjects continued on, or were switched to, the HP diet for another 44 weeks.

Results.—At 8 weeks, weight and WC decreased by ~10% and ~5% with the LCD and HP diet, respectively. Both diets significantly improved plasma glucose, low-density lipoprotein (LDL), SHBG, IIEF-5, SDI and IPSS scores, and endothelial function (increased FMD, reduced soluble E-selectin). Erectile function, sexual desire, and urinary symptoms improved by a similar degree with both diets. CRP and IL-6 decreased with the HP diet. At 52 weeks, reductions in weight, WC, and CRP were maintained. IIEF-5, SDI, and IPSS scores improved further.

Conclusions.—Diet-induced weight loss induces rapid improvement of sexual, urinary, and endothelial function in obese diabetic men. A high-protein, carbohydrate-reduced, low-fat diet also reduces systemic inflammation and sustains these beneficial effects to 1 year.

▶ Esposito et al have published numerous articles touting the virtues of the Mediterranean diet coupled with exercise for the management of vascular disease and erectile problems in obese men with the metabolic syndrome.[1] While there are clear-cut benefits to healthful eating and physical activity, lifestyle change remains difficult; this is hardly surprising given the ubiquity of cheap, unhealthful food choices that are engineered to appeal to consumers. Healthy living is not easy and it's not inexpensive.

It is the external costs of unhealthy living that so often go unnoticed. Positive lifestyle change will almost certainly reap substantial savings in reduced health care costs, increased productivity, and better quality of life. Convincing the public at large and policy makers of this truth remains a challenge but perhaps one of the more important ones facing health care providers. Data are yet another useful motivator that we should be using to encourage people to take steps toward healthier living.

It is worth mentioning that men in both treatment groups (meal replacement and portion reduction) experienced improvements in their sexual function, so drastic and sudden change is not necessary for long-term results; indeed, drastic changes are hard to live with, and few people can stay on such interventions for the long term required to permanently improve their metabolic parameters.

A. W. Shindel, MD

Reference

1. Esposito K, Giugliano F, Di Palo C, et al. Effect of lifestyle changes on erectile dysfunction in obese men: a randomized controlled trial. *JAMA.* 2004;291:2978-2984.

Treating stuttering priapism
Kheirandish P, Chinegwundoh F, Kulkarni S (Newham Univ Hosp, London, UK)
BJU Int 108:1068-1072, 2011

Stuttering priapism is an uncommon recurrent form of ischaemic priapism consisting of episodes of unwanted, painful erections that typically last for <3 h. It occurs repeatedly with intervening periods of detumescence. If these episodes are not treated, it may evolve into a classic ischaemic priapism and eventually lead to irreversible corporal fibrosis with permanent erectile dysfunction. A comprehensive literature search was conducted in August 2010 using the PubMed database, MEDLINE and generic search engines.

The search terms used to source information on this topic were, stuttering priapism (44 hits) and recurrent priapism (161 hits). Although there are numerous publications on this topic the majority of them are small trials and case reports. We identified 117 case reports, 28 reviews, 37 anecdotal reports, 22 small size clinical trials and one in vitro work. Our understanding of the underlying pathophysiology of stuttering priapism has improved in recent years. Further multicentre randomized clinical trials are required to evaluate the efficacy of different treatment options and to define safe and effective management strategies for patients with low-flow recurrent priapism.

▶ Priapism remains one of the more frustrating problems with which urologists must contend. Incomplete understanding of the pathophysiology of the disorder limits our options for prevention and leaves us primarily with reactive strategies involving administration of adrenergic agents and/or surgical shunts.

This mini-review provides a concise if somewhat limited synopsis of the current state of the art with respect to our understanding and management of stuttering priapism. Although the information is not original and is too vague to clearly guide treatment decisions, it does provide a sense of where we stand and what options exist for management of patients with recurrent priapism episodes. Androgen ablation appears to be the favored option and has the greatest number of publications. Other therapies are mentioned briefly; because most of these are derived from case reports or small series, it is unclear what utility is to be gained by these other options, including terbutaline, pseudoephedrine, digoxin, gabapentin, and PDE5 inhibitors.

A. W. Shindel, MD

Prediction of Erectile Function Following Treatment for Prostate Cancer

Alemozaffar M, Regan MM, Cooperberg MR, et al (Beth Israel Deaconess Med Ctr and Harvard Med School, Boston, MA; Dana-Farber Cancer Inst and Harvard Med School, Boston, MA; Univ of California, San Francisco; et al)
JAMA 306:1205-1214, 2011

Context.—Sexual function is the health-related quality of life (HRQOL) domain most commonly impaired after prostate cancer treatment; however, validated tools to enable personalized prediction of erectile dysfunction after prostate cancer treatment are lacking.

Objective.—To predict long-term erectile function following prostate cancer treatment based on individual patient and treatment characteristics.

Design.—Pretreatment patient characteristics, sexual HRQOL, and treatment details measured in a longitudinal academic multicenter cohort (Prostate Cancer Outcomes and Satisfaction With Treatment Quality Assessment; enrolled from 2003 through 2006), were used to develop models predicting erectile function 2 years after treatment. A community-based cohort (community-based Cancer of the Prostate Strategic Urologic

Research Endeavor [CaPSURE]; enrolled 1995 through 2007) externally validated model performance. Patients in US academic and community-based practices whose HRQOL was measured pretreatment (N = 1201) underwent follow-up after prostatectomy, external radiotherapy, or brachytherapy for prostate cancer. Sexual outcomes among men completing 2 years' follow-up (n = 1027) were used to develop models predicting erectile function that were externally validated among 1913 patients in a community-based cohort.

Main Outcome Measures.—Patient-reported functional erections suitable for intercourse 2 years following prostate cancer treatment.

Results.—Two years after prostate cancer treatment, 368 (37% [95% CI, 34%-40%]) of all patients and 335 (48% [95% CI, 45%-52%]) of those with functional erections prior to treatment reported functional erections; 531 (53% [95% CI, 50%-56%]) of patients without penile prostheses reported use of medications or other devices for erectile dysfunction. Pretreatment sexual HRQOL score, age, serum prostate-specific antigen level, race/ethnicity, body mass index, and intended treatment details were associated with functional erections 2 years after treatment. Multivariable logistic regression models predicting erectile function estimated 2-year function probabilities from as low as 10% or less to as high as 70% or greater depending on the individual's pretreatment patient characteristics and treatment details. The models performed well in predicting erections in external validation among CaPSURE cohort patients (areas under the receiver operating characteristic curve, 0.77 [95% CI, 0.74-0.80] for prostatectomy; 0.87 [95% CI, 0.80-0.94] for external radiotherapy; and 0.90 [95% CI, 0.85-0.95] for brachytherapy).

Conclusion.—Stratification by pretreatment patient characteristics and treatment details enables prediction of erectile function 2 years after prostatectomy, external radiotherapy, or brachytherapy for prostate cancer.

▶ This manuscript makes an attempt to create nomograms with which to predict the likelihood of erectile function recovery after prostate cancer treatment, including both radiation and surgery. Relevant factors for the models include age, prostate cancer grade, prostate-specific antigen, race, body mass index, and nerve-sparing status. The analysis is strengthened in that the model was externally validated and showed good predictive power in 2 separate large data sets of prostate cancer patients. This may be a useful tool to counsel patients on their likelihood of sexual function recovery.

Unfortunately, the authors did not create a numeric system that would enable easy incorporation of all of these variables into a single predictive model. These data may still be of utility when counseling patients, but this conversation will require either assessment of all the various models presented herein and generation of a subjective composite estimate or selection of 1 or 2 models that seem the most salient to a given clinical situation.

A. W. Shindel, MD

Long-term oral treatment with BAY 41-2272 ameliorates impaired corpus cavernosum relaxations in a nitric oxide-deficient rat model

Claudino MA, da Silva FH, Mónica FZT, et al (Univ of Campinas (UNICAMP), Brazil)

BJU Int 108:116-122, 2011

Objective.—• To investigate the potential beneficial effects of 4-week oral treatment with 5-cyclopropyl-2-[1-(2-fluoro-benzyl)-1Hpyrazolo [3,4-b]pyridin-3-yl]-pyrimidin-4-ylamine (BAY 41-2272), a nitric oxide (NO)-independent soluble guanylate cyclase activator, on impaired rat corpus cavernosum relaxations in NO-deficient rats.

Material and Methods.—• Male Wistar rats were divided into four groups: Control, N (G)-nitro-L- arginine methyl ester (L-NAME; 20 mg/rat/day), BAY 41-2272 (20 mg/kg/day) and L-NAME + BAY 41-2272.

• Rats were treated with L-NAME concomitantly with BAY 41-2272 for 4 weeks.

• Concentration—response curves to acetylcholine (ACh) and sodium nitroprusside (SNP), along with the nitrergic relaxations (1—32 Hz) were obtained in rat corpus cavernosum (RaCC).

• The RaCC contractile responses to the α_1-adrenoceptor agonist phenylephrine (PE) were obtained.

Results.—• Acetylcholine (0.01—1000 µmol/L) produced concentration-dependent relaxing responses in RaCC that were significantly enhanced ($P < 0.05$) in BAY 41-2272-treated rats.

• The ACh-induced relaxations were largely reduced in L-NAME-treated rats, and cotreatment with BAY 41-2272 failed to significantly modify these impaired relaxations.

• The SNP-induced relaxations were modified neither by L-NAME nor by cotreatment with BAY 41-2272.

• The nitrergic relaxations were significantly amplified in BAY 41-2272-treated rats (at 16 and 32 Hz). A significant reduction in the nitrergic relaxations was observed in L-NAME-treated rats, an effect largely restored by co-treatment with BAY 41-2272.

• The contractile RaCC responses produced by PE (0.001—100 µmol/L) were significantly higher ($P < 0.05$) in L-NAME-treated rats, and co-treatment of L-NAME with BAY 41-2272 nearly restored these enhanced contractile responses.

Conclusion.—• Four-week therapy with BAY 41-2272 prevents the impaired corpus cavernosum relaxations of rats treated chronically with L-NAME, indicating that accumulation of cyclic guanosine monophosphate into erectile tissue counteracts the NO deficiency.

▶ The nitric oxide guanylate cyclase cyclic GMP (cGMP) pathway has been clearly elucidated as one of the primary effectors of erectile function in men. Knowledge of this pathway and how to exploit it via selective inhibitors of PDE5 (the enzyme responsible for breaking down cGMP) has revolutionized the management of erectile dysfunction (ED). However, men with poor initial generation of nitric oxide (NO; eg, cavernous nerve injury or diabetic neuropathy) typically do not respond well to PDE5 inhibitors because of a lack of substrate.

This interesting study demonstrates how a non-NO-dependent mechanism for activation of guanylate cyclase might salvage PDE5 refractory men or even serve as a novel new monotherapy for ED. Using a variety of treatment modalities, the authors demonstrated how the guanylate cyclase activator BAY 41-2272 led to relaxation of rat cavernosal tissue even in the setting of NOS inhibition. As proof of concept, this is an important study that may lead to a marked improvement in our ability to care for patients with impairment of NO-mediated cavernosal muscle relaxation.

A. W. Shindel, MD

Critical Analysis of the Relationship Between Sexual Dysfunctions and Lower Urinary Tract Symptoms Due to Benign Prostatic Hyperplasia

Gacci M, Eardley I, Giuliano F, et al (Univ of Florence, Italy; St James Univ Hosp, Leeds, England; Raymond Poincaré Hosp, Garches, France; et al)

Eur Urol 60:809-825, 2011

Context.—This review focuses on the relationship among sexual dysfunction (SD), lower urinary tract symptoms (LUTS) due to benign prostatic hyperplasia (BPH), and related therapies.

Objective.—We reviewed the current literature to provide an overview of current data regarding epidemiology and pathophysiology of SD and LUTS. Moreover, we analysed the impact of currently available therapies of LUTS/BPH on both erectile dysfunction (ED) and ejaculatory dysfunction and the effect of phosphodiesterase type 5 inhibitors (PDE5-Is) in patients with ED and LUTS.

Evidence Acquisition.—We conducted a Medline search to identify original articles, reviews, editorials, and international scientific congress abstracts by combining the following terms: *benign prostatic hyperplasia, lower urinary tract symptoms, sexual dysfunction, erectile dysfunction, and ejaculatory dysfunction.*

Evidence Synthesis.—We conducted a comprehensive analysis of more relevant general population—based and BPH/LUTS or SD clinic-based trials and evaluated the common pathophysiologic mechanisms related to both conditions. In a further step, the overall impact of current BPH/LUTS therapies on sexual life, including phytotherapies, novel drugs, and surgical procedures, was scrutinized. Finally, the usefulness of PDE5-Is in LUTS/BPH was critically analysed, including preclinical and clinical research data as well as possible mechanisms of action that may contribute to the efficacy of PDE5-Is with LUTS/BPH.

Conclusions.—Community-based and clinical data demonstrate a strong and consistent association between LUTS and ED, suggesting that elderly men with LUTS should be evaluated for SD and vice versa. Pathophysiologic hypotheses regarding common basics of LUTS and SD as discussed in the literature are (1) alteration of the nitric oxide (NO)—cyclic guanosine monophosphate (cGMP) pathway, (2) enhancement of RhoA—Rho-kinase (ROCK) contractile signalling, (3) autonomic adrenergic hyperactivity, and (4) pelvic atherosclerosis. The most important sexual adverse effects of medical therapies are ejaculation disorders after the use of some α-blockers and sexual desire impairment, ED, and ejaculatory disorders after the use of α-reductase inhibitors. Minimally invasive, conventional, and innovative surgical treatments for BPH may induce both retrograde ejaculation and ED. PDE5-Is have demonstrated significant improvements in both LUTS and ED in men with BPH; combination therapy with PDE5-Is and α1-adrenergic blockers seems superior to PDE5-I monotherapy.

▶ This critical analysis dissects the relationship between lower urinary tract symptoms (LUTS) and erectile dysfunction (ED) in men from epidemiological, pathophysiological, and therapeutic contexts. A very nice review of how benign prostatic hyperplasia (BPH) treatment may influence sexual function is included; a somewhat shorter review on how ED treatments may improve urinary function is also included.

The conditions are commonly comorbid, and it is tempting to speculate that some of the same physiological processes may lead to both. That said, correlation does not imply causation; the conditions may simply share risk factors (particularly old age). It is also possible that a man who is experiencing one set of problems (urinary or sexual) may view the overall health of his entire genitourinary system in a more negative light; the strong association between subjective measures of ED and LUTS is not replicated by objective associations between ED and urine flow rate, postvoid residual, and other concerns.

Fundamentally, both conditions are important and occur through similar or related mechanisms. Treatment of one condition may improve the other. However, careful and meticulous data are required to prove that the changes in subjective LUTS are driven by genuine changes in urological parameters and not by simple improvements in sexual life and satisfaction.

A. W. Shindel, MD

Survivors of endometrial cancer: Who is at risk for sexual dysfunction?
Onujiogu N, Johnson T, Seo S, et al (Univ of Wisconsin School of Medicine and Public Health, Madison)
Gynecol Oncol 123:356-359, 2011

Objective.—Our goal was to determine the prevalence of sexual dysfunction and identify risk factors associated with sexual morbidity in patients with early stage endometrial cancer.

Methods.—This prospective trial included patients with stage I-IIIa endometrial cancer, without evidence of disease, and one to five years out from primary surgical treatment. Patients who received chemotherapy were excluded. The Female Sexual Function Index (FSFI) was used to measure our primary endpoint of sexual function. Other patient reported outcome indices included: Functional Assessment of Cancer Therapy-Endometrial (FACT-En), Center for Epidemiology Studies Depression scale (CES-D), and Menopausal Rating Scale (MRS).

Results.—Of the 72 women treated for early stage endometrial cancer, 65% were married, 69% had a sexual partner, the mean age was 60, 86% had stage I disease, and 18% received radiation therapy. The median score for the FSFI was 16.6 (0—32.8; scores below 26 are diagnostic for sexual dysfunction). Eighty nine percent of the patients had a score below 26. There was a moderate correlation between the total FSFI score and FACT-En scores but not with CES-D or MRS. Histologic grade, relationship status, mental health, and diabetes significantly correlated with total FSFI scores in multivariate analysis.

Conclusion.—This patient population commonly thought to be at low risk actually suffers from severe sexual dysfunction. The four risk factors revealed by multivariate analysis need to be studied in greater detail in order to appropriately target patients and develop meaningful interventions.

▶ This report details female sexual function as assessed by the Female Sexual Function Index (FSFI) in a population of women after treatment for early-stage endometrial cancer. This analysis is limited in that the FSFI is not necessarily designed to ascertain sex-related distress; however, it is noteworthy that the mean value for FSFI in the initial validation study was 30, and this population scored well below that mark. It is implied that sexual function is often impaired in women who are status—posttreatment for endometrial cancer. On multivariable analysis, more aggressive cancers, lack of regular partner, higher blood sugar, and poor mental health were associated with greater risk of low FSFI scores. Pain with sexual activity appeared to be the most prevalent concern in this population.

Limitations include the lack of preoperative data and absence of a control group of similar women without history of gynecological malignancy; it would have been interesting to compare whether hysterectomy for malignant disease portends a worse sexual prognosis than hysterectomy for benign conditions. Clearly there is a need for more detailed investigation of what problems these women face and how to best address them.

A. W. Shindel, MD

Minimal Clinically Important Differences in the Erectile Function Domain of the International Index of Erectile Function Scale
Rosen RC, Allen KR, Ni X, et al (New England Res Insts, Inc, Watertown, MA; Lilly USA, LLC, Indianapolis, IN)
Eur Urol 60:1010-1016, 2011

Background.—Despite widespread adoption of the six-item erectile function (EF) domain of the International Index of Erectile Function (IIEF) as a clinical trial end point, there are currently no objective data on what constitutes a minimal clinically important difference (MCID) in the EF domain.

Objective.—Estimate the MCID for the IIEF EF domain.

Design, Setting, and Participants.—Anchor-based MCIDs were estimated using data from 17 randomized, double-blind, placebo-controlled, parallel-group clinical trials of the phosphodiesterase type 5 inhibitor (PDE5-I) tadalafil for 3345 patients treated for 12 wk.

Measurements.—The anchor for the MCID is the minimal improvement measure calculated using change from baseline to 12 wk on IIEF question 7: "Over the past 4 weeks, when you attempted sexual intercourse how often was it satisfactory for you?" MCIDs were developed using analysis of variance (ANOVA)— and receiver operating characteristic (ROC)—based methods in a subset of studies ($n = 11$) by comparing patients with and without minimal improvement ($n = 863$). MCIDs were validated in the remaining six studies ($n = 377$).

Results and Limitations.—The ROC-based MCID for the EF domain was 4, with estimated sensitivity and specificity of 0.74 and 0.73, respectively. MCIDs varied significantly ($p < 0.0001$) according to baseline ED severity (mild: 2; moderate: 5; severe: 7). MCIDs consistently distinguished between patients in the validation sample classified as no change or minimally improved overall and by geographic region, ED etiology, and age group. MCIDs did not differ by age group, geographic region, or ED etiology. Current analyses were based on 17 clinical trials of tadalafil. Results need to be replicated in studies using other PDE5-Is or in non-pharmacologic intervention studies.

Conclusions.—The contextualization of treatment-related changes in terms of clinically relevant improvement is essential to understanding treatment efficacy, to interpreting results across studies, and to managing patients effectively. This analysis provides, for the first time, anchor-based estimates of MCIDs in the EF domain score of the IIEF.

▶ Reporting of sexual function outcomes in trials of new therapies for erectile dysfunction (ED) often relies on mean scores on the erectile function domain of the International Index of Erectile Function (IIEF-EF) or the closely related Sexual Health Inventory for Men (SHIM). But what does a 1-point change in IIEF-EF/SHIM mean? What about a 4-point change? Or a 10-point change? When is it enough for a patient to notice?

This article looks at 17 double-blind placebo-controlled trials of ED therapy with tadalafil using the single-item question on overall satisfaction with sexual intercourse as an "anchor" to assess clinically meaningful change. Although the larger 6- or 5-item IIEF or SHIM may contain more data, the single-item satisfaction questionnaire does permit concise assessment of how a man feels about his sexual function.

The authors conclude that a change of 4 points constitutes a clinically relevant change. This relationship held across age, ED etiology, and geographic regions. This number must be taken with the important caveat that men with severe ED (scores in the 6–10 range on IIEF-EF) may not be contented with a 4-point change because this may not translate into a meaningful improvement in ability to reliably achieve erections sufficient for satisfactory intercourse. Similarly, men with mild ED might be satisfied with a relatively smaller change.

Although not perfect, this new minimally important clinical change number does permit a bit more objectivity for assessing reported changes in the literature.

A. W. Shindel, MD

Combination of BAY 60-4552 and Vardenafil Exerts Proerectile Facilitator Effects in Rats With Cavernous Nerve Injury: A Proof of Concept Study for the Treatment of Phosphodiesterase Type 5 Inhibitor Failure
Oudot A, Behr-Roussel D, Poirier S, et al (Pelvipharm, Orsay, France; et al)
Eur Urol 60:1020-1026, 2011

Background.—Radical prostatectomy (RP) is frequently responsible for erectile dysfunction (ED). Post-RP patients often show a failure to respond to phosphodiesterase type 5 (PDE5) inhibitors.

Objective.—The acute effect of BAY 60-4552, the soluble guanylate cyclase (sGC) stimulator, and vardenafil were evaluated alone or in combination on erectile responses to electrical stimulation of the cavernous nerve (ES CN) in rats with cavernous nerve (CN) crush injury—induced ED.

Design, Setting, and Participants.—Male adult Sprague-Dawley rats underwent laparotomy (sham, $n = 10$) or bilateral CN crush injury ($n = 56$). After 3 wk of recovery, erectile function was evaluated under urethane anaesthesia following ES CN at different frequencies.

Measurements.—The acute effects of intravenous (IV) injection of vehicle, vardenafil 0.03 mg/kg, BAY 60-4552 0.03 mg/kg or 0.3 mg/kg, or a BAY 60-4552 0.03 mg/kg plus vardenafil 0.03 mg/kg combination were evaluated in CN-crushed rats.

Results and Limitations.—Bilateral CN crush injury followed by a 3-wk recovery period decreased erectile responses to ES CN by about 50%. In CN-crushed rats, IV vardenafil 0.03 mg/kg and BAY 60-4552 (0.03 or 0.3 mg/kg) increased erectile responses to ES CN to the same extent: Δ intracavernosal pressure/mean arterial pressure (ICP/MAP) at 10 Hz ES CN was $21 \pm 1\%$ after vehicle, $25 \pm 3\%$ ($p < 0.001$) after vardenafil, and $26 \pm 5\%$ and $27 \pm 5\%$ after BAY 60-4552 0.03 mg/kg ($p < 0.01$) and 0.3 mg/kg ($p < 0.001$), respectively. The combination of vardenafil with BAY 60-4552 in CN-crushed rats totally restored erectile responses to ES CN equivalent to sham rats (ΔICP/MAP at 10 Hz ES CN: $34 \pm 4\%$ after BAY 60-4552/vardenafil combination vs $39 \pm 4\%$ in sham rats; not significant).

Conclusions.—The present study supports the concept that the combined administration of a sGC stimulator, BAY 60-4552, and vardenafil provides synergistic beneficial effects and might therefore salvage patients who experience treatment failures with PDE5 inhibitors after RP.

▶ The nitric oxide/cGMP pathway has been clearly elucidated as one of the primary effectors of erectile function in men. Knowledge of this pathway and how to exploit it via selective inhibitors of PDE5 (the enzyme responsible for breaking down cGMP) has revolutionized the management of erectile dysfunction (ED). However, men with poor initial generation of NO (cavernous nerve injury or diabetic neuropathy, for instance) typically do not respond well to PDE5 inhibitors because of a lack of substrate. This is the second study in recent months that shows how a non—NO-dependent mechanism for activation of guanylate cyclase might salvage PDE5 refractory men or even serve as a novel new monotherapy for ED. This study reports on outcomes in an in vivo model of rats with cavernous nerve crush injury and resultant impairment of penile erection. Rats that received this treatment showed improved erectile response to cavernous nerve stimulation; this is of some interest, as the guanylate cyclase activator should theoretically be able to work even in the absence of nerve input. Further work is warranted to determine how much efficacy this interesting drug might have in humans with ED of various causes.

A. W. Shindel, MD

Satisfying Sexual Events as Outcome Measures in Clinical Trial of Female Sexual Dysfunction

Kingsberg SA, Althof SE (Univ Hosps Case Med Ctr Cleveland, OH; Case Western Reserve Univ School of Medicine, Cleveland, OH)
J Sex Med 8:3262-3270, 2011

Introduction.—Assessing the sexual response in women with female sexual dysfunctions (FSDs) in clinical trials remains difficult. Part of the challenge is the development of meaningful and valid end points that capture the complexity of women's sexual response.

Aim.—The purpose of this review is to highlight the shortcomings of daily diaries and the limitations of satisfying sexual events (SSEs) as primary end points in clinical trials of women with hypoactive sexual desire disorder (HSDD) as recommended by the Food and Drug Administration (FDA) in their draft guidance on standards for clinical trials in women with FSD.

Methods.—Clinical trials in women with HSDD using SSEs as primary end points were reviewed.

Main Outcome Measures.—The agreement between three outcome measures (SSEs, desire, and distress) was assessed to illustrate to what degree improvements in SSEs were in agreement with improvements in sexual desire and/or personal distress.

Results.—Nine placebo-controlled randomized trials in women with HSDD were reviewed: seven with transdermal testosterone and two with flibanserin. In four trials, all using transdermal testosterone 300 µg/day had agreement between changes in SSEs, desire, and distress. In five studies (testosterone 300 µg/day, n = 2; testosterone 150 µg/day, n = 1; flibanserin n = 2), changes in SSEs did not correlate with changes in desire and/or distress and vice versa. It should be noted that in the flibanserin trials, SSEs did correlate with desire assessed using the Female Sexual Function Index but not when it was assessed using the eDiary.

Conclusions.—Findings in the literature do not uniformly support the recommendations from the FDA draft guidance to use diary measures in clinical trials of HSDD as primary end points. Patient-reported outcomes appear to be better suited to capture the multidimensional and more subjective information collected in trials of FSD.

▶ It is understandable that the tools used to quantify sexual dysfunction in men must be distinct from those used in studies of female sexual dysfunction (FSD). However, a tally of "satisfying sexual events" (SSE) does not completely encompass the sexual experience for women (or men for that matter).

In June 2010, flibanserin was rejected as a treatment for hypoactive sexual desire disorder (HSDD) in women by the US Food and Drug Administration based primarily on studies in which the principal efficacy endpoint was SSE. In this study, Kingsberg and Althof articulate that SSE may have little to do with sexual desire nor with the construct of the HSDD diagnosis.

It is of particular interest that SSE was not a criterion in the evaluation of drugs for the management of erectile dysfunction in men; Kingsberg and Althof make note of this in their commentary. It is important that sexual medicine professionals advocate for standards that are universal and fair; the basic standards by which a drug for sexual problems in women are evaluated should not fundamentally differ from the standards used for sexual problems in men.

A. W. Shindel, MD

Exercise Training Improves the Defective Centrally Mediated Erectile Responses in Rats with Type I Diabetes

Zheng H, Mayhan WG, Patel KP (Univ of Nebraska Med Ctr, Omaha)
J Sex Med 8:3086-3097, 2011

Introduction.—Erectile dysfunction is a serious and common complication of diabetes mellitus. Apart from the peripheral actions, central mechanisms are also responsible for the penile erection.

Aim.—The goal of the present study was to determine the impact of exercise training (ExT) on the centrally mediated erectile dysfunction in streptozotocin (STZ)-induced type I diabetic (T1D) rats.

Methods.—Male Sprague—Dawley rats were injected with STZ to induce diabetes mellitus. Three weeks after STZ or vehicle injections, rats were assigned to either ExT (treadmill running for 3—4 weeks) or sedentary groups to produce four experimental groups: control + sedentary, T1D + sedentary, control + ExT, and T1D + ExT.

Main Outcome Measure.—After 3—4 weeks ExT, central N-methyl-D-aspartic acid (NMDA) or sodium nitroprusside (SNP)-induced penile erectile responses were measured. Neuronal nitric oxide synthase (nNOS) expression in the paraventricular nucleus (PVN) of the hypothalamus was measured by using histochemistry, real time polymerase chain reaction (PCR) and Western blot approaches.

Results.—In rats with T1D, ExT significantly improved the blunted erectile response, and the intracavernous pressure changes to NMDA (50 ng) microinjection within the PVN (T1D + ExT: 3.0 ± 0.6 penile erection/rat; T1D + sedentary: 0.5 ± 0.3 penile erection/rat within 20 minutes, $P < 0.05$). ExT improved erectile dysfunction induced by central administration of exogenous nitric oxide (NO) donor, SNP in T1D rats. Other behavior responses including yawning and stretching, induced by central NMDA and SNP microinjection were also significantly increased in T1D rats after ExT. Furthermore, we found that ExT restored the nNOS mRNA and protein expression in the PVN in T1D rats.

Conclusions.—These results suggest that ExT may have beneficial effects on the erectile dysfunction in diabetes through improvement of NO bioavailability within the PVN. Thus, ExT may be used as therapeutic modality to up-regulate nNOS within the PVN and improve the central component of the erectile dysfunction in diabetes mellitus.

▶ Exercise has known vascular benefits; in work from a variety of authors these benefits have been shown to extend to penile circulation and improve erectile function. Indeed, the only treatment to date that has shown long-term efficacy in reversal of erectile dysfunction is diet and lifestyle change. In this study, it is suggested that central mechanisms may play a role in some of these changes.

Diabetic animals were randomized to daily treadmill exercise. Penile hemodynamic response to central nervous system injection of erectogenic agents was improved in the animals in the exercise arm. These changes were associated with histological differences in brain nuclei relevant to sexual functioning.

This novel finding implies that the benefits of exercise extend beyond circulation and to the central nervous system. Although lifestyle change is difficult, increasing evidence support its role in the long-term treatment plan for men with erectile dysfunction.

A. W. Shindel, MD

Erectile Dysfunction and Risk of Cardiovascular Disease: Meta-Analysis of Prospective Cohort Studies
Dong J-Y, Zhang Y-H, Qin L-Q (Soochow Univ, Suzhou, China)
J Am Coll Cardiol 58:1378-1385, 2011

Objectives.—Our goal was to evaluate the association between erectile dysfunction (ED) and risk of cardiovascular disease (CVD) and all-cause mortality by conducting a meta-analysis of prospective cohort studies.

Background.—Observational studies suggest an association between ED and the incidence of CVD. However, whether ED is an independent risk factor of CVD remains controversial.

Methods.—The PubMed database was searched through January 2011 to identify studies that met pre-stated inclusion criteria. Reference lists of retrieved articles were also reviewed. Two authors independently extracted information on the designs of the studies, the characteristics of the study participants, exposure and outcome assessments, and control for potential confounding factors. Either a fixed- or a random-effects model was used to calculate the overall combined risk estimates.

Results.—Twelve prospective cohort studies involving 36,744 participants were included in the meta-analysis. The overall combined relative risks for men with ED compared with the reference group were 1.48 (95% confidence interval [CI]: 1.25 to 1.74) for CVD, 1.46 (95% CI: 1.31 to 1.63) for coronary heart disease, 1.35 (95% CI: 1.19 to 1.54) for stroke, and 1.19 (95% CI: 1.05 to 1.34) for all-cause mortality. Sensitivity analysis restricted to studies with control for conventional cardiovascular risk factors yielded similar results. No evidence of publication bias was observed.

Conclusions.—This meta-analysis of prospective cohort studies suggests that ED significantly increases the risk of CVD, coronary heart disease, stroke, and all-cause mortality, and the increase is probably independent of conventional cardiovascular risk factors.

▶ This meta-analysis analyzes 12 prospective cohort studies on mortality associated with erectile dysfunction (ED). Using careful and thorough inclusion criteria, the authors determine that prevalent ED is indeed an independent risk factor for cardiovascular and all-cause mortality, independent of its known association with cardiovascular risk factors common to both ED and cardiac disease. This analysis is strengthened by inclusion of only prospective cohort studies (thereby reducing the odds of reverse causality, ie, cardiovascular disease causing ED) and sensitivity analyses that attempted to ascertain the presence of publication bias.

The association between ED and cardiovascular disease is indisputable. The real value in these data is to conjure questions of whether ED, as an independent risk factor, portends some systemic condition other than overt vascular disease (depression, hypogonadism, systemic inflammation, etc), which may explain the connection between ED and cardiovascular morbidity/mortality.

Physicians, including urologists, too often ignore or dismiss concerns about erectile function in their male patients. Data such as these argue that we do patients multiple disservices by not inquiring about sexual function—first by ignoring the serious and morbid condition of sexual dysfunction and second by missing an important sign of increased mortality risk.

A. W. Shindel, MD

The Importance of Sexual Self-Disclosure to Sexual Satisfaction and Functioning in Committed Relationships
Rehman US, Rellini AH, Fallis E (Univ of Waterloo, Ontario, Canada; Univ of Vermont, Burlington)
J Sex Med 8:3108-3115, 2011

Introduction.—Past research indicates that sexual self-disclosure, or the degree to which an individual is open with his or her partner about sexual preferences, is a key aspect of sexual satisfaction and that partner's lack of knowledge about one's sexual preferences is associated with persistent sexual dysfunction.

Aims.—To replicate and extend past research by examining (i) how one's own levels of sexual self-disclosure are related to one's own sexual health (after controlling for partner's levels of sexual self-disclosure); (ii) how one's partner's levels of sexual self-disclosure are associated with one's own sexual health (after controlling for one's own levels of sexual self-disclosure); and (iii) whether gender moderates the associations between sexual self-disclosure and sexual health.

Main Outcome Measures.—Scores from the Golombok Rust Inventory of Sexual Satisfaction and the Sexual Communication Satisfaction Scale.

Methods.—A cross-sectional dyadic study using a convenience sample of 91 heterosexual couples in long-term committed relationships. Data were analyzed using the Actor–Partner Interdependence Model.

Results.—One's own level of sexual self-disclosure is positively associated with one's own sexual satisfaction, $\beta = -0.24, t(172.85) = -3.50, P < 0.001$. Furthermore, partner's level of sexual self-disclosure is associated with men's sexual satisfaction but not with women's sexual satisfaction, $\beta = -0.45$, $t(86.81) = -4.06, P < 0.001$ and $\beta = 0.02, t(87.00) = 0.20$, ns, respectively. The association between own self-disclosure and sexual problems is stronger for women as compared with men, $\beta = -0.72, t(87.00) = -6.31, P < 0.001$ and $\beta = -0.24, t(86.27) = -3.04, P < 0.01$, respectively.

Conclusions.—Our results demonstrate that sexual self-disclosure is significantly associated with sexual satisfaction and functioning for both men and women, albeit in different ways. Our findings underscore the importance of sexual self-disclosure and highlight the importance of the interpersonal level of analysis in understanding human sexuality.

▶ It's not exactly novel to conclude that sexual satisfaction is dependent on the ability to engage in activities that are sexually fulfilling at a frequency that varies from person to person and from time to time. There is a diverse array of sexual preferences; what is satisfying for one person may be unpleasant or even repugnant to another. Within the bounds of consenting interactions between adults of sound mind, it is my opinion that no sexual act is intrinsically wrong.

This article attempts to objectively characterize this relationship. A group of heterosexual couples were queried about their degree of sexual self-disclosure. Sexual satisfaction of both the index subjects and their partners was then compared with this value. It was determined that sexual satisfaction is positively related to degree of sexual self-disclosure for both the index subjects and for the index subjects' partners, although the nature of this relationship showed some interesting gender differences. Particularly, women with higher levels of sexual self-disclosure tended to have less sexual dysfunction and partners who endorsed greater overall sexual satisfaction.

What does this mean? Simply put, open and honest communication is important. This idea is given lip service by most practitioners, but in my opinion, it needs to receive greater attention as the most fundamental precept in management of sexual problems. All too often, men and women come to the office to discuss sexual concerns that they have either not discussed or discussed only sparingly with their significant other. Sexual compatibility is an important part of relationships and should be a topic of communication. I'll add the corollary that openness about genuine sexual preference is also important for partner selection; disagreements about sexual frequency and/or activity are a major source of stress for long-term dyads. Upfront communication early in the relationship may better equip individuals to select partners with whom they can share long-term stable relationships.

A. W. Shindel, MD

The Effect of Lifestyle Modification and Cardiovascular Risk Factor Reduction on Erectile Dysfunction: A Systematic Review and Meta-analysis
Gupta BP, Murad MH, Clifton MM, et al (Mayo Clinic, Rochester, MN)
Arch Intern Med 171:1797-1803, 2011

Background.—Erectile dysfunction (ED) shares similar modifiable risks factors with coronary artery disease (CAD). Lifestyle modification that targets CAD risk factors may also lead to improvement in ED. We conducted a systematic review and meta-analysis of randomized controlled trials evaluating the effect of lifestyle interventions and pharmacotherapy for cardiovascular (CV) risk factors on the severity of ED.

Methods.—A comprehensive search of multiple electronic databases through August 2010 was conducted using predefined criteria. We included randomized controlled clinical trials with follow-up of at least 6 weeks of lifestyle modification intervention or pharmacotherapy for CV risk factor reduction. Studies were selected by 2 independent reviewers. The main outcome measure of the study is the weighted mean differences in the International Index of Erectile Dysfunction (IIEF-5) score with 95% confidence intervals (CIs) using a random effects model.

Results.—A total of 740 participants from 6 clinical trials in 4 countries were identified. Lifestyle modifications and pharmacotherapy for CV risk factors were associated with statistically significant improvement in sexual function (IIEF-5 score): weighted mean difference, 2.66 (95% CI, 1.86-3.47). If the trials with statin intervention (n = 143) are excluded, the remaining 4 trials of lifestyle modification interventions (n = 597) demonstrate statistically significant improvement in sexual function: weighted mean difference, 2.40 (95% CI, 1.19-3.61).

Conclusion.—The results of our study further strengthen the evidence that lifestyle modification and pharmacotherapy for CV risk factors are effective in improving sexual function in men with ED.

▶ This meta-analysis investigated lifestyle change (diet and exercise) as a means to improve erectile function. Also included is medical management of hyperlipidemia via HMG-CoA reductase inhibitors (statins); in this article, both of the statin studies used atorvastatin. The authors identified 6 clinical trials in 4 countries; the conclusion from all published data was that increased exercise and reduction in weight were both helpful at reducing the burden of ED in men.

Publication of a meta-analysis on ED outcomes in a prestigious journal such as *Annals of Internal Medicine* emphasizes the growing body of knowledge on the importance of mitigating vascular disease in the prevention of ED. Certainly use of drug therapy can play an important role in this, but a more fundamental conclusion is that men should eat more healthfully and exercise more regularly. Modern Western lifestyles are not conducive to vascular health and it may be necessary as medical practitioners (urologists or otherwise) to intervene on behalf of our patients' well-being by advising them to eat better and exercise more.

A. W. Shindel, MD

Evaluation of Endothelial Function with Brachial Artery Ultrasound in Men with or without Erectile Dysfunction and Classified as Intermediate Risk According to the Framingham Score

Averbeck MA, Colares C, de Lira GHS, et al (Federal Univ of Health Sciences of Porto Alegre, Brazil; Dom Vicente Scherer Hosp, Porto Alegre, Brazil)
J Sex Med 9:849-856, 2012

Introduction.—Flow-mediated vasodilation (FMD) of the brachial artery is a noninvasive tool used for endothelial function evaluation. There is increasing evidence that endothelial dysfunction is a common etiological factor for erectile dysfunction (ED) and cardiovascular events.

Aim.—To evaluate endothelial function with a high-resolution ultrasound device, to assess FMD in men diagnosed with ED and without clinical evidence of significant atherosclerotic disease, classified as "intermediate risk" according to the Framingham risk score (FRS).

Methods.—This is a case-control study that included 52 consecutive men. In all men with ED evaluated by a score less than 22 on International Index of Erectile Function-5 questionnaire (IIEF-5), clinical parameters such as blood pressure, waist circumference, hip circumference, body mass index, lipid profile, fasting glucose, and serum total testosterone were obtained. These parameters were compared with those men without diagnosis of ED (IIEF-5 score ≥ 22) (age-matched, also classified as "intermediate risk" according to the FRS). All underwent brachial artery ultrasound for assessment of FMD, as a noninvasive method to evaluate endothelial function. Statistical analysis was performed considering a $P < 0.05$.

Main Outcome Measures.—Endothelium-dependent FMD was evaluated in the right brachial artery with a high-resolution ultrasound machine following reactive hyperemia.

Results.—Thirty-four men were included in the ED group, and 18 were included in the group without ED. The mean ages were 59.61 ± 9.87 and 56.18 ± 10.93, respectively ($P = 0.27$). Clinical and laboratory evaluations were similar between men with and without ED ($P > 0.05$) except for waist circumference that was greater in patients with ED (mean $= 100.85$ cm vs.

96.05; $P < 0.05$). The percentage of FMD was higher in men without ED when compared with those with ED (mean FMD 11.33 ± 6.08% vs. 4.24 + 7.06%, respectively; $P = 0.001$).

Conclusions.—Men without established atherosclerotic disease presenting with ED demonstrated a worse endothelial function.

▶ This case-control study examines brachial artery flow-mediated dilation, an assessment of endothelial reactivity after restriction of peripheral blood flow to the arm for a period of 5 minutes followed by measurement of flow after release. This technique is an accepted one for testing vascular reactivity and overall endothelial health.

Fifty-two men without prior diagnoses of vascular disease were divided into 2 groups based on subjective erectile function, dichotomized as a score of 22 or greater versus 21 or less (no erective dysfunction [ED] vs ED, respectively) on the 5-item International Index of Erectile Function Scale. Cases were selected from men who presented for sexual dysfunction, whereas controls were selected from men who presented for prostate cancer screening. Flow-mediated dilation was markedly superior in the "no ED" group, despite similar parameters between groups on a variety of other vascular parameters; in fact, the only biomarker that differed between groups was waist circumference.

What do these data mean? Fundamentally, they indicate that endothelial reactivity may be an independent predictor of ED risk. On a more functional level, it begs the question of whether this type of noninvasive testing could take the place of penile Doppler ultrasound, the current standard of care in assessment of penile hemodynamics. This flow-mediated dilation methodology is simple and potentially less invasive; whether it would compare favorably to penile Doppler is an interesting research question.

A. W. Shindel, MD

Low-Intensity Extracorporeal Shock Wave Therapy—A Novel Effective Treatment for Erectile Dysfunction in Severe ED Patients Who Respond Poorly to PDE5 Inhibitor Therapy

Gruenwald I, Appel B, Vardi Y (Rambam Healthcare Campus, Haifa, Israel)
J Sex Med 9:259-264, 2012

Introduction.—Low-intensity shock wave therapy (LI-ESWT) has been reported as an effective treatment in men with mild and moderate erectile dysfunction (ED).

Aim.—The aim of this study is to determine the efficacy of LI-ESWT in severe ED patients who were poor responders to phosphodiesterase type 5 inhibitor (PDE5i) therapy.

Methods.—This was an open-label single-arm prospective study on ED patients with an erection hardness score (EHS) ≤2 at baseline. The protocol comprised two treatment sessions per week for 3 weeks, which were repeated after a 3-week no-treatment interval. Patients were followed at 1 month (FU1), and only then an active PDE5i medication was provided for an additional month until final follow-up visit (FU2).

At each treatment session, LI-ESWT was applied on the penile shaft and crus at five different anatomical sites (300 shocks, 0.09 mJ/mm^2 intensity at 120 shocks/min).

Each subject underwent a full baseline assessment of erectile function using validated questionnaires and objective penile hemodynamic testing before and after LI-ESWT.

Main Outcome Measures.—Outcome measures used are changes in the International Index of Erectile Function-erectile function domain (IIEF-ED) scores, the EHS measurement, and the three parameters of penile hemodynamics and endothelial function.

Results.—Twenty-nine men (mean age of 61.3) completed the study. Their mean IIEF-ED scores increased from 8.8 ± 1 (baseline) to 12.3 ± 1 at FU1 ($P = 0.035$). At FU2 (on active PDE5i treatment), their IIEF-ED further increased to 18.8 ± 1 ($P < 0.0001$), and 72.4% ($P < 0.0001$) reached an EHS of ≥3 (allowing full sexual intercourse). A significant improvement ($P = 0.0001$) in penile hemodynamics was detected after treatment and this improvement significantly correlated with increases in the IIEF-ED ($P < 0.05$). No noteworthy adverse events were reported.

Conclusions.—Penile LI-ESWT is a new modality that has the potential to treat a subgroup of severe ED patients. These preliminary data need to be reconfirmed by multicenter sham control studies in a larger group of ED patients.

▶ The quest for identification of treatment modalities to actually reverse erectile dysfunction continues. In this pilot article, the authors demonstrate that application of low-intensity shock waves to the penis enhances response to erectogenic therapy. At baseline, these men had erections of insufficient rigidity for penetrative sexual activity. At follow-up, a substantial number had improved their erectile responses, and this was confirmed by ultrasound measurement of penile blood flow.

Low-intensity shock waves are distinct from their higher-energy counterparts, which are used for treatment of urinary stones. This type of treatment can often be applied without the need for anesthesia. The mechanism of action is at this time unclear, although there has been published evidence that these treatments may induce production of trophic or growth factors or recruit stem cells to the region of interest.

As pilot data, these findings are very compelling. However, the lack of randomization and blinding makes these data preliminary at best. Rigorous and well-designed follow-up trials are required to ascertain how much of the observed effect may be related to placebo.

A. W. Shindel, MD

Exercise is Associated with Better Erectile Function in Men Under 40 as Evaluated by the International Index of Erectile Function
Hsiao W, Shrewsberry AB, Moses KA, et al (Emory Univ, Atlanta, GA)
J Sex Med 9:524-530, 2012

Introduction.—Studies have shown an association between erectile dysfunction and sedentary lifestyle in middle-aged men, with a direct correlation between increased physical activity and improved erectile function. Whether or not this relationship is present in young, healthy men has yet to be demonstrated.

Aim.—The aim of this study was to assess the association between physical activity and erectile function in young, healthy men.

Main Outcome Measures.—The primary end points for our study were: (i) differences in baseline scores of greater than one point per question for the International Index of Erectile Function (IIEF); (ii) differences in baseline scores of greater than one point per question for each domain of the IIEF; (iii) exercise energy expenditure; and (iv) predictors of dysfunction as seen on the IIEF.

Methods.—The participants were men between the ages of 18 and 40 years old at an academic urology practice. Patients self-administered the Paffenbarger Physical Activity Questionnaire and the IIEF. Patients were stratified by physical activity into two groups: a sedentary group ($\leq 1,400$ calories/week) and an active group (>1,400 calories/week). Men presenting for the primary reason of erectile dysfunction or Peyronie's disease were excluded.

Results.—Seventy-eight patients had complete information in this study: 27 patients (34.6%) in the sedentary group ($\leq 1,400$ kcal/week) and 51 patients (65.4%) in the active group (>1,400 kcal/week). Sedentary lifestyle was associated with increased dysfunction in the following domains of the IIEF: erectile function (44.4% vs. 21.6%, $P = 0.04$), orgasm function (44.4% vs. 17.7%, $P = 0.01$), intercourse satisfaction (59.3% vs. 35.3%, $P = 0.04$), and overall satisfaction (63.0% vs. 35.3%, $P = 0.02$). There was a trend toward more dysfunction in the sedentary group for total score on the IIEF (44.4% vs. 23.5%, $P = 0.057$), while sexual desire domain scores were similar in both groups (51.9% vs. 41.2%, $P = 0.37$).

Conclusions.—We have demonstrated that increased physical activity is associated with better sexual function measured by a validated questionnaire in a young, healthy population. Further studies are needed on the long-term effects of exercise, or lack thereof, on erectile function as these men age.

▶ Several studies have indicated that sedentary, middle-aged men are at increased risk of prevalent or incident erectile dysfunction (ED). A smaller selection of trials has indicated that initiation of exercise regimens may reduce the risk of ED or even reverse the condition if it is already present. These are compelling data, but, as the authors of this article point out, it is not clear what relevance they have to younger men without the diagnosis of ED.

These authors report that men who had less than 1400 kcal of energy expenditure per week were significantly more likely to have low scores on the International Index of Erectile Function domains for erectile function (IIEF-EF), orgasmic function, intercourse satisfaction, and overall satisfaction. These relationships held after controlling for race, body mass index, age, blood pressure, and several medical conditions known to be associated with ED. Desire did not appear to be influenced by physical activity.

This small study (n = 78) does not really prove much, and the means used to categorize sexual dysfunction (score of 8 or less out of 10, or 12 or less out of 15) have not been validated; it is hard to know whether these men had genuine sexual dysfunction or not, particularly since the IIEF-EF was primarily validated in older men (in fairness, a number of studies since initial validation have indicated that the IIEF-EF probably works in young men too).

I certainly would not mind using this article as evidence for the benefits of exercise in men of all ages. Aside from improving sexual function, exercise may help men live longer and better lives, so I think it is in our best interests as practitioners to sanction it.

A. W. Shindel, MD

Chronic Oral Administration of the Arginase Inhibitor 2(S)-amino-6-boronohexanoic acid (ABH) Improves Erectile Function in Aged Rats

Segal R, Hannan JL, Lu X, et al (Johns Hopkins Med Institutions, Baltimore, MD; et al)
J Androl 2012 [Epub ahead of print]

Arginase expression and activity has been noted to be heightened in conditions associated with erectile dysfunction, including aging. Previously, arginase inhibition by chronic administration of the arginase inhibitor 2-S-amino-6-boronohexanoic acid (ABH) has been shown to improve endothelial dysfunction in aged rats. The objective of this study was to assess whether chronic oral ABH administration affects cavernosal erectile function. Rats were divided into 4 groups: young control, young treated with arginase inhibitor, aged control, and aged treated with arginase inhibitor. Arginase activity was measured and presented as a proportion of young untreated rats. In vivo erectile responses to cavernous nerve stimulation (CNS) were measured in all cohorts. The cavernous nerve (CN) was stimulated with a graded electrical stimulus, and the intracavernosal/mean arterial pressure (ICP/MAP) ratios and total ICP were recorded. Arginase activity was elevated in the aged rats compared to young controls; however, arginase activity was significantly decreased in aged rats treated with ABH. With the addition of ABH, erectile responses improved in the aged rats ($P < 0.05$). Oral inhibition of arginase with ABH results in improved erectile function in aged rats, resulting in erectile hemodynamics similar to young rats. This represents the first documentation of systemic arginase inhibition positively affecting corporal cavernosal function.

▶ Nitric oxide (NO) is currently regarded as the principal neurotransmitter involved in the vasodilatory effects leading to penile erection. All current oral pharmacotherapies for erectile dysfunction (ED) work on the downstream effector cyclic guanosine monophosphate (cGMP); ergo, there is great potential for development of alternative therapies that take advantage of the NO/cGMP pathway.

Arginine is the precursor to NO. Hence, enhancement of arginine concentration has been touted as a naturopathic approach to enhance endothelial reactivity and sexual response. In this study, the authors demonstrate that aging rats have increased activity of the enzyme arginase, which in turn tends to decrease the amount of arginine available for conversion to NO. Inhibition of arginase activity via the compound 2-S-amino-6-boronohexanoic (ABH) acid in a group of these aged rats led to normalization of penile hemodynamics in aged rats relative to younger control rats.

The potential for synergic use of drugs such as ABH with phosphodiesterase type 5 inhibitors may markedly improve the management of ED in men with neuropathic etiologies for ED, such as radical prostatectomy, diabetes, and other neurodegenerative conditions.

A. W. Shindel, MD

Does Current Scientific and Clinical Evidence Support the Use of Phosphodiesterase Type 5 Inhibitors for the Treatment of Premature Ejaculation? A Systematic Review and Meta-analysis
Asimakopoulos AD, Miano R, Agrò EF, et al (Univ of Tor Vergata, Rome, Italy)
J Sex Med 2012 [Epub ahead of print]

Introduction.—Premature ejaculation (PE) is a highly prevalent and complex syndrome that remains poorly defined and inadequately characterized. Pharmacotherapy represents the current basis of lifelong PE treatment.

Aim.—The goal of this study was to assess the role of phosphodiesterase type 5 inhibitors (PDE5-Is) in the treatment of patients with PE without associated erectile dysfunction (ED).

Main Outcome Measure.—The posttreatment intravaginal ejaculatory latency time was used as the primary end point of efficacy.

Methods.—A systematic review of the literature was performed by electronically searching the MedLine database for peer-reviewed articles regarding the mechanism of action and the clinical trials of PDE5 in the management of PE. A meta-analysis of these clinical studies was performed to pool the efficacy.

Results.—Twenty-nine articles that examined the supposed mechanisms of action and 14 articles that reported data from clinical studies were reviewed. The PDE5 may exert their influence by increasing the levels of nitric oxide both centrally (reducing sympathetic drive) and peripherally (leading to smooth-muscle dilatation of the seminal tract). These drugs may also induce peripheral analgesia to prolong the duration of the erection, increase confidence, improve the perception of ejaculatory control and overall sexual satisfaction, and decrease the postorgasmic refractory time for achieving a second erection after ejaculation. Concerning the efficacy, the meta-analysis shows an overall positive effect for the use of PDE5 as monotherapy or as components of a combination regimen in the treatment of PE. The major limitations of the published literature included poor study design, the absence of solid methodology, which was characterized by the lack of a unique PE definition, and the lack of appropriate endpoints for outcome evaluation of a placebo control arm and of Institutional Review Board approval.

Conclusion.—There is inadequate, partial basic, and clinical evidence to support the use of PDE5 for the treatment of PE.

▶ This systematic review attempts to ascertain whether current evidence supports the use of phosphodiesterase type 5 inhibitors (PDE5Is) for premature ejaculation (PE). PDE5Is are the only oral pharmacotherapy that are currently FDA approved for the management of a sexual concern in human patients, and it is, hence, not surprising that PDE5I might be prescribed for all manner of sexual ills, not just erectile dysfunction, for which it is clearly indicated in appropriately selected patients. The authors are able to conclude in this review that there is some fragmentary evidence, based on both basic science and clinical study, to support the use of PDE5Is.

There is some biological rationale for the use of PDE5Is in PE, and, on a very simplistic level, reduction of the refractory period and/or optimization of erectile hardness may play a role in helping men to adapt to (if not genuinely treat) PE. These drugs are generally safe for appropriately screened patients; ergo, there seems little risk in a trial of PDE5Is for PE. Nevertheless, inadequacies of the existing data make it clear that the search for a true, proven therapy designed specifically for PE is still required. Research in this vein must continue.

A. W. Shindel, MD

Adipose tissue-derived stem cell-seeded small intestinal submucosa for tunica albuginea grafting and reconstruction
Ma L, Yang Y, Sikka SC, et al (Tulane Univ Health Sciences Ctr, New Orleans, LA; et al)
Proc Natl Acad Sci U S A 109:2090-2095, 2012

Porcine small intestinal submucosa (SIS) has been widely used in tunica albuginea (TA) reconstructive surgery. Adipose tissue-derived stem cells (ADSCs) can repair damaged tissue, augment cellular differentiation, and stimulate release of multiple growth factors. The aim of this rat study was to assess the feasibility of seeding ADSCs onto SIS grafts for TA reconstruction. Here, we demonstrate that seeding syngeneic ADSCs onto SIS grafts (SIS-ADSC) resulted in significant cavernosal tissue preservation and maintained erectile responses, similar to controls, in a rat model of bilateral incision of TA, compared with sham-operated animals and rats grafted with SIS graft (SIS) alone. In addition to increased TGF-β1 and FGF-2 expression levels, cross-sectional studies of the rat penis with SIS and SIS-ADSC revealed mild to moderate fibrosis and an increase of 30% and 40% in mean diameter in flaccid and erectile states, respectively. SIS grafting induced transcriptional up-regulation of iNOS and down-regulation of endothelial NOS, neuronal NOS, and VEGF, an effect that was restored by seeding ADCSs on the SIS graft. Taken together, these data show that rats undergoing TA incision with autologous SIS-ADSC grafts maintained better erectile function compared with animals grafted with SIS alone. This study suggests that SIS-ADSC grafting can be successfully used for TA reconstruction procedures and can restore erectile function.

▶ This article assesses the utility of adipose-derived stem cells (ADSC) as seed material on an acellular graft used in reconstruction of the tunica albuginea of the penis. Impregnation of the graft material with ADSC led to superior functional outcomes relative to unseeded grafts in similarly treated animals. These gains were associated with improvements in smooth muscle and endothelial content, nitric oxide synthase expression, and reductions in markers of fibrosis.

Exogenous graft materials have several desirable features in comparison with autologous options. However, these materials tend to produce more inflammation and/or integrate less well into biological systems. Use of ADSC, a plentiful and easily accessed source of stem cells, in conjunction with nonautologous graft material combines the best of both worlds in many respects and represents an appealing alternative to current treatment options. Whether this type of material might be useful in other applications is an intriguing question worthy of further research.

A. W. Shindel, MD

Does Low Intensity Extracorporeal Shock Wave Therapy Have a Physiological Effect on Erectile Function? Short-Term Results of a Randomized, Double-Blind, Sham Controlled Study

Vardi Y, Appel B, Kilchevsky A, et al (Rambam Healthcare Campus, Haifa, Israel)
J Urol 187:1769-1775, 2012

Purpose.—We investigated the clinical and physiological effect of low intensity extracorporeal shock wave therapy on men with organic erectile dysfunction who are phosphodiesterase type 5 inhibitor responders.

Materials and Methods.—After a 1-month phosphodiesterase type 5 inhibitor washout period, 67 men were randomized in a 2:1 ratio to receive 12 sessions of low intensity extracorporeal shock wave therapy or sham therapy. Erectile function and penile hemodynamics were assessed before the first treatment (visit 1) and 1 month after the final treatment (followup 1) using validated sexual function questionnaires and venooc-clusive strain gauge plethysmography.

Results.—Clinically we found a significantly greater increase in the International Index of Erectile Function-Erectile Function domain score from visit 1 to followup 1 in the treated group than in the sham treated group (mean ± SEM 6.7 ± 0.9 vs 3.0 ± 1.4, $p = 0.0322$). There were 19 men in the treated group who were initially unable to achieve erections hard enough for penetration (Erection Hardness Score 2 or less) who were able to achieve erections sufficiently firm for penetration (Erection Hardness Score 3 or greater) after low intensity extracorporeal shock wave therapy, compared to none in the sham group. Physiologically penile hemodynamics significantly improved in the treated group but not in the sham group (maximal post-ischemic penile blood flow 8.2 vs 0.1 ml per minute per dl, $p < 0.0001$). None of the men experienced discomfort or reported any adverse effects from the treatment.

Conclusions.—This is the first randomized, double-blind, sham con-trolled study to our knowledge that shows that low intensity extracorporeal shock wave therapy has a positive short-term clinical and physiological effect on the erectile function of men who respond to oral phosphodiesterase type 5 inhibitor therapy. The feasibility and tolerability of this treatment, coupled with its potential rehabilitative characteristics, make it an attractive new therapeutic option for men with erectile dysfunction.

▶ This work is really interesting. Shock wave therapy enjoyed a brief period of interest as a potential treatment for Peyronie disease, but results were discour-aging. This latest wave of interest in shock wave application to the penis is directed not toward resolving scar tissue but rather toward stimulating angiogen-esis with the intent of improving circulation and subsequent erectile capacity.

In this study, there was evidence of improved endothelial reactivity of the penis via flow-mediated dilation postobstruction. Although not as compelling as Doppler ultrasound data, this evidence is interesting. There was also a subjec-tive improvement in erectile hardness in several men in the treatment group versus none in the sham group. Men enrolled in the study had International Index of Erectile Function—Erectile Function domain scores of 19 or greater, indicative of mild to moderate or mild erectile dysfunction at baseline. The authors made efforts to blind the subjects with respect to their treatment group; they report that the sounds and vibrations of the devices are similar in the sham and the treatment devices and that the procedure itself is painless. I have a little bit of trouble believing that there is not even delayed pain after application of multiple shock waves to the penis, but I'll accept that the blinding efforts were as good as could be hoped for.

In the end, there are methodological problems here, but this effort is appre-ciated as a novel and innovative idea for management of erectile dysfunction. These pilot data seem to indicate that more extensive studies with more robust end points and methodology are warranted.

A. W. Shindel, MD

Penile revascularization in vasculogenic erectile dysfunction (ED): long—term follow—up
Kayigil O, Okulu E, Aldemir M, et al (Clinic of Ankara Ataturk Training and Res Hosp, Turkey)
BJU Int 109:109-115, 2012

Objective.—● To determine the overall long-term success of penile revascularization surgery in the treatment of vasculogenic erectile dysfunction (ED) and also to investigate the effect of risk factors on the results of a modified Furlow—Fisher technique.

Patients and Methods.—● Between 1999 and 2010, 125 men with a mean (SD, range) age of 43.2 (11.3, 23—69) years underwent penile revascularization surgery. In all, 110 men completed the long-term follow-up with a mean follow-up of 73.2 months.

● Diagnostic evaluations, penile colour Doppler ultrasonography, corpus cavernosum electromyography, and cavernosometry, were performed in all the men before surgery.

● The efficacy of the surgery was assessed as improvement or failure according to the change in the five-item version of the International Index of Erectile Function (IIEF-5). A ≥5 point increase in the IIEF-5 score during the latest patient visit after surgery compared with that before surgery was regarded as improvement (surgical success).

Results.—● The mean (SD) IIEF-5 score was 7.3 (3.2) before surgery and at the end of the follow-up period it was 16.8 (3.1).

● The success rates were 81.8% at 3 months, 77.2% at 1 year, 70% at 2 years, 66.3% at 3 years and 63.6% at 5 years after surgery in the men who achieved a no-ED threshold score of >26 in the IIEF-15.

● The success rate was the highest in the men with no risk factors (92.8%).

● Seven patients (6.36%) showed signs of glans hypervascularization as a major complication.

Conclusions.—● Penile revascularization surgery has not been widely used by urologists probably due to the technical difficulties and the use of phosphodiesterase type 5 inhibitors.

● However, with reported high rates of noncompliance or failure of oral pharmacotherapy it seems likely that this surgery will become more popular in the near future.

▶ This case series represents the second largest report of outcomes of penile revascularization for erectile dysfunction. The report consists of 125 men (mean age, 43 years; range, 23-69 years). It is interesting that 71% of these men had primarily venoocclusive disease as determined by cavernosometry. This is unusual because most experts recommend revascularization for cases of traumatic and isolated trauma to the cavernous artery rather than for diffuse failure of venous occlusion.

This report is limited by its heterogeneous outcomes and by the general vagaries of retrospective chart-review type research. The unresolved question is why penile revascularization has not been more popular. The authors of this study speculate that technical challenges and novel pharmacotherapy have driven this effect. However, published series of results remain few and far between, and it is hard to avoid speculating, based on this study, that outcomes are often disappointing, so they are not published. In my opinion, penile revascularization remains an experimental option that may be useful in selected, healthy patients; it will remain as such until more definitive results are available.

A. W. Shindel, MD

Peripheral neuropathy: an underdiagnosed cause of erectile dysfunction
Valles-Antuña C, Fernandez-Gomez J, Fernandez-Gonzalez F (Hospital Universitario Central de Asturias, Oviedo, Spain)
BJU Int 108:1855-1859, 2011

Objectives.—• To assess the prevalence of peripheral neuropathy in patients with erectile dysfunction (ED).

• To evaluate the reliability of clinical tests such as the five-item version of the International Index of Erectile Function (IIEF-5) and the Neuropathy Symptom Score (NSS) classification system in predicting the concurrence of peripheral neuropathy.

Patients and Methods.—• We studied 90 patients who were consecutively recruited from the Department of Andrology of the Central Hospital of Asturias.

• Anamnesis included questions about risk factors related to ED.

• The severity of ED was classified according to IIEF-5 scores and symptoms of peripheral neuropathy were assessed using the NSS.

• Neurophysiological tests included electromyography, nerve conduction studies, evoked potentials from pudendal and tibial nerves as well as bulbocavernosus reflex.

• Small fibre function was assessed using quantitative sensory tests and sympathetic skin response. Statistical analysis was performed using the SPSS-11 program.

Results.—• Patients with more severe symptoms of peripheral neuropathy showed lower (worse) IIEF-5 scores ($P = 0.015$) and required more aggressive therapies ($P < 0.001$).

• Neurophysiological exploration confirmed neurological pathology in 68.9% of patients, of whom 7.8% had myelopathy and 61.1% peripheral neuropathy.

• Polyneuropathy was found in 37.8% of the patients, of whom 8.9% had pure small fibre polyneuropathy, and pudendal neuropathy was diagnosed in 14.4%.

• No association between neurophysiological diagnosis and IIEF-5 score was detected, but a statistical association was found between neuropathy and NSS scores.

Conclusions.—• Up to now, the impact of peripheral neuropathy in the pathogenesis of ED has been underestimated. The combination of anamnesis and an *ad hoc* neurophysiological protocol showed its high prevalence and provided a more accurate prognosis.

• In future, clinical practice should optimize the assessment of pelvic small fibre function.

▶ The authors of this interesting article investigate neuropathy as a contributing factor in erectile dysfunction (ED). It was determined that more severe neuropathic symptoms were associated with greater odds of ED and also with greater odds of abnormality on neurophysiological testing. Interestingly, ED was not significantly associated with abnormalities of objective neurophysiological data.

The lack of association between objective neurophysiological data and erectile function scores is an important caveat to these data. My sense from this is that while neuropathy may be associated with ED, this study does not establish the causal change. It is possible that decreased sensation or generally poorer health from neuropathic symptoms contributes to declines in erectile capacity.

Although compelling, the question remains "What to do with these data?" There is no clearly proven therapy to reverse neuropathic changes, although there are several promising candidate drugs. Whether these might have utility in management of ED is an intriguing concept that may be worth further study.

A. W. Shindel, MD

Recruitment of Intracavernously Injected Adipose-Derived Stem Cells to the Major Pelvic Ganglion Improves Erectile Function in a Rat Model of Cavernous Nerve Injury

Fandel TM, Albersen M, Lin G, et al (Univ of California, San Francisco)
Eur Urol 61:201-210, 2012

Background.—Intracavernous (IC) injection of stem cells has been shown to ameliorate cavernous-nerve (CN) injury-induced erectile dysfunction (ED). However, the mechanisms of action of adipose-derived stem cells (ADSC) remain unclear.

Objectives.—To investigate the mechanism of action and fate of IC injected ADSC in a rat model of CN crush injury.

Design, Setting, and Participants.—Sprague-Dawley rats ($n = 110$) were randomly divided into five groups. Thirty-five rats underwent sham surgery and IC injection of ADSC ($n = 25$) or vehicle ($n = 10$). Another 75 rats underwent bilateral CN crush injury and were treated with vehicle or ADSC injected either IC or in the dorsal penile perineural space. At 1, 3, 7 ($n = 5$), and 28 d ($n = 10$) postsurgery, penile tissues and major pelvic ganglia (MPG) were harvested for histology. ADSC were labeled with 5-ethynyl-2-deoxyuridine (EdU) before treatment. Rats in the 28-d groups were examined for erectile function prior to tissue harvest.

Measurements.—IC pressure recording on CN electrostimulation, immunohistochemistry of the penis and the MPG, and number of EdU-positive (EdU+) cells in the injection site and the MPG.

Results and Limitations.—IC, but not perineural, injection of ADSC resulted in significantly improved erectile function. Significantly more EdU+ ADSC appeared in the MPG of animals with CN injury and IC injection of ADSC compared with those injected perineurally and those in the sham group. One day after crush injury, stromal cell-derived factor-1 (SDF-1) was upregulated in the MPG, providing an incentive for ADSC recruitment toward the MPG. Neuroregeneration was observed in the group that underwent IC injection of ADSC, and IC ADSC treatment had beneficial effects on the smooth muscle/collagen ratio in the corpus cavernosum.

Conclusions.—CN injury upregulates SDF-1 expression in the MPG and thereby attracts intracavernously injected ADSC. At the MPG, ADSC exert neuroregenerative effects on the cell bodies of injured nerves, resulting in enhanced erectile response.

▶ The authors of this article have a long record of research into adipose-derived stem cell (ADSC) therapy for urologic indications, most specifically erectile dysfunction. This article reports on improvement of penile hemodynamics as well as a number of histological benefits from injection of ADSC into the cavernosa of the penis in rats subjected to cavernous nerve injury. Furthermore, there was apparent migration of ADSC to the major pelvic ganglion (MPG); the authors attribute this to upregulation of a stem cell homing factor SDF-1 in the MPG, which was detected as early as 1 day after cavernous nerve crush.

It will be interesting to determine if ADSC migration can be blocked by downregulation of the homing factor SDF-1; this will be required to prove definitively that this mechanism is driving cell migration. The authors report an interesting association between SDF-1 expression and ADSC localization, but further study is required to prove this relation is the driving factor for these observed results.

A. W. Shindel, MD

Association between smoking cessation and sexual health in men
Harte CB, Meston CM (Univ of Texas at Austin)
BJU Int 109:888-896, 2012

Objective.—• To provide the first empirical investigation of the association between smoking cessation and indices of physiological and subjective sexual health in men.

Subjects and Methods.—• Male smokers, irrespective of erectile dysfunction status, who were motivated to stop smoking ('quitters'), were enrolled in an 8-week smoking cessation programme involving a nicotine transdermal patch treatment and adjunctive counselling.

• Participants were assessed at baseline (while smoking regularly), at mid-treatment (while using a high-dose nicotine transdermal patch), and at a 4-week post-cessation follow-up.

- Physiological (circumferential change via penile plethysmography) and subjective sexual arousal indices (continuous self-report), as well as self-reported sexual functioning were assessed at each visit.

Results.—• Intent-to-treat analyses indicated that, at follow-up, successful quitters ($n = 20$), compared with those who relapsed ($n = 45$), showed enhanced erectile tumescence responses, and faster onset to reach maximum subjective sexual arousal.

- Although successful quitters displayed across-session enhancements in sexual function, they did not show a differential improvement compared with unsuccessful quitters.

Conclusions.—• Smoking cessation significantly enhances both physiological and self-reported indices of sexual health in long-term male smokers, irrespective of baseline erectile impairment.

- It is hoped that these results may serve as a novel means to motivate men to stop smoking.

▶ This is a very important study. It is no mystery that tobacco use takes a toll on the vascular system, and tobacco cessation may help reverse this. This study provides real-world proof that men can take charge of their erectile dysfunction (ED) and improve their sexual function by stopping cigarette smoking. Men who were successfully able to quit had improvements in penile engorgement and subjective sexual arousal in response to erotic stimuli. The reduction in diagnosable ED based on the International Index of Erectile Function scoring was not significant, but this does not detract from the importance of the other clinical endpoints of this study.

Smoking cessation is very difficult, and there is no one way to do it. However, data do suggest that each instance of provider counseling on smoking cessation leads to a small but finite percentage of patients attempting to quit. We should be relentless on our efforts to inform patients about the health risks of tobacco use and the myriad benefits of tobacco cessation. Sexual medicine specialists will do their patients a great service if they incorporate this counseling into their standard patient assessment. This may require partnering with tobacco cessation specialists or community resources for smokers who wish to quit. This is fertile ground for public health research.

A. W. Shindel, MD

A Randomized, Double-Blind, Placebo-Controlled Evaluation of the Safety and Efficacy of Avanafil in Subjects with Erectile Dysfunction
Goldstein I, McCullough AR, Jones LA, et al (Alvarado Hosp, San Diego, CA; Albany College of Medicine, NY; Urology San Antonio Res, TX; et al)
J Sex Med 9:1122-1133, 2012

Introduction.—Phosphodiesterase type 5 (PDE5) inhibitors have become standard treatment for erectile dysfunction (ED).

Aim.—To prospectively evaluate the safety and efficacy of avanafil, a novel PDE5 inhibitor, in men with mild to severe ED.

Methods.—In this multicenter, double-blind, Phase 3 trial, 646 subjects were randomized to receive avanafil (50 mg, 100 mg, 200 mg) or placebo throughout a 12-week treatment period. Subjects were instructed to take study drug 30 minutes prior to initiation of sexual activity. At least a 12-hour separation time between doses was required; no restrictions were placed on food or alcohol intake.

Main Outcome Measures.—Improvement in erectile function (EF) was measured by Sexual Encounter Profile questions 2 and 3 (SEP2 and SEP3) and by the EF domain of the International Index of Erectile Function (IIEF) questionnaire.

Results.—Mean change in percentage of successful sexual attempts (SEP2 and SEP3) and IIEF-EF domain score significantly favored all doses of avanafil over placebo ($P \leq 0.001$). Secondary analyses demonstrated achievement of successful intercourse by subjects within 15 minutes of dosing. Of the 300 sexual attempts made during this interval, 64% to 71% were successful in avanafil-treated subjects compared with 27% in placebo-treated subjects. Successful intercourse was also demonstrated >6 hours post dosing, with 59% to 83% of the 80 sexual attempts successful in avanafil-treated subjects compared with 25% of placebo-treated subjects. The most commonly reported adverse events in subjects taking avanafil included headache, flushing, and nasal congestion; there were no drug-related serious adverse events.

Conclusion.—Following 12 weeks of avanafil treatment without food or alcohol restrictions, significant improvements in sexual function were observed with all 3 doses of avanafil compared with placebo. Successful intercourse was observed as early as 15 minutes and >6 hours after dosing in some subjects. Avanafil was generally well tolerated for the treatment of ED.

▶ These authors report on outcomes of avanafil, a novel PDE5 inhibitor, in the management of erectile dysfunction (ED) in men over a 3-month randomized controlled trial. As would be expected, this drug improved erectile function at all doses with significant differences versus placebo in all of the standard parameters used in ED trials.

The pharmacokinetics of this drug (onset with 15 minutes and duration of more than 6 hours in some patients) may make it appealing to some patients, although both of these findings have been reported with the currently available PDE5i. Of potentially greater interest is more selectivity (in vitro) for PDE5; this *may* translate to a lower incidence of side effects in human patients. However, treatment-emergent adverse events were not uncommon in the treatment arm (38% vs 26% in placebo), so it seems premature to hope that this drug will have a markedly different side effects profile, and additional data are required.

A more fundamental question is whether a new PDE5i is what we need. The proliferation of "me too" drugs may lead to incremental improvements in treatment across medical specialties, but drugs exploiting the same mechanism are seldom "game changers." It would be of greater interest to investigate alternative targets along the NO/cGMP pathway (eg, guanylate cyclase) and downstream modulators of intracellular calcium content in smooth muscle.

A. W. Shindel, MD

Couples' Reasons for Adherence to, or Discontinuation of, PDE Type 5 Inhibitors for Men with Erectile Dysfunction at 12 to 24-Month Follow-Up after a 6-Month Free Trial
Conaglen HM, Conaglen JV (Univ of Auckland, Hamilton, New Zealand)
J Sex Med 9:857-865, 2012

Introduction.—The history of treatments for erectile dysfunction (ED) has involved a repeated pattern of uptake, followed by abandonment of the various therapies in the medium term. Even effective and simple to use medications are not necessarily continued; discontinuation rates range between 15% and 60%. Despite the association between partner sexual function and men's use of PDE5, no previous studies have reported any contact with partners of men taking PDE5 for their ED. This study involved both partners in couples followed up at least 1 year after treatment of ED.

Aim.—The study sought clarification of factors influencing adherence to, or discontinuation of, oral ED medications from couples. We hypothesized that many factors contribute to decision making about ED medication use at >12 months.

Main Outcome Measures.—The main outcome measures of this article were interviews and International Index of Erectile Function-erectile function domain.

Methods.—A total of 155 interviews were conducted seeking details of frequency of usage and preference for the drugs available; reasons for that choice, or for discontinuation of use, were also sought.

Results.—Of men interviewed, 71% were using PDE5 at 18 months. Most men interviewed were using the oral medications either 1−2×/week or 1−2×/month. Forty-four percent of men who had decreased their use of the medications reported less need for them. Thirty-four men said the main reason they were using less medication was cost. "Partner issues" from the men's perspective were seldom reported in this study. However, for a number of women, "partner issues" meant a range of problems from separation to alcohol abuse, lack of communication, and lack of confidence, or fear of failure.

Conclusions.—This is the first study to ask couples why they decided to continue or stop using PDE5 when followed up. Female partners provided a different perspective on "partner issues" often cited as reasons for discontinuing PDE5 use. It was also clear that discontinuation did not mean couples were no longer sexually active.

▶ Phosphodiesterase type 5 inhibitors (PDE5I) have a significant failure rate that is in many cases related to inadequate efficacy of the medication. However, the psychosocial complexities of sexuality probably play an important role in many, if not all, cases of sexual dysfunction, and this may have profound effects on treatment efficacy.

In this study, 155 interviews were conducted with men who had erectile dysfunction and with their female partners; this cohort had previously been enrolled in a study of PDE5I, and most (~80%) had expressed a desire to continue with therapy. A substantial number of interviewees (about one-third) had ceased using the drugs (partner had ceased using in the case of female interviewees). Commonly reported reasons for medication discontinuation by men were medical illness and cost, whereas for female partners, issues (emotional distance and psychosocial disturbance) and cost figured most prominently. Only 1 of the male subjects reported that he discontinued treatment because of lack of efficacy.

It is clear from these data that simple prescription is not enough. It is to be hoped that lower-cost alternatives will soon be available. Providers must also keep in mind the necessity of couple's sexual counseling as an adjunct to pharmacotherapy, particularly in situations in which there has been prolonged cessation of sexual activity.

A. W. Shindel, MD

A systematic review of sexual concerns reported by gynecological cancer survivors

Abbott-Anderson K, Kwekkeboom KL (Univ of Wisconsin-Madison)
Gynecol Oncol 124:477-489, 2012

Objective.—To identify physical, psychological and social sexual concerns reported by gynecological (GYN) cancer survivors.

Methods.—A systematic review of the literature was conducted using CINAHL, PubMed and PsycInfo databases. Reference lists from articles provided additional relevant literature. Only research articles from peer-reviewed journals were included. A total of 37 articles were located; 34 explored women's sexual concerns following gynecological cancer diagnosis and treatment and 3 tested interventions for sexual concerns in women with gynecological cancer.

Results.—Sexual concerns were identified across all dimensions of sexuality. Common concerns in the physical dimension were dyspareunia, changes in the vagina, and decreased sexual activity. In the psychological dimension, common concerns were decreased libido, alterations in body image, and anxiety related to sexual performance. And in the social dimension, common concerns were difficulty maintaining previous sexual roles, emotional distancing from the partner, and perceived change in the partner's level of sexual interest. Of the three psychoeducational intervention studies, two reported improvements in physical aspects of sexual function, and one reported improved knowledge, but without resolution of sexual concerns.

Conclusion.—Gynecological cancer survivors experience a broad range of sexual concerns after diagnosis and treatment, but the majority of studies emphasized physical aspects of sexuality, and may not adequately represent women's psychological and social sexual concerns. Health care providers should remain mindful of psychological and social sexual concerns when caring for gynecologic cancer survivors. Future research should systematically evaluate the full range of sexual concerns in large, representative samples of GYN cancer survivors and develop and test interventions to address those concerns.

▶ A great deal of time and attention is devoted to the recovery of sexual function in men after radical prostatectomy. It is interesting that relatively little attention is paid to similar outcome measures when assessing survivors of gynecologic cancer.

This article summarizes published, peer-reviewed articles concerning recovery of sexual function after management of gynecologic malignancy. None of the concerns highlighted in this review are in and of themselves novel or even unexpected, given the nature of gynecologic cancer treatment.

However, it is telling that only 3 articles meeting the criteria for this review included interventions to mitigate the effects of cancer treatment on women's sexual function; furthermore, all of these interventions were psychological or educational. This is interesting in that 33 of the 34 studies included in the review identified physical sexual concerns.

The importance of psychological and knowledge-based interventions in cases of sexual concerns cannot be overemphasized, but complete neglect of biomedical factors does not do justice to this large population of female patients. The lack of current understanding is a reason but not an excuse for the continued disparity in attention to the biological aspects of sexuality in women, including women who have been or are being treated for cancer.

A. W. Shindel, MD

10-Year Analysis of Adverse Event Reports to the Food and Drug Administration for Phosphodiesterase Type-5 Inhibitors
Lowe G, Costabile RA (Ohio State Univ Med Ctr, Columbus; Univ of Virginia Health System, Charlottesville)
J Sex Med 9:265-270, 2012

Introduction.—To ensure public safety all Food and Drug Administration (FDA)-approved medications undergo postapproval safety analysis. Phosphodiesterase type-5 inhibitors (PDE5-i) are generally regarded as safe and effective.

Aim.—We performed a nonindustry-sponsored analysis of FDA reports for sildenafil, tadalafil, and vardenafil to evaluate the reported cardiovascular and mortality events over the past 10 years.

Methods.—Summarized reports of adverse events (AEs) for each PDE5-i were requested from the Center for Drug Evaluation and Research within the FDA. These data are available under the Freedom of Information Act and document industry and nonindustry reports of AEs entered into the computerized system maintained by the Office of Surveillance and Epidemiology.

Main Outcome Measure.—The data were analyzed for the number of AE reports, number of objective cardiovascular events, and reported deaths.

Results.—Overall, 14,818 AEs were reported for sildenafil. There were 1,824 (12.3%) reported deaths, and reports of cardiovascular AEs numbered 2,406 (16.2%). Tadalafil was associated with 5,548 AEs and 236 deaths were reported. Vardenafil was associated with 6,085 AEs and 121 reports of deaths. The percentage of reported severe cardiovascular disorders has stabilized at 10% to 15% of all AE reports for sildenafil and tadalafil and 5% to 10% for vardenafil. Only 10% of AE reports sent to the FDA for PDE5-i were from pharmaceutical manufacturers.

Conclusion.—Reports of deaths associated with PDE5-i remain around 5% of total reported events. Despite inherent limitations from evaluating FDA reports of AEs, it is important that these reports be reviewed outside pharmaceutical industry support in order to provide due diligence and transparency.

▶ This important study investigates reports made to the US Food and Drug Administration concerning adverse events resulting from phosphodiesterase type-5 inhibitors (PDE5-i) over a 10-year period. This phase IV study is important to assess the incidence of rare adverse outcomes that may be related to these drugs. However, such a database is limited in some respects by possible attribution of negative outcomes to the drugs when some other unknown variable was operative.

The authors determined that a significant number of adverse events purported to be related to PDE5-i include death. The most likely etiology in the majority of these cases was cardiovascular, and it is not too much of a stretch to hypothesize that many of these deaths may be related to sexual exertion in deconditioned men. This brings up the important point that doctors should pay some heed to their patients' levels of fitness and cardiac health prior to facilitating sexual activity. This is not meant as a way of dissuading patients from engaging in sexual activity or castigating PDE5-i as lethal drugs. However, it is wise to remind patients that sex is work and their hearts must be strong enough to handle the potential exertion.

A. W. Shindel, MD

A Pivotal Role of Lumbar Spinothalamic Cells in the Regulation of Ejaculation via Intraspinal Connections

Staudt MD, Truitt WA, McKenna KE, et al (The Univ of Western Ontario, London, Ontario, Canada; Indiana Univ-Purdue Univ Indianapolis; Northwestern Univ, Chicago, IL)
J Sex Med 2011 [Epub ahead of print]

Introduction.—A population of lumbar spinothalamic cells (LSt cells) has been demonstrated to play a pivotal role in ejaculatory behavior and comprise a critical component of the spinal ejaculation generator. LSt cells are hypothesized to regulate ejaculation via their projections to autonomic and motor neurons in the lumbosacral spinal cord.

Aim.—The current study tested the hypothesis that ejaculatory reflexes are dependent on LSt cells via projections within the lumbosacral spinal cord.

Methods.—Male rats received intraspinal injections of neurotoxin saporin conjugated to substance P analog, previously shown to selectively lesion LSt cells. Two weeks later, males were anesthetized and spinal cords were transected. Subsequently, males were subjected to ejaculatory reflex paradigms, including stimulation of the dorsal penile nerve (DPN), urethrogenital stimulation or administration of D3 agonist 7-OH-DPAT. Electromyographic recordings of the bulbocavernosus muscle (BCM) were analyzed for rhythmic bursting characteristic of the expulsion phase of ejaculation. In addition, a fourth commonly used paradigm for ejaculation and erections in unanesthetized, spinal-intact male rats was utilized: the ex copula reflex paradigm.

Main Outcome Measures.—LSt cell lesions were predicted to prevent rhythmic bursting of BCM following DPN, urethral, or pharmacological stimulation, and emissions in the ex copula paradigm. In contrast, LSt cell lesions were not expected to abolish erectile function as measured in the ex copula paradigm.

Results.—LSt cell lesions prevented rhythmic contractions of the BCM induced by any of the ejaculatory reflex paradigms in spinalized rats. However, LSt cell lesions did not affect erectile function nor emissions determined in the ex copula reflex paradigm.

Conclusions.—These data demonstrate that LSt cells are essential for ejaculatory, but not erectile reflexes, as previously reported for mating animals. Moreover, LSt cells mediate ejaculation via projections within the spinal cord, presumably to autonomic and motor neurons.

▶ The authors of this study investigated a population of lumbar spinothalamic neurons using elegant techniques of nerve injury. It was determined in this study that these neurons play a critical role in ejaculation induced by any one of a number of separate stimuli. However, lesion of these neurons did not disrupt penile erection, suggesting a very specific function for these neurons in the sexual activity of rats.

Ejaculation disorders are less prevalent and potentially less disabling than erectile dysfunction, but they remain a very bothersome and poorly understood condition. There has been much recent progress in ascertaining central nervous system contributions to this process. It is not currently clear how this particular discovery may be applied to human men, but as understanding of ejaculation increases, it is reasonable to hope that new therapies may be developed that may improve sexual function in men with ejaculatory or orgasmic disorders. These treatments may have additional ramifications for male fertility, particularly in cases of an ejaculation related to sympathetic chain disruption resulting from neuropathy or retroperitoneal surgery.

A. W. Shindel, MD

A Randomized Double-Blind, Placebo-Controlled Multicenter Study to Evaluate the Efficacy and Safety of Two Doses of the Tramadol Orally Disintegrating Tablet for the Treatment of Premature Ejaculation Within Less Than 2 Minutes

Bar-Or D, for the Tramadol ODT Study Group (Swedish Med Ctr, Englewood, CO; et al)
Eur Urol 61:736-743, 2012

Background.—Premature ejaculation (PE) is a widely observed male sexual dysfunction with a major impact on quality of life for many men and their sexual partners.

Objective.—To assess the safety of tramadol orally disintegrating tablet (ODT) (Zertane) and its efficacy in prolonging intravaginal ejaculation latency time (IELT) and improving Premature Ejaculation Profile (PEP) scores.

Design, Setting, and Participants.—We conducted an integrated analysis of two identical 12-wk randomized double-blind, placebo-controlled phase 3 trials across 62 sites in Europe. Healthy men 18–65 yr of age with a history of lifelong PE according to the *Diagnostic and Statistical Manual of Mental Disorders, 4th Edition, Text Revision*, and an IELT ≤120 s were included. There were 604 intent-to-treat subjects included in the analysis.

Intervention.—Subjects were randomized to receive 1:1:1 placebo ($n = 200$), 62 mg tramadol ODT ($n = 206$), or 89 mg tramadol ODT ($n = 198$).

Measurements.—We measured overall change and fold increase in median IELT and the mean change in all four measures of the PEP. Differences across treatment groups were analyzed using Wilcoxon rank-sum tests, analysis of variance, and chi-square analyses.

Results and Limitations.—Tramadol ODT resulted in significant increases in median IELT compared with placebo; increases were 0.6 min (1.6 fold), 1.2 min (2.4 fold), and 1.5 min (2.5 fold) for placebo, 62 mg tramadol ODT, and 89 mg tramadol ODT, respectively ($p < 0.001$ for all comparisons). Men saw significantly greater improvement in all four measures of the PEP in both doses compared with placebo ($p < 0.05$ for all comparisons). Tramadol ODT was well tolerated; study discontinuation occurred in 0%, 1.0%, and 1.6% of subjects in placebo, 62 mg, and 89 mg tramadol ODT groups, respectively. Limitations include study inclusion for men with IELT up to 120 s.

Conclusions.—On-demand 62 mg tramadol ODT is an effective treatment for PE in a low and safe therapeutic dose and provides a new option for managing mild to severe PE.

Trial Registration.—ClinicalTrials.gov identifiers NCT00983151 and NCT00983736; http://clinicaltrials.gov/.

▶ This study is a synopsis of 2 randomized controlled investigations of tramadol orally dissolving tablets for management of lifelong premature ejaculation (PE). The groups randomized to therapy with on-demand tramadol had significantly increased ejaculation latency relative to the group randomized to placebo. This effect was associated with significantly greater scores on the Premature Ejaculation Profile, a validated instrument for assessment of ejaculation-related satisfaction or distress.

The mechanism of action of tramadol in the management of PE is unclear; this drug affects numerous central nervous system receptors, so the specific pathway(s) involved is unclear. While the mechanism may not have immediate relevance to the patient himself, further elucidation of the mechanism may permit refinement and improvement of this treatment effect. Consideration must also be given to the potential for addiction to this medication.

Finally, it is worth noting that the mean ejaculation latency in the treatment groups remains low, at about a minute and a half. This is a marked improvement over where these men started, but careful counseling is required when addressing patients' expectations because it is likely that most men with PE would prefer a greater prolongation of ejaculation than these drugs are able to provide.

A. W. Shindel, MD

Measuring erectile function after radical prostatectomy: comparing a single question with the International Index of Erectile Function

Tal R, Rabbani F, Scardino PT, et al (Memorial Sloan Kettering Cancer Ctr, NY)
BJU Int 109:414-417, 2012

Objective.—• To present a single-question institutional erectile function scale, which was developed at Memorial Sloan-Kettering Cancer Center (MSKCC) before the availability of the International Index of Erectile Function (IIEF), and to compare its performance with the IIEF. Erectile function status assessment after radical prostatectomy is a significant challenge both for research purposes and in clinical practice. Recently, there has been a shift away from complex questionnaire use such as the IIEF and regression to single-item assessment of erectile function.

Patients and Methods.—• Our erectile function score, a single question 5-point score based on physician—patient interview, was applied to 276 patients with prostate cancer after radical prostatectomy. Based on the erectile function score, patients were grouped into five groups. The mean IIEF score and the mean score of questions 3 and 4 of the IIEF were calculated and compared across the groups.

• Each score group was compared with the preceding group and tested for significant difference. The erectile function domain of the IIEF and the institutional score were tested for correlation.

Results.—• The complete erectile function domain score from the IIEF was available for 170 patients and scores from questions 3 and 4 were available for 220 patients. The institutional erectile function score categorized the subjects into distinct groups based on erectile function status.

• The institutional erectile function score was highly correlated with the IIEF erectile function domain score ($r = -0.692$, $P < 0.001$) and with the questions 3 and 4 combined score ($r = -0.678$, $P < 0.001$).

Conclusions.—• The MSKCC erectile function scale is a practical, readily administered method to assess erectile function in patients with prostate cancer after radical prostatectomy.

• The erectile function score, as determined by this scale, is highly correlated with the IIEF erectile function domain score.

▶ The International Index of Erectile Function (IIEF) has been used extensively in research and clinical practice. It is a very useful and well-validated instrument; however, it remains somewhat burdensome for patients and is often left uncompleted on intake forms. It may not be practical for everyday use by practicing urologists not involved in research.

This article, from a prominent sexual function research institution, addresses outcome measures after radical prostatectomy. In this study, a single-item score for erectile dysfunction (determined based on patient interview) was compared with the validated measures of IIEF EF domain and specifically to the IIEF questions relating to the ability to attain and maintain erection sufficient for penetrative sexual activity (IIEF-3 and IIEF-4, respectively). It was determined that the single item correlated very well with the more extensive measures, suggesting that this single item may be a more wieldy approach to assessing sexual response.

A single item will, of course, not address subtleties and nuances that may be better detected by more extensive questioning. However, these are useful data that may help streamline patient flow and/or research outcomes in certain settings.

A. W. Shindel, MD

Pelvic Ring Injury Is Associated With Sexual Dysfunction in Women
Vallier HA, Cureton BA, Schubeck D (MetroHealth Med Ctr, Cleveland, OH)
J Orthop Trauma 26:308-313, 2012

Objectives.—Previous studies have reported a negative effect of pelvic trauma on genitourinary and reproductive function of women. However, fracture pattern, injury severity, and final fracture alignment have not been well studied. The purpose of this project was to describe sexual function in women after pelvic ring injury.

Design.—Cohort study: a prospective collection of sexual function data for women with prior pelvic ring injury versus control groups of uninjured women and other women from the orthopaedic trauma clinic.

Setting.—Level I trauma center.

Patients/Participants.—One hundred eighty-seven women younger than age 55 years with pelvic ring injury, including 101 B-type (61-B1: n = 25, B2: n = 69, B3: n = 7) and 86 C-type (61-C1: n = 56, C2: n = 18, C3: n = 12) fractures. Four had open fractures, and 23 had associated genitourinary injury.

Intervention.—Seventy-four were treated operatively. Surgical treatment was percutaneous in 62: iliosacral screws (n = 58), external fixation (n = 4), or both (n = 19). Open reduction and internal fixation was performed for the pubis symphysis (n = 27), sacroiliac joint (n = 2), and posterior ileum (n = 3).

Main Outcome Measurements.—Sexual function questionnaires were completed for 92 patients (49%) with minimum 12 months and mean 46 months follow-up.

Results.—Forty-eight patients (56%) reported pain with intercourse. Their mean Musculoskeletal Function Assessment was 44.3 versus 20.9 without dyspareunia ($P < 0.0001$). Seventy-eight percent of patients with B-type fractures and 43% of patients with C-type fractures had dyspareunia ($P = 0.002$). Dyspareunia occurred after 91% of anteroposterior compression injuries ($P = 0.02$) and in 79% with a symphyseal disruption treated with plate fixation ($P = 0.005$). All patients with bladder ruptures (n = 5) reported dyspareunia. Sacral fracture or sacroiliac injury, type of posterior treatment, and residual malalignment of the posterior ring were not associated with dyspareunia. Fourteen patients each had associated femur fractures and/or tibia fractures. Seventeen of them had pain during intercourse ($P = 0.19$ for association of femoral or tibial fractures with dyspareunia).

Conclusions.—Dyspareunia is common in women after pelvic ring fracture. Women with pelvic ring injury are more likely to report dyspareunia than other female patients with musculoskeletal trauma. Dyspareunia was related to anteroposterior compression and B-type injuries. Symphyseal plate fixation is also associated with dyspareunia. Pain with intercourse was also noted in all patients with a history of bladder rupture. Poor functional outcomes as measured by Musculoskeletal Function Assessment scores were reported in women with dyspareunia.

Level of Evidence.—Prognostic Level III. See Instructions for Authors for a complete description of levels of evidence.

▶ This is a retrospective report on sexual function outcomes in women who have suffered pelvic fracture at a mean follow-up of 46 months postinjury. The authors focus on dyspareunia outcomes in the abstract section. Although it is hardly surprising that women (like men) often suffer sexual sequelae of major pelvic traumas, this article does add to the literature by characterizing the type of injury most prone to sexual problems. Crush injuries appeared most prone to dyspareunia in women; interestingly, there was a lower prevalence of dyspareunia in type C injuries (complete disruption of the posterior sacroiliac complex) versus type B injuries (partial disruption of the posterior sacroiliac complex).

The authors compare the injured cohort to a control population of gynecology outpatients without documented sexual concerns or prior major injury to the lower trunk and a second control population with orthopedic injuries not involving the lower trunk. Interestingly, almost the entire population of uninjured controls (96%) reported pelvic pain with intercourse compared to 65% and 71% of the pelvic fracture and nonpelvic injury groups, respectively. The authors' rather general definition of dyspareunia (pain in any of a number of locations during intercourse) is semantically not quite accurate. Future studies of this nature would benefit from closer involvement with dedicated sexual health specialists to obtain more meaningful and nuanced results.

A. W. Shindel, MD

Molecular and Functional Characterization of *ORAI* and *STIM* in Human Corporeal Smooth Muscle Cells and Effects of the Transfer of Their Dominant-Negative Mutant Genes into Diabetic Rats

Sung HH, Kam SC, Lee JH, et al (Sungkyunkwan Univ School of Medicine, Seoul, South Korea; Gyeongsang Natl Univ, Jinju, South Korea; et al)
J Urol 187:1903-1910, 2012

Purpose.—We investigated the molecular identity and functional activity of *STIM1* and *ORAI* in human cavernous smooth muscle. We also determined whether transferring dominant negative mutants of the *STIM1* or *ORAI* gene would correct diabetes related erectile dysfunction in a rat model.

Materials and Methods.—Reverse transcriptase-polymerase chain reaction was done to identify *ORAI* and *STIM* in human cavernous smooth muscle. For the in vivo study intracavernous pressure, blood pressure and their ratio were assessed after cavernous nerve stimulation to diabetic rats transfected with pcDNA encoding the $ORAI1^{DN}$ or the $STIM1^{DN}$ gene.

Results.—ORAI (1, 2 and 3) and STIM (1 and 2) were identified in human cavernous smooth muscle cells. After $[Ca^{2+}]$ depletion by thapsigargin and cyclopiazonic acid we recorded store operated Ca^{2+} entry in human cavernous smooth muscle cells. Entry was decreased by the store operated Ca^{2+} channel blockers La^{3+} and SKF96365. Mean ± SE intracavernous pressure/blood pressure in rats with $ORAI1^{DN}$ or $STIM1^{DN}$ gene transfer was 78.8% ± 2.2% and 77.1% ± 1.2% in 11 and 10, respectively. This result was significantly higher than that in 10 diabetic controls (51.0% ± 3.7%) and similar to that in 9 normal controls (85.8% ± 2.6%). Using reverse transcriptase-polymerase chain reaction we confirmed transgene expression in rat cavernous tissue.

Conclusions.—Transfer of $ORAI^{DN}$ or $STIM1^{DN}$ genes restored erectile function in diabetic rats. It might be applicable to develop new therapy for erectile dysfunction.

▶ Gene therapy for erectile dysfunction was a much anticipated future avenue for development in the mid-2000s. Unfortunately, publications on successful gene therapy applications have been few and far between, and there has been greater interest in recent years in stem cell therapies.

This article examines two molecules (*STIM1* and *ORAI*) that seem to regulate calcium efflux into the cytoplasm from the sarcoplasmic reticulum as a means to ameliorate diabetes-associated penile hemodynamic impairment in rats. These genes are expressed in both human and rat cavernous tissue. Knock down of gene function by transfection of a dominant mutant gene construct for *STIM1* and *ORAI* partially ameliorated impaired penile hemodynamics in rats with streptozotocin-induced diabetes (a model system for type 1 diabetes).

Whether this sort of treatment would be practical or safe in humans is an important question, but as a completely novel target for future therapies (direct regulation of calcium vs preservation of cyclic guanosine monophosphate activity with phosphodiesterase-5 inhibitors), this is a discovery worth noting.

A. W. Shindel, MD

Erectile Dysfunction in Young Surgically Treated Patients With Lumbar Spine Disease: A Prospective Follow-up Study
Siddiqui MA, Peng B, Shanmugam N, et al (Singapore General Hosp)
Spine 37:797-801, 2012

Study Design.—This is a prospective study.

Objective.—The prevalence of erectile dysfunction (ED) in patients younger than 50 years with fracture-unrelated lumbar spine disease requiring surgical decompression without other risk factors for ED is evaluated.

Summary of Background Data.—There is little literature documenting ED in young patients with atraumatic lumbar spine disease.

Methods.—All male patients younger than 50 years who underwent lumbar spine surgery during June 2006 to November 2007 without risk factors for ED were included. Patient demographics, neurological dysfunction, visual analogue scale (VAS) for back and leg pain, Oswestry Disability Index (ODI), North American Spine Society score for neurogenic symptoms (NS), and the International Index of Erectile function (IIEF-5) scores were recorded preoperatively, at 1, 3, and 6 months.

Results.—There were 61 patients with mean age 38.4 years (SD = 7.0; range, 20–49). Most of patients had (43 or 70.5%) prolapsed intervertebral disc with discectomy being the commonest operation. Mean VAS scores, ODI, and NS improved significantly postoperatively. However, the mean IIEF-5 scores did not. Preoperatively, there was no correlation between ED and VAS scores on back pain ($P = 0.70$), leg pain ($P = 0.91$), ODI ($P = 0.93$), or NS ($P = 0.51$). At 6 months, patients with NS > 70 had an increased risk of ED ($P = 0.03$). Eighty percent of patients with NS > 70 had ED compared with 30% of patients with NS ≤ 70. There was, however, no correlation between ED with ODI ($P = 0.38$) and VAS scores on back pain ($P = 0.20$) or leg pain ($P = 0.08$) at 6 months.

Conclusion.—The incidence of ED in patients younger than 50 years with nonfracture-related lumbar spine disease undergoing surgery without risk factors was 34.3%. Despite improvement in VAS, ODI, and NS scores postoperatively, ED did not improve. Patients with NS > 70 postoperatively were more likely to have ED reflecting possible permanent nerve damage from lumbar spine pathology.

▶ This article examines erectile function and pain scores in a cohort of men younger than 50 who underwent spinal surgery. There was no significant change in the International Index of Erectile Function (IIEF-5) scores after surgery, despite improvement in a number of pain metrics and, more interestingly, a significant improvement on a separate metric for "improvement in sexual life." The authors posit that this may be because of "lumbar nerve damage." Lumbar neurons are not clearly linked to sexual function, at least not to the extent of the sacral neurons. This causes one to question their conclusions, but closer analysis reveals more fundamental flaws with this study.

The baseline mean IIEF-5 score was normal at about 22; hence, although 34% met the numeric score for erectile dysfunction (ED), it seems most likely that the vast majority of the ED subjects had mild symptoms and hence substantial further improvements in erectile function were unlikely. The heterogeneous population of subject also complicates interpretation. Finally, in the conclusion the authors state "there is no literature documenting the prevalence of ED in patients as young as 20 years, without other known risk factors for ED, to compare against."

The bottom line is that this study was not well planned nor well executed to detect the difference of interest, and the authors did a poor job of reviewing relevant literature. This is an interesting topic that does merit further investigation and consideration, but I do not believe this study adds much.

A. W. Shindel, MD

Sexual Activity and Cardiovascular Disease: A Scientific Statement From the American Heart Association
Levine GN, on behalf of the American Heart Association Council on Clinical Cardiology, Council on Cardiovascular Nursing, Council on Cardiovascular Surgery and Anesthesia, and Council on Quality of Care and Outcomes Research
Circulation 125:1058-1072, 2012

Background.—The components of quality of life for both men and women with cardiovascular disease (CVD) include sexual activity. This also applies to elderly patients. However, diminished sexual activity and function often occur in patients with CVD and can be related to anxiety and depression. Data relevant to sexual activity and heart disease were synthesized and summarized to develop recommendations and support physician and other healthcare professional communication with heart disease patients concerning sexual activity. Most of the data are drawn from studies of men, which may influence their applicability.

Recommendations.—Patients with CVD who wish to engage in sexual activity should have a complete history and physical examination before beginning such activity. If their symptoms are stable and their functional capacity is good, patients usually have a low risk of adverse cardiovascular events accompanying sexual activity. If symptoms are unstable or severe, treatment should be undertaken to stabilize them before beginning sexual activity. Exercise testing can provide insight into the safety of sexual activity in patients whose risk is indeterminate or unclear.

Usually cardiovascular medications do not cause erectile dysfunction (ED). Concern about the potential impact of medications that can improve the patient's symptoms and survival should not be sufficient cause to withhold such medications. Many patients with stable CVD can safely take phosphodiesterase-5 (PDE5) inhibitors, which can be effective. However, nitrate use is an absolute contraindication to PDE5 inhibitor use.

Patients with CVD who experience anxiety and depression may also develop reduced or impaired sexual activity. One important component of recovery that is seldom used is sexual counseling of CVD patients and their partners.

Conclusions.—Research is needed on sexual activity related to specific cardiovascular conditions, especially in women and older adults. Pharmacotherapy, device and surgical intervention, registries, and longitudinal studies of patients with CVD should include information on sexual activity and function. Interventions to improve sexual activity in patients with CVD, including sexual counseling, are needed.

▶ The availability of effective and easily tolerated therapy for erectile dysfunction has made sexual intercourse possible for many men with vascular comorbidities. The exertional toll of sexual activity does increase the risk of cardiac ischemia in the short term and is an important consideration when considering.

This review and consensus statement summarizes the current data on sexual activity and cardiac risk. The authors conclude that assessment of cardiac risk is an important consideration when considering initiation of therapy to restore sexual capacity. As a basic rule of thumb, exercise tolerance of 3 to 5 METS (approximately the same as walking at a speed of 3 to 4 miles per hour) without symptoms of angina or other indication of cardiopulmonary insufficiency is likely indicative of ability to tolerate the metabolic demands of sexual activity.

Unfortunately, the majority of recommendations contained in this document are based on level C evidence (consensus opinions, case studies, evaluation of limited populations). While this does not take away from their value as guide lines for providers, it is worthwhile to keep these recommendations in mind when counseling patients on management of sexual concerns.

A. W. Shindel, MD

Prostate, Baldness Drugs Linked to Sexual Dysfunction
Kuehn BM
JAMA 307:1903, 2012

Background.—Medications containing the active ingredient finasteride show a possible relationship to sexual dysfunction and infertility. These drugs are used to treat male baldness or an enlarged prostate. The US Food and Drug Administration (FDA) is recommending changes to these drugs' labels to reflect these possible side effects.

Labeling Changes.—The labels of Propecia and Proscar were updated in 2011 to reflect the possibility that users may experience erectile dysfunction even after discontinuing the drug. The newer labeling change adds that several other sexual adverse effects may also occur in association with these agents. Both have been associated with male infertility and poor semen quality, although such symptoms improve after men stop taking these medications. Men who take Proscar may experience reduced libido during and after drug use. Those who take Propecia may suffer libido disorders, ejaculation disorders, and orgasm disorders both during and after using this drug.

Evidence.—No clear causal relationship has been found between the reported adverse effects and use of these agents. The Adverse Events Reporting System of the FDA received 421 reports of sexual dysfunction from patients taking Propecia and 131 reports from patients taking Proscar between 1998 and 2011.

Conclusions.—The FDA urges physicians to discuss the potential risks of both Propecia and Proscar with their patients. It is important to weigh the risks and benefits of each of these treatments.

▶ A chorus of irate patients and a core of very dedicated and passionate providers have reported serious and, in some cases, long-lasting sexual side effects in men treated with 5 α-reductase inhibitors, commonly utilized to treat benign prostatic hyperplasia and, in the case of finasteride, male pattern baldness. The groundswell of opinion has motivated the US Food and Drug Administration to change their labeling, including more explicit warnings about the potential for a variety of adverse andrologic outcomes.

This class has been associated with changes in ejaculate volume, libido, and erectile function nearly since their inception. These new warnings primarily address side effects that are durable after cessation of the drug therapy and now include warnings about long-term degradation of semen quality, which may or may not be reversible.

A clear causal pathway for these syndromes has not been elucidated, although a number of theories have been promulgated.[1] Ergo, these new warning labels should not necessarily prompt massive changes in practice. However, providers and their patients are now beholden to more stringent standards of discussion on the potential risks of these drugs. As finasteride is often used by young men without other conditions that may predispose to erectile dysfunction, the potential for serious and long-lasting side effects is a serious one that merits mention.

A. W. Shindel, MD

Reference

1. Traish AM, Hassani J, Guay AT, Zitzmann M, Hansen ML. Adverse side effects of 5α-reductase inhibitors therapy: persistent diminished libido and erectile dysfunction and depression in a subset of patients. *J Sex Med.* 2011;8:872-884.

10 STD

Evidence of Human Papillomavirus Vaccine Effectiveness in Reducing Genital Warts: An Analysis of California Public Family Planning Administrative Claims Data, 2007–2010
Bauer HM, Wright G, Chow J (Ctr for Infectious Diseases, Richmond, CA)
Am J Public Health 102:833-835, 2012

Because of the rapid development of genital warts (GW) after infection, monitoring GW trends may provide early evidence of population-level human papillomavirus (HPV) vaccine effectiveness. Trends in GW diagnoses were assessed using public family planning administrative data. Between 2007 and 2010, among females younger than 21 years, these diagnoses decreased 35% from 0.94% to 0.61% ($P_{\text{trend}} < .001$). Decreases were also observed among males younger than 21 years (19%); and among females and males ages 21-25 (10% and 11%, respectively). The diagnoses stabilized or increased among older age groups. HPV vaccine may be preventing GW among young people.

▶ Quadrivalent human papilloma virus (HPV) vaccine is now approved (2006) for use in men and women for the prevention of genital warts. As of 2010, nearly 50% of women had received at least 1 of the scheduled 3 vaccination doses. Because genital warts develop rapidly after infection, monitoring of genital wart incidence is a pretty good surrogate for the effectiveness of the new vaccine. The data show a clear decline in the incidence of warts in younger women. It is possible that the decreases could be spurious and related to the accuracy of the ICD-9 coding. In the long term, the more important analysis is evaluation of reduction of HPV-related cancers.

D. E. Coplen, MD

11 Urinary Reconstruction

Annual Endoscopy and Urine Cytology for the Surveillance of Bladder Tumors After Enterocystoplasty for Congenital Bladder Anomalies
Higuchi TT, Fox JA, Husmann DA (Mayo Clinic, Rochester, MN)
J Urol 186:1791-1795, 2011

Purpose.—It is currently recommended that patients with congenital bladder anomalies managed by enterocystoplasty undergo annual surveillance with urine cytology and endoscopy. We reviewed our experience with this protocol and suggest modifications based on this experience.

Materials and Methods.—A total of 65 patients 10 years or more after enterocystoplasty were placed on an annual surveillance protocol consisting of interval medical history, renal-bladder ultrasound, serum B12, electrolytes, creatinine, urinalysis, urine cytology and endoscopy.

Results.—Of the 65 patients 50 (77%) with enterocystoplasty (ileal in 40 and colonic in 10) remain on the protocol. Median age at the initiation of surveillance was 28 years (range 24 to 40) with a median time from augmentation of 15 years (range 12 to 29). During the first 5 years of surveillance 26 of 250 cytology results (10.5%) were suspicious for cancer. Further evaluation revealed no evidence of malignancy. Specificity for cytology was 90% with unknown sensitivity. Of 250 surveillance endoscopic evaluations 4 lesions (1.6%) were identified and biopsied/removed. Pathological evaluation revealed 1 adenomatous polyp, 1 squamous metaplasia and 2 nephrogenic adenomas. Due to the low event rate and high cost routine cytology and endoscopy were discontinued after each patient completed 5 years of followup and annual evaluations were maintained. No tumors developed during the median surveillance interval of 15 years (range 12 to 20). Currently median patient age is 42 years (range 36 to 59) and median time since augmentation is 27 years (range 23 to 40).

Conclusions.—Due to the low incidence of malignancy, lack of proven benefit and enhanced cost containment we recommend that annual surveillance endoscopy and cytology be discontinued.

▶ Substitution of intestine into the urinary tract (bladder augmentation, continent neobladder, etc) may be an independent risk factor for the development of cancer. Over the past 10 years, there have been reports of gastric tumors (after gastrocystoplasty), gastrointestinal tumors (colocystoplasty), and transitional cell carcinoma after intestinal bladder augmentation. The tumors have been reported at younger ages, implying some relationship to chronic inflammation from bacterial colonization, abnormal cell signaling between intestinal and bladder epithelium, and repeated trauma from catheterization. The incidence of malignancy is estimated to be between 1.5% to 2% per decade.

The most appropriate screening in children and young adults after enterocystoplasty is unknown. The authors' prospective series evaluates the utility of ultrasound, urinary cytology, and endoscopy in 50 patients with a history of enterocystoplasty for neurogenic bladder (36), exstrophy (9), and posterior urethral valves (5). The sensitivity of urinary cytology for malignancy in this population cannot be determined because there were no cancers in the study population (even though 10% of cytologies were suspicious for malignancy). Cystoscopy revealed abnormalities in a very small number of patients. Although annual follow-up of these patients is required to prevent upper tract deterioration and identify metabolic derangements, there is little evidence to support annual endoscopy. The authors changed their evaluation and screening criteria to those shown in the Table. This seems a reasonable approach, and, although more cost-effective, there is no evidence that either approach is better with regard to early detection of malignancy in this patient population.

D. E. Coplen, MD

Ureteral Substitution With Reconfigured Colon: Long-Term Followup
Lazica DA, Ubrig B, Brandt AS, et al (Univ of Witten/Herdecke, Wuppertal, Germany)
J Urol 187:542-548, 2012

Purpose.—Long defects in the mid and upper ureter are not amenable to end-to-end reconstruction. Therefore, we present the long-term results of our technique with reconfigured colon segments.

Materials and Methods.—Between June 1998 and July 2008, 14 patients underwent ureteral replacement at our institution with reconfigured colon. In 4 patients the substitute was anastomosed to the skin as a modified colon conduit. In 10 patients it was interposed with anastomosis to the ureter in 4, to the bladder in 5 and to the afferent loop of an ileal bladder substitute in 1.

Results.—At a median followup of 52.4 months (range 7 to 136) excellent renal function was confirmed in 10 of 14 patients. Now at a median followup of 95.8 months (range 38 to 136) 6 patients are alive, all without an indwelling stent and with no sign of obstruction of the ureteral replacement. Metabolic disorders, mucus obstruction and stricture or adhesive ileus were absent during followup. In this series death was unrelated to the procedure. In 7 patients 11 specific reinterventions were necessary including 4 cases of prolonged stenting after surgery, 3 which required secondary drainage, 3 cases of urinary tract infection at 4 weeks and 3 and 112 months, and 1 acute bowel obstruction due to peritoneal carcinosis.

Conclusions.—Reconfigured colon segments can be used successfully to replace long ureteral defects. The advantages are use in patients with impaired renal function and lack of small intestine, proximity of the colon to the ureter, optimal cross-sectional diameter of the graft and less intraperitoneal surgical trauma than with ileal substitutes.

▶ The authors interpose a narrowed segment of the large intestine in patients with long ureteral defects. Although the authors did not calibrate the size of the reconfigured channel, a 3- to 4-cm segment would be about 30 French. The postoperative imaging shows that there is nonuniform dilation of the segments. Mercaptoacetyltriglycine-3 scintigraphy showed improved transit and no evidence of obstruction in the studied patients. It is unclear if the reconfigured segment transports urine more efficiently than a nontapered ileum or colon. Obstructive complications were related to recurrent malignancy. Colonic mucus did not seem to be a problem. The reconfiguration increases the complexity of reconstruction, and although the authors show efficacy, they do not show that this approach is better than an ileal ureter.

D. E. Coplen, MD

Long-term Renal Function After Urinary Diversion by Ileal Conduit or Orthotopic Ileal Bladder Substitution

Jin X-D, Roethlisberger S, Burkhard FC, et al (Univ of Bern, Switzerland)
Eur Urol 61:491-497, 2012

Background.—Data on long-term renal function are scarce for ileal conduit diversion (ICD) and even rarer for orthotopic ileal bladder substitution (BS).

Objective.—Explore the changes in renal function of patients who lived ≥10 yr with an ICD or BS and determine the risk factors contributing to renal function deterioration.

Design, Setting, and Participants.—Fifty consecutive ICD patients and 111 consecutive BS patients who lived ≥10 yr after undergoing surgery between January 1985 and December 2000 were retrospectively analyzed.

Measurements.—The glomerular filtration rate (GFR) was calculated with the Modification of Diet in Renal Disease (MDRD) equation before and 10 yr after surgery. *Decreased renal function* was defined as a decrease in GFR > 10 ml/min per 1.73 m^2 in 10 yr.

Results and Limitations.—Median GFR values in patients with ICD or BS decreased from 65.5 (range: 23—90) to 57 (range: 7—100) ml/min per 1.73 m^2 and from 68 (range: 33—106) to 66 (range: 16—100) ml/min per 1.73 m^2, respectively. Eighteen ICD patients (36%) and 23 BS patients (21%) had deteriorating renal function. Seven of 12 ICD patients with obstruction (ureteroileal stricture, stomal stenosis/parastomal hernia) (58%) had renal function deterioration, as did 17 of 46 BS patients with obstruction (ureteroileal/nipple stricture and/or bladder outlet obstruction) (37%). Logistic regression analysis confirmed that obstruction was the leading, and an independent, risk factor for renal function deterioration for both ICD patients $(p = 0.045)$ and BS patients $(p = 0.002)$. Patients with diabetes or hypertension were significantly more likely to have deterioration of renal function if they had ICD $(p = 0.002$ and $p = 0.05$, respectively). The limitation of the study is its retrospective nature and its composition that included many patients who did not survive 10 yr.

Conclusions.—Urinary tract obstruction was the leading cause of long-term renal function impairment, regardless of whether the patient had ICD or BS. ICD patients with predisposing risk factors, such as diabetes or hypertension, were at increased risk for impaired renal function.

▶ The authors in this article compare renal function (calculated glomerular filtration rate) 10 years after ileal conduit diversion (ICD) or neobladder construction (bladder substitution) performed after cystectomy for bladder cancer. The causes of renal dysfunction are multifactorial. Two-thirds of the patient population had died prior to 10-year follow-up. Approximately half of these deaths were related to malignancy, but 4% of the deaths were directly related to the diversion. The cause of death was not available in 25% of patients, so it is conceivable that complications of urinary diversion alone were greater than noted. As would be anticipated, obstruction at the ureteroileal anastomosis was most highly associated with deterioration of renal function. Close follow-up and prompt relief of obstruction (typically surgical revision) is necessary. ICD stomal obstruction and bladder outlet obstruction in the neobladder were also issues, but these are not necessarily surgical issues. Attention to conduit and bladder drainage (voiding vs clean intermittent catheterization) is imperative after diversion. Chronic bacteriuria was associated with renal function deterioration. In the absence of fevers, hydronephrosis, or obstruction, this is somewhat surprising, and I would not recommend routine use of prophylactic antibiotics in these patients.

D. E. Coplen, MD

12 Laparoscopy

Analysis of Robotic-assisted Laparoscopic Pyeloplasty for Primary Versus Secondary Repair in 119 Consecutive Cases
Niver BE, Agalliu I, Bareket R, et al (New York Univ School of Medicine; Albert Einstein College of Medicine, Bronx, NY; Wake Forest Univ School of Medicine, Winston-Salem, NC)
Urology 79:689-694, 2012

Objective.—To analyze the outcomes of our robotic-assisted pyeloplasty series for primary ureteropelvic junction obstruction (UPJO) and compare them with our series of robotic-assisted pyeloplasty for secondary UPJO. The repair of secondary UPJO can pose additional challenges to surgeons. Robotic assistance could aid in these repairs.

Methods.—Using an institutional review board-approved database, we reviewed 119 consecutive patients who had undergone robotic-assisted laparoscopic pyeloplasty at our institution during an 8-year period (May 2002 to February 2010). Data were collected in a combined retrospective and prospective manner. The patients were stratified into primary repair and secondary repair for the primary analysis. The patients were also stratified into those with stones and those without stones for the secondary analysis. We compared the demographic, operative, postoperative, and radiographic outcomes. Student's *t* test and Pearson's chi-square correlation were used for statistical analysis of continuous and categorical variables, respectively.

Results.—Of the original 119 patients, data were available for 117. Of the 117 patients, 97 had undergone primary pyeloplasty repair and 20 had undergone secondary pyeloplasty repair. Radiographic data were available for 84 patients with primary repair and 17 patients with secondary repair. The radiographic success rate was 96.1% and 94.1%, respectively. No statistically significant differences were found in the patient demographics, operative data, or postoperative or radiographic outcomes for the primary analysis. Additionally, no differences were found in the outcomes for patients with concomitant stone disease.

Conclusion.—These data represent the largest single-center report of its kind. These data strongly suggest that robotic-assisted laparoscopic pyeloplasty is a safe and durable option for secondary UPJO repair.

▶ The authors report on 20 robotic pyeloplasties performed after prior surgery for ureteropelvic junction obstruction (UPJO). All of the patients had a prior endopyelotomy, and only 5 had a prior pyeloplasty (unsure if the endopyelotomy was performed before or after the pyeloplasty). Eighty percent of the patients had a crossing vessel (known crossing vessel is a contraindication to endopyelotomy) identified at the time of secondary surgery. The authors do not report on the magnitude of scarring in the secondary group, but because the operating time was the same in both groups, the prior surgery did not seem to affect the surgery or outcomes (follow-up is only 23 months, but failure after pyeloplasty typically occurs early). On that basis, it is not clear if robotic assistance was needed to facilitate the reoperative repair or if a pure laparoscopic approach would have achieved the same results. Endopyelotomy has only 60% success when used primarily. However, it successfully relieves obstruction in more than 95% of cases when performed after prior dismembered pyeloplasty. This improved success is related to elimination of the crossing vessel and reconstruction of a dependent, funneled ureteral position at the time of pyeloplasty. Even though the authors report excellent results with a secondary robotic pyeloplasty, endopyelotomy should strongly be considered as a minimally invasive alternative.

D. E. Coplen, MD

13 Neurogenic Bladder/ Urinary Diversion

Long-Term Urological Impact of Fetal Myelomeningocele Closure
Clayton DB, Tanaka ST, Trusler L, et al (Vanderbilt Univ, Nashville, TN)
J Urol 186:1581-1585, 2011

Purpose.—Between 1997 and 2002 a large number of fetal myelomeningocele closures were performed at our institution. Previously early reports showed little improvement in neonatal bladder function after fetal back closure. We evaluated the long-term urological impact of this procedure.

Materials and Methods.—Using a combination of retrospective review and survey questionnaire we reviewed the records of 28 patients in whom fetal myelomeningocele closure was done at our institution between 1997 and 2002. The areas addressed included medical management for neurogenic bladder and bowel, need for lower urinary tract reconstruction and functional bladder assessment by videourodynamics. Parameters after fetal myelomeningocele closure were compared to those of 33 age and sex matched patients with myelomeningocele who underwent standard postnatal closure.

Results.—We reviewed the records of 28 patients after fetal myelomeningocele closure. At a mean age of 9.6 years 23 used clean intermittent catheterization to manage the bladder, 24 required a bowel regimen to manage constipation and 6 underwent lower urinary tract reconstruction with enterocystoplasty and a catheterizable bladder channel. Videourodynamics performed in 14 patients at a mean age of 7.4 years revealed decreased bladder capacity in 71%, detrusor overactivity in 35% and increased detrusor pressure in 25%. Compared to age and sex matched children who underwent postnatal closure we noted no significant differences in bladder management, urinary tract surgery or urodynamics.

Conclusions.—Neurogenic bowel and bladder management continues to be a significant issue for patients after fetal myelomeningocele closure. After fetal surgery patients should be followed closely, similar to patients who undergo postnatal closure.

▶ The Management of Myelomeningocele Study (MOMS trial) is a National Institutes of Health—funded randomized trial evaluating the effect of prenatal closure on hydrocephalus and the need for VP shunt placement. The authors report urologic outcomes on a select group of children undergoing in utero closure prior to the onset of MOMS trial enrollment. During a 5-year period, 177 closures were performed at Vanderbilt, but urologic follow-up is available in only 28 of the children. Eighty-three percent of children required clean intermittent catheterization and some form of bowel regimen (retrograde or antegrade enema). The authors do not delineate their indications for intervention, but only 4 children had urinary continence without clean intermittent catheterization or anticholinergics. The figure shows bowel and bladder management is no different in 33 age-matched children undergoing postnatal closure during the same time period at Vanderbilt. This report is a highly select subset. It is possible that highly functioning patients did not adhere to follow-up recommendations. Fetal closure does not eliminate the need for medical and surgical management of neurogenic bladder.

D. E. Coplen, MD

Phase IIb/III Dose Ranging Study of Tamsulosin as Treatment for Children With Neuropathic Bladder
Homsy Y, Arnold P, Zhang W (Univ of South Florida, Tampa, FL; Boehringer Ingelheim Pharmaceuticals, Inc, Ridgefield, CT)
J Urol 186:2033-2039, 2011

Purpose.—We evaluated the efficacy and safety of tamsulosin hydrochloride in children with increased detrusor leak point pressure associated with neuropathic bladder.

Materials and Methods.—In a double-blind, randomized, placebo controlled trial patients with detrusor leak point pressure 40 cm H_2O or greater were stratified by age (2 to less than 5 years, 5 to less than 10 years, 10 to 16 years) and concomitant anticholinergic use, and were randomized to receive various doses of tamsulosin or placebo. A 2-week titration was followed by a 12-week maintenance treatment period. Primary end point was response, ie detrusor leak point pressure less than 40 cm H_2O from 2 evaluations on the same day at week 14. Secondary end points included detrusor leak point pressure change from baseline, hydronephrosis and hydroureter responses, change in catheterization volumes and adverse events.

Results.—A total of 161 patients received 1 or more treatment doses between January 2008 and February 2009, and 135 were evaluable for the primary end point. A total of 51 patients (37.8%) were detrusor leak point pressure responders, with no statistically significant difference in response rates between each tamsulosin dose and placebo. Adjusting for stratification variables, mean detrusor leak point pressure changes from baseline to week 14 for placebo and low, medium and high dose groups were −11.4, −17.6, −4.6 and −14.3 cm H_2O, respectively. In 141 evaluable patients hydroureter/hydronephrosis improvement rates were 7.1% and 5.7% in left and right kidneys (hydroureter), respectively, and 14.9% and 14.2% in left and right kidneys (hydronephrosis), respectively. No group experienced decreases in median post-void residual volume at week 14. Drug related adverse event incidences were 4.9% (placebo) and 5.8% (tamsulosin).

Conclusions.—Tamsulosin was well tolerated but not efficacious in this pediatric population with neuropathic bladder.

▶ A leak point pressure greater than 40 cm H_2O increases the chance of pressure-related renal injury in children with neurogenic bladder. Standard management includes anticholinergics to decrease storage pressures (and increase bladder capacity) and intermittent catheterization prior to bladder pressure reaching 40 cm H_2O. When a child has a small capacity, high-pressure bladder, the required frequency of clean intermittent catheterization may not be feasible. Other options include urethral dilation, external sphincteric injection of botulinum toxin, and pharmacologic manipulation of external sphincteric tone as secondary management choices. In females, aggressive dilation of the external sphincter has been found to decrease outlet resistance and increase functional bladder capacity. The potential for urethral trauma precludes the use of dilation in males. Botulinum toxin has efficacy but use is currently off-label in the United States. Alpha-antagonists reduce bladder outlet resistance, improve urine flow, and decrease PVR in males with BPH. The authors evaluate tamsulosin in a heterogeneous population. Response was defined as a decrease in detrusor leak point pressure (DLPP) to less than 40 cm H_2O. The magnitude of decrease in DLPP was not considered. In some patients, the pressure that places the upper tracts at risk may be greater than 40 cm H_2O. Consequently, this study may underestimate a clinically significant response.

D. E. Coplen, MD

Ventriculoperitoneal Shunt Infections After Bladder Surgery: is Mechanical Bowel Preparation Necessary?
Casperson KJ, Fronczak CM, Siparsky G, et al (Univ of Colorado School of Medicine, Aurora; Univ of Chicago Med Ctr, IL)
J Urol 186:1571-1575, 2011

Purpose.—We investigated whether children with a ventriculoperitoneal shunt who undergo mechanical bowel preparation before bladder reconstruction with bowel have a lower rate of infection than children who do not undergo preoperative bowel preparation.

Materials and Methods.—We performed an institutional review board approved, retrospective chart review of the incidence of ventriculoperitoneal shunt infections after bladder reconstruction using bowel and compared infection rates using Fisher's exact test. Mean ± SD followup was 2.9 ± 2.3 years.

Results.—Between 2003 and 2009, 31 patients with a ventriculoperitoneal shunt underwent bladder reconstruction using bowel, of whom 19 (61%) and 12 (39%) did and did not undergo mechanical bowel preparation, respectively. There was no significant difference in gender or age at surgery between the 2 groups. Infection developed in 3 children (9.6%)

within 2 months postoperatively, including 2 (10.5%) with and 1 (8.3%) without bowel preparation (2-tailed $p = 1.0$).

Conclusions.—There was no significant difference in the shunt infection rate between patients with a ventriculoperitoneal shunt who did and did not undergo preoperative bowel preparation. Our results add to the current literature suggesting that bowel preparation is unnecessary even in patients with a ventriculoperitoneal shunt.

▶ Prior studies have found no definite benefit of mechanical bowel preparation with regard to wound infection, postoperative ileus, and length of hospital stay. There is no evidence that a bowel preparation necessarily causes harm. This is a nonrandomized evaluation of mechanical bowel preparation prior to urinary tract reconstruction. The incidence of shunt infections was not different between the 2 groups, but the patient numbers are very small. Only half of the patients had a bowel resection (only 2 of these were colonic). Several also had manipulation of the appendix (appendicocecostomy and appendicovesicostomy). The appendix and colon were manipulated in a smaller number of children who did not have a bowel preparation. This may be a selection bias. Given that the urinary tract was violated in all patients, it is surprising that urine cultures were not obtained preoperatively in any case. Once the bladder is open, infected urine can percolate in the abdominal cavity and lead to a shunt infection. I do find that the chance of gross fecal contamination is small in this population. Given the magnitude of the constipation in these patients, an adequate cleanout is difficult, and I have often thought that a marginal effort at cleanout is no better or worse than no cleanout.

D. E. Coplen, MD

Complications After Use of Gastric Segments for Lower Urinary Tract Reconstruction
Castellan M, Gosalbez R, Bar-Yosef Y, et al (Univ of Miami, FL)
J Urol 187:1823-1827, 2012

Purpose.—We retrospectively reviewed our experience with the use of gastric segments for lower urinary tract reconstruction with an emphasis on long-term complications.

Materials and Methods.—A total of 29 patients underwent reconstruction of the lower urinary tract using gastric segments between 1993 and 2000. Diagnoses included neurogenic bladder (21), cloacal exstrophy (5), solitary kidney/ectopic ureter (1), posterior urethral valves (1) and rhabdomyosarcoma of prostate (1). Gastric segment was used as gastrocystoplasty (21), composite gastroenteric cystoplasty (6), demucosalized gastrocystoplasty (1) and continent gastric reservoir (1).

Results.—Mean followup was 13.9 years (range 9 to 16.5). Complications were seen in 15 (51.7%) patients. Seven patients had the hematuria-dysuria syndrome, which was intractable in 1 and necessitated excision of the gastric patch. Due to severe complications necessitating major reoperations 3 patients underwent re-augmentation with enteric segments without excision of the gastric tissue (composite). One patient who underwent demucosalized gastrocystoplasty had excision of the gastric tissue and re-augmentation with enteric segment due to contraction of the gastric patch. A stone developed in 1 patient with a composite gastroenteric reservoir. Malignancy developed in the reservoir in 3 patients 11, 12 and 14 years after gastrocystoplasty, and all 3 died of metastasis.

Conclusions.—We do not recommend the use of gastric segments for reconstruction of the lower urinary tract due to the high incidence of reoperations and complications. In patients in whom gastric segments were used in the past for lower urinary tract reconstruction, regular surveillance and close followup are strongly advocated.

▶ The use of gastric segments in urinary tract reconstruction was popularized in the 1990s. Initially, this was primarily used in children with acidosis, renal insufficiency, or short gut physiology. Because the stomach does not produce mucus and the acid secretion decreases the incidence of bacteriuria, the indications were expanded to all children with neurogenic bladder. The stomach has thicker muscle than the small and large intestines, and implantation of continent catheterizable channels is more successful. In sensate bladders, the acidosis causes significant pain. The low urinary pH is associated with hematuria in up to 50% of patients. These symptoms may not respond to H2 blockers. If continence is not perfect, the acidic urine can cause significant skin irritation or breakdown. Unfortunately, this study also reports on 3 patients with metastatic gastric adenocarcinoma 10 or more years after reconstruction. Gastric segments should be a last option in urinary tract reconstruction.

D. E. Coplen, MD

Cost-effectiveness analysis of sacral neuromodulation and botulinum toxin A treatment for patients with idiopathic overactive bladder

Leong RK, de Wachter SGG, Joore MA, et al (Maastricht Univ Med Ctr, the Netherlands)
BJU Int 108:558-564, 2011

Objective.—To assess and compare the costs and effects value of either starting with sacral neuromodulation (SNM) or botulinum toxin A (BTX) treatment in patients with refractory idiopathic overactive bladder from a societal perspective.

Materials and Methods.—An economic model comparing SNM with BTX was developed. A clinical relevant effect (i.e. success) was defined as 50% or greater reduction in incontinence episodes or urgency frequency symptoms. Information on the clinical effectiveness of the two treatments and on the course of the disease with the two treatments were based primarily on published literature and, when required, on expert opinion. Both treatments were assumed to be performed under general anaesthesia and, for SNM treatment, first-stage tined lead test was used. All costs were based on national data from the year 2008. Analyses from the societal perspective were conducted for a 5-year duration. Costs were discounted at 4% and effects at 1.5%. In addition, different modelling scenarios were used to see determine any changes in the results obtained.

Results.—Starting with SNM resulted in a higher quality adjusted life year (QALY) gain (difference of 0.23) and a higher cost (difference of € 6428) compared to starting with BTX. The corresponding incremental cost-effectiveness ratio was € 27 991/QALY. The probability of this ratio being cost effective (e.g. under € 40 000/QALY) is 88%. SNM starts to be cost-effective after 4 years. SNM was not cost-effective in some other scenarios, such as when BTX was conducted under local anaesthesia or when peripheral nerve evaluation or bilateral testing was used for SNM.

Conclusions.—Starting with SNM, treatment is cost-effective after 5 years compared to BTX. However, in some scenarios, such as the use of local anaesthesia for BTX treatment and SNM peripheral nerve evaluation or bilateral test, SNM was not cost-effective.

▶ Several studies have looked at the relative cost-effectiveness of these 2 treatments for idiopathic overactive bladder. Most of these studies, including this one, are limited by the lack of long-term data for the use of Botox in idiopathic overactive bladder. Although the results of this analysis suggest that botulinum toxin A injection is initially cost-effective, after a period of 4 to 5 years, sacral neuromodulation becomes more cost-effective. However, there are several significant limitations of this article including, most important, cost assumptions that can vary considerably on a national basis. This study was done in the Netherlands, and thus the cost assumptions would be very different in the United States, which would no doubt affect the conclusions. Furthermore, it was assumed in this study that botulinum toxin A was injected under general anesthesia, which is not standard of care in the United States. If the botulinum toxin injection was assumed to be done under local anesthesia or the sacral neuromodulation procedure was done using a peripheral nerve evaluation (instead of a staged approach), then the conclusions in this study might be considerably different. It is important to note that botulinum toxin A is not approved for treatment of idiopathic overactive bladder in the United States, although it is approved for neurogenic detrusor overactivity.

E. S. Rovner, MD

Efficacy of Botulinum Toxin A Injection for Neurogenic Detrusor Overactivity and Urinary Incontinence: A Randomized, Double-Blind Trial
Herschorn S, Gajewski J, Ethans K, et al (Univ of Toronto, Ontario, Canada; Dalhousie Univ, Halifax, Nova Scotia, Canada; Univ of Manitoba, Winnipeg, Canada; et al)
J Urol 185:2229-2235, 2011

Purpose.—We determined the efficacy of onabotulinumtoxinA for neurogenic detrusor overactivity secondary to spinal cord injury or multiple sclerosis.

Materials and Methods.—In a prospective, double-blind, multicenter study 57 patients 18 to 75 years old with neurogenic detrusor overactivity secondary to spinal cord injury or multiple sclerosis and urinary incontinence (defined as 1 or more occurrences daily) despite current antimuscarinic treatment were randomized to onabotulinumtoxinA 300 U (28) or placebo (29) via cystoscopic injection at 30 intradetrusor sites, sparing the trigone. Patients were offered open label onabotulinumtoxinA 300 U at week 36 and followed a further 6 months while 24 each in the treatment and placebo groups received open label therapy. The primary efficacy parameter was daily urinary incontinence frequency on 3-day voiding diary at week 6. Secondary parameters were changes in the International Consultation on Incontinence Questionnaire and the urinary incontinence quality of life scale at week 6. Diary and quality of life evaluations were also done after open label treatment.

Results.—The mean daily frequency of urinary incontinence episodes was significantly lower for onabotulinumtoxinA than for placebo at week 6 (1.31 vs 4.76, $p < 0.0001$), and for weeks 24 and 36. Improved urodynamic and quality of life parameters for treatment vs placebo were evident at week 6 and persisted to weeks 24 to 36. The most common adverse event in each group was urinary tract infection.

Conclusions.—In adults with antimuscarinic refractory neurogenic detrusor overactivity and multiple sclerosis onabotulinumtoxinA is well tolerated and provides clinically beneficial improvement for up to 9 months.

▶ This small but well-done Canadian trial demonstrated that botulinum toxin A is effective and safe for the treatment of neurogenic detrusor overactivity. This study supports the increasing body of evidence for this therapy in patients with neurogenic detrusor overactivity—related urinary incontinence. The intradetrusor injection of botulinum toxin at a dose of 200 units is approved in the United States for neurogenic detrusor overactivity. This study used a higher dose of 300 units. Urinary retention requiring intermittent catheterization, which, in this neurogenic patient population might be considered by some to be a desirable outcome, occurred in 5 of the 9 patients in the botulinum toxin-A group and only 2 of the 9 in the placebo group. Quite remarkable in this study is the strikingly low placebo response with respect to both voiding diary parameters and urodynamic parameters. The broad difference between efficacy in the active arm versus the placebo arm of this trial suggests an excellent therapeutic effect in the treatment of refractory neurogenic detrusor overactivity—associated urinary incontinence.

E. S. Rovner, MD

Functional Outcomes After Management of End-stage Neurological Bladder Dysfunction With Ileal Conduit in a Multiple Sclerosis Population: A Monocentric Experience

Legrand G, Rouprêt M, Comperat E, et al (Univ Paris VI, France; Université de Versailles St Quentin en Yvelines, Paris, France)
Urology 78:937-941, 2011

Objective.—To assess the outcome of cutaneous noncontinent urinary diversion (CNCUD) for neurogenic bladder management in multiple sclerosis (MS) patients.

Methods.—We retrospectively reviewed the charts of our MS patients who underwent surgery for CNCUD between 1994 and 2009. To assess the impact of urinary problems on health-related quality of life (HRQOL), a Qualiveen questionnaire was completed by the patients (scale $0 =$ no impact of urinary problems and $4 =$ high adverse impact).

Results.—Overall, 53 patients with a median age of 51 years were included in the study. The mean Expanded Disability Status Scale score before surgery was 7.48 ± 1.02 (range 6.5-9). The mean duration of follow-up was 73 months (range 6-168). The complication rate was 55%. Minor postoperative complications (Clavien grades I-II) occurred in 23 cases, and major complications (Clavien grades III-IV) occurred in 6 cases. The mean creatinine levels before surgery and at the last follow-up were 0.63 ± 0.2 mg/dL and 0.73 ± 0.53 mg/dL, respectively. The mean overall HRQOL scores before surgery and at last follow-up, and which assess the impact of the urinary problems on the patient, were 2.1 ± 1.18 and 1.16 ± 0.63 ($P =.02$), respectively.

Conclusion.—Cystectomy and CNCUD are indicated in MS-impaired patients who are refractory to medical treatment and they can result in disappearance of neurological bladder symptoms. CNCUD appears to be the procedure of choice to improve the quality of life of selected patients, despite the fact that it is associated with high perioperative morbidity.

▶ Neurogenic voiding dysfunction secondary to multiple sclerosis is a widespread and challenging clinical condition for both the patient and the physician. Although the vast majority of these individuals will not require urinary diversion, a small number eventually will. This case series represents an honest appraisal of outcomes with urinary diversion in a debilitated, end-stage population of individuals with neuropathic bladder dysfunction secondary to multiple sclerosis. Clearly, urinary diversion in this patient population is not a simple or benign undertaking. Complication rates are high. Options are limited in this patient population and the "take home" point of this article suggests that such reconstructive surgery should be reserved only for those who absolutely need it.

E. S. Rovner, MD

Efficacy and Safety of OnabotulinumtoxinA in Patients with Urinary Incontinence Due to Neurogenic Detrusor Overactivity: A Randomised, Double Blind, Placebo-Controlled Trial

Cruz F, Herschorn S, Aliotta P, et al (Hospital São João & Universidade Do Porto, Portugal; Univ of Toronto, Canada; Ctr for Urologic Res of Western New York, Williamsville; et al)
Eur Urol 60:742-750, 2011

Background.—Neurogenic detrusor overactivity (NDO) frequently results in urinary incontinence (UI) which impairs quality of life (QOL) and puts the upper urinary tract at risk.

Objective.—To assess the effects of onabotulinumtoxinA (BOTOX®, Allergan, Inc.) on UI, urodynamic variables, and QOL in incontinent patients with NDO.

Design, Setting, and Participants.—This multicentre, randomised, double-blind, placebo-controlled study enrolled patients with multiple sclerosis (MS; $n = 154$) or spinal cord injury (SCI; $n = 121$) with UI due to NDO (≥ 14 UI episodes per week).

Intervention.—Patients received 30 intradetrusor injections of onabotulinumtoxinA 200 U ($n = 92$), 300 U ($n = 91$), or placebo ($n = 92$), avoiding the trigone.

Measurements.—Primary end point was change from baseline in UI episodes per week (week 6). Secondary end points included urodynamics (maximum cystometric capacity [MCC], maximum detrusor pressure during first involuntary detrusor contraction [$P_{detmaxIDC}$]), and Incontinence Quality of Life (I-QOL) total score. Adverse events (AEs) were assessed.

Results and Limitations.—At baseline, mean UI episodes per week (33.5) were similar across groups. At week 6, onabotulinumtoxinA 200 U and 300 U significantly reduced UI episodes per week (-21.8 and -19.4, respectively) compared with placebo (-13.2; $p < 0.01$); onabotulinumtoxinA benefit was observed by the first posttreatment study visit at week 2. Improvements in MCC, $P_{detmaxIDC}$, and I-QOL at week 6 were significantly greater with both onabotulinumtoxinA doses than with placebo ($p < 0.001$). Benefits were observed in both the MS and SCI populations. The median time to patient request for retreatment was the same for both onabotulinumtoxinA doses (42.1 wk) and greater than placebo (13.1 wk; $p < 0.001$). Most frequent AEs were localised urologic events (urinary tract infections and urinary retention, which were dose related in patients not using clean intermittent catheterisation [CIC] at baseline). Significant increases in postvoid residual were observed in patients not using CIC prior to treatment, and 12%, 30%, and 42% of patients in the placebo, 200-U, and 300-U groups, respectively, initiated CIC posttreatment.

Conclusions.—OnabotulinumtoxinA significantly reduced UI and improved urodynamics and QOL in MS and SCI patients with NDO. Both doses were well tolerated with no clinically relevant differences in efficacy or duration of effect between the two doses (http://www.clinicaltrials.gov; NCT00461292).

▶ This represents 1 of the 2 pivotal studies submitted to the FDA for approval of onabotulinumtoxinA in the United States for treatment of neurogenic detrusor overactivity. This study included only patients with urodynamically demonstrable detrusor overactivity and with relevant neurological lesions, and it included only patients who were reasonably highly functioning individuals with multiple sclerosis or spinal cord injury. Whether these results are applicable to other types of neurogenic detrusor overactivity—related incontinence, such as that resulting from Parkinson disease, lumbosacral disk disease, or stroke, is unclear. At both doses (200 units and 300 units), the drug was clearly superior to placebo, but the higher dose was associated with an increased risk for requiring intermittent catheterization without corresponding improvement in efficacy, suggesting that the therapeutic index for the 200-unit dose is superior to that of the 300-unit dose. The improvements in urodynamic parameters were striking at both doses, and there was essentially no response in those in the placebo group. These data are strongly supportive of onabotulinumtoxinA as a treatment for individuals with urinary incontinence due to neurogenic detrusor overactivity who are unresponsive to antimuscarinics.

E. S. Rovner, MD

14 Neurogenic Reconstruction

Extravesical Implantation of a Continent Catheterizable Channel
VanderBrink BA, Kaefer M, Cain MP, et al (Nationwide Children's Hosp, Columbus, OH)
J Urol 185:2572-2575, 2011

Purpose.—Extravesical ureteral reimplantation provides results equivalent to those of the open technique with the advantage of less postoperative morbidity from a large cystotomy. Surgical series describing the technique and efficacy of extravesical implantation of continent catheterizable channel are lacking. We reviewed our results to determine the efficacy of this technique with an emphasis on continence and the need for revision.

Materials and Methods.—We reviewed the records of 394 patients who underwent a bladder continent catheterizable channel procedure from 1999 to 2009. Operative records describing an extravesical technique were noted. Briefly, a 3 to 6 cm incision is made in the detrusor and seromuscular flaps are created. The continent catheterizable channel is laid in the tunnel and the flaps are brought anterior to the channel and sutured to each other. Fixation of the bladder wall to the abdominal wall preserves tunnel length and minimizes the risk of angulation. The type of continent catheterizable channel, stomal continence and the need for revision were recorded.

Results.—The extravesical implantation technique of a continent catheterizable channel was done in 84 of 394 patients (21%). The channel was an appendix in 47 cases and Monti ileovesicostomy in 37. Stomal continence was achieved in 79 of 84 cases (94%). At a mean followup of 45 months 22 patients (26%) required a total of 30 surgical revisions, of which most were skin level or endoscopic procedures at a mean of 26 months after channel creation.

Conclusions.—The extravesical technique for continent catheterizable channel implantation is effective. If intravesical surgery is not necessary, avoidance of a large cystotomy and longer operative time may expedite postoperative recovery when using an extravesical implantation technique to create a continent catheterizable channel.

▶ Implantation of a continent catheterizable channel (CCC) into the native bladder is preferred when compared with implantation into a bowel segment. Intestinal segments tend to thin with distension, and, over time, the antireflux mechanism becomes solely dependent on the length of the channel. An extravesical implantation technique has the advantage of assuring a fixed and non-angulated pathway into the bladder. The bladder is distended, and accurate positioning of the submucosal trough can be planned. (The color pictures in the manuscript are excellent.)

Once position is determined, I like to mature the abdominal stoma prior to connecting the channel to the bladder. This allows skin anastomosis without any tension. With retraction of the channel into the abdominal cavity, the stoma is very nicely concealed.

The authors describe using the extravesical technique only when the bladder is not opened for other procedures (ureteral reimplantation, bladder augmentation, bladder neck reconstruction), but the extravesical approach can be performed after these procedures have been completed and the bladder has been closed.

Postoperative endoscopic inspection of the bladder and bladder neck are much easier when the channel is placed on the anterolateral wall compared with a posterior wall.

D. E. Coplen, MD

15 Vesicoureteral Reflux

Prospective Blinded Laboratory Assessment of Prophylactic Antibiotic Compliance in a Pediatric Outpatient Setting
Yiee JH, Baskin LS, Patel N, et al (Univ of California, Los Angeles; Univ of California, San Francisco)
J Urol 187:2176-2181, 2012

Purpose.—Prophylactic antibiotics are commonly used to prevent urinary tract infections in children with conditions such as vesicoureteral reflux. Patient compliance with antibiotics is salient, given the effects that noncompliance can have on development of antibiotic resistance and outcomes of clinical trials. Prior series have shown variable compliance (17% to 70%). However, no study has used objective methods. We hypothesized that direct measurement of urine antibiotic levels can reveal poor compliance.

Materials and Methods.—During a pediatric urology clinic visit patients 0 to 18 years old taking trimethoprim prophylaxis for any urological diagnosis were invited to participate in the study. They were unaware of any potential urine testing before the visit. Urine was sent for chromatography to quantify trimethoprim levels. Parents also completed a compliance self-assessment.

Results.—Of patients invited to participate 97% consented (54 patients). Of the patients 91% were compliant based on urine levels. Factors not associated with compliance included age, gender, self-report of compliance, duration of time on antibiotics, insurance status and history of breakthrough infection, surgery, pyelonephritis or hospitalization.

Conclusions.—This study demonstrates the highest compliance reported for children taking prophylactic antibiotics to prevent urinary tract infection. We attribute this unexpected result to the discussion by specialists of 1 problem for the duration of an office visit. All education in this study was part of clinical care. Thus, our results should be generalizable to non-study environments. Future studies should confirm whether this high level of compliance can be achieved by nephrologists and pediatricians. If such compliance cannot be achieved at nonsurgical clinics, then early referral to a pediatric urologist may be warranted.

▶ Antibiotic prophylaxis has been routinely used in the medical management of vesicoureteral reflux. Recent placebo-controlled trials question the efficacy of prophylaxis, but 1 variable not assessed in many studies is parental compliance with administration. Analysis of a pharmacy dataset in the United States showed poor compliance based on medication refills,[1] although children with "breakthrough" infections participating in the Australian Prevention of Recurrent urinary tract Infection in children with Vesicoureteric reflux and Normal renal Tracts trial had bacteria resistant to the prophylactic Bactrim, suggesting that patients were taking the medication.[2] Based on a single urine sample obtained at a follow-up office visit (compliance equals any detectable trimethoprim), these authors show a very high compliance rate. A single positive urine test indicates that medication was taken in the prior 24 to 48 hours but does not necessarily mean that parents are giving medication on a regular basis. It is possible that parents gave the medicine because they remembered they were going to see the doctor. It is likely that directed counseling regarding the importance of therapy will improve compliance. The Randomized Intervention for Children with Vesicoureteral Reflux trial controls for compliance, so this trial will hopefully give more information on the efficacy of antibiotic prophylaxis that can be relayed to parents.

D. E. Coplen, MD

References

1. Copp HL, Nelson CP, Shortliffe LD, et al. Compliance with antibiotic prophylaxis in children with vesicoureteral reflux: results from a national pharmacy claims database. *J Urol.* 2010;183:1994-1999.
2. Craig JC, Simpson JM, Williams GJ, et al. Antibiotic prophylaxis and recurrent urinary tract infection in children. *N Engl J Med.* 2009;361:1748-1759.

Incidence of Febrile Urinary Tract Infections in Children after Successful Endoscopic Treatment of Vesicoureteral Reflux: A Long-Term Follow-Up

Hunziker M, Mohanan N, D'Asta F, et al (Natl Children's Hosp, Dublin, Ireland)
J Pediatr 160:1015-1020, 2012

Objective.—To evaluate the incidence of febrile urinary tract infection (UTI) after successful endoscopic correction of intermediate and high-grade vesicoureteral reflux (VUR).

Study Design.—Medical records of 1271 consecutive children (male, 411; female, 903) who underwent successful endoscopic correction of VUR were reviewed. Factors potentially influencing postoperative UTIs, such as history of presentation, age, sex, grade of VUR, renal scarring, and agent used for the endoscopic injection, were analyzed.

Results.—Febrile UTI developed in 73 children (5.7%) after successful endoscopic correction of VUR. Thirty-nine children had a single episode of UTI, and 34 children had two or more episodes at 1 month to 5.9 years (median, 1 year) after correction of VUR. With multivariate analysis, female sex ($P < .001$), history of preoperative bladder/bowel dysfunction (BBD; $P = .005$), and BBD after endoscopic correction ($P = .001$) were revealed to be the most important independent risk factors for a febrile UTI after successful correction of VUR.

Conclusions.—The incidence of febrile UTIs after successful correction of intermediate and high grade VUR is low. Female sex and BBD were the most important risk factors in the development of febrile UTI. Our data supports the importance of assessing bladder and bowel habits in older children with febrile UTIs after endoscopic correction of VUR.

▶ The primary goals of reflux management are prevention of renal scarring and recurrent urinary tract infections (UTIs). Ureteral reimplantation is known to decrease the incidence of febrile urinary tract infections. The incidence of cystitis does not decrease predominantly secondary to dysfunctional elimination. Endoscopic subureteric injection to correct reflux was developed in Ireland in the 1980s. It is now a widely accepted minimally invasive management of vesicoureteral reflux. The authors report a very low incidence of febrile UTI. The incidence was ascertained by parental reporting and may underestimate that actual frequency. Cystitis was not evaluated. Children with dysfunctional voiding were more likely to have a febrile UTI, but the prevalence of dysfunctional voiding was very low (4%) in the study population. Successful endoscopic correction of reflux is as effective as ureteral reimplantation in the prevention of febrile UTI.

D. E. Coplen, MD

16 Male Incontinence/ Voiding Dysfunction

Behavioral Versus Drug Treatment for Overactive Bladder in Men: The Male Overactive Bladder Treatment in Veterans (MOTIVE) Trial

Burgio KL, Goode PS, Johnson TM II, et al (Birmingham/Atlanta Geriatric Res, AL; et al)

J Am Geriatr Soc 59:2209-2216, 2011

Objectives.—To compare the effectiveness of behavioral treatment with that of antimuscarinic therapy in men without bladder outlet obstruction who continue to have overactive bladder (OAB) symptoms with alpha-blocker therapy.

Design.—The Male Overactive Bladder Treatment in Veterans (MOTIVE) Trial was a two-site randomized, controlled, equivalence trial with 4-week alpha-blocker run-in.

Setting.—Veterans Affairs Medical Center outpatient clinics.

Participants.—Volunteer sample of 143 men aged 42 to 88 who continued to have urgency and more than eight voids per day, with or without incontinence, after run-in.

Interventions.—Participants were randomized to 8 weeks of behavioral treatment (pelvic floor muscle exercises, urge suppression techniques, delayed voiding) or drug therapy (individually titrated, extended-release oxybutynin, 5−30 mg/d).

Measurements.—Seven-day bladder diaries and a validated urgency scale were used to calculate changes in 24-hour voiding frequency, nocturia, urgency, and incontinence. Secondary outcomes were global patient ratings and American Urological Association Symptom Index.

Results.—Mean voids per day decreased from 11.3 to 9.1 (−18.8%) with behavioral treatment and 11.5 to 9.5 (−16.9%) with drug therapy. Equivalence analysis indicated that posttreatment means were equivalent ($P < .01$). After treatment, 85% of participants rated themselves as much better or better; more than 90% were completely or somewhat satisfied, with no between-group differences. The behavioral group showed greater reductions in nocturia (mean = −0.70 vs −0.32 episodes/night; $P = .05$). The drug group showed greater reductions in maximum urgency scores (mean = −0.44 vs −0.12; $P = .02$). Other between-group differences were nonsignificant.

Conclusion.—Behavioral and antimuscarinic therapy are effective when added to alpha-blocker therapy for OAB in men without outlet obstruction. Behavioral treatment is at least as effective as antimuscarinic therapy.

▶ This was a trial conducted in men who continued to experience overactive bladder (OAB) symptoms despite α-blocker therapy. All men with OAB symptoms were treated with tamsulosin for 4 weeks and then reassessed to ensure they still met symptom inclusion criteria before being enrolled in the study. Those with postvoid residual volumes greater than 150 cc were excluded. Approximately 30% of men experienced sufficient symptom improvement with an α-blocker alone, and they were no longer study candidates. All of the patients continued α-blockers throughout the study. The symptom improvements observed in this trial are equivalent to those observed in similar clinical trials in women. This may not be surprising, but it has not been previously documented.

J. Q. Clemens, MD

A Single Center Prospective Study: Prediction of Postoperative General Quality of Life, Potency and Continence After Radical Retropubic Prostatectomy

Treiyer A, Anheuser P, Bütow Z, et al (St Antonius Hosp, Eschweiler, Germany)

J Urol 185:1681-1685, 2011

Purpose.—We investigated the importance of patient and tumor characteristics to predict continence, potency, and physical and mental health 1 year after radical prostatectomy.

Materials and Methods.—This prospective study included 236 patients who underwent open radical retropubic prostatectomy at a single institution between January 2005 and October 2007. We used validated questionnaires, including the Short Form General Health Survey, the International Index of Erectile Function and the International Consultation of Incontinence Questionnaire, to evaluate postoperative health related quality of life, erectile function and continence, respectively. Questionnaires were completed at months 3, 6 and 12 postoperatively.

Results.—At 1-year followup 75%, 73%, 75% and 26% of patients had returned to baseline physical health, mental health, continence and potency, respectively. Mental health recovered more slowly than physical health. Preoperative prostate specific antigen less than 20 ng/ml, nerve sparing technique, no intraoperative or postoperative complications, no adjuvant treatment and attendance at a postoperative rehabilitation program were significant factors that positively influenced the outcome in regard to health related quality of life, and postoperative potency and continence ($p < 0.05$).

Conclusions.—Predictors can be used when counseling patients who are preparing themselves for radical retropubic prostatectomy. This study highlights the mental impact of this surgery on these patients. We propose that men should undergo a combined mental and physical counseling program before surgery to predict postoperative health related quality of life, potency and continence after radical retropubic prostatectomy.

▶ It is critically important to preoperatively counsel patients with prostate cancer considering surgical treatment regarding postoperative outcomes. Although somewhat dated by the emergence of minimally invasive surgical techniques, this well-done prospective study of open radical retropubic prostatectomy performed by experienced surgeons suggests that return to preoperative baseline mental health, continence, and potency is not optimal. This study, using validated questionnaires in a prospective fashion at a minimum follow-up of 1 year, had only an 8% dropout rate (lost to follow-up), and thus the results are fairly robust. Perhaps most sobering in the data reported is that only 26% of the patients achieved the "trifecta" of no biochemical recurrence and postoperative recovery of continence and potency. This is not dissimilar to other studies in the literature that have looked at this type of outcome parameter. Ultimately, it is this trifecta that patients may be expecting postoperatively and, if not achieved, leads to disappointed and unhappy patients. Do robotic prostatectomy or other modified techniques for radical prostatectomy result in better outcomes? This remains unclear.

E. S. Rovner, MD

Treatment of Post-Prostatectomy Incontinence With Male Slings in Patients With Impaired Detrusor Contractility on Urodynamics and/or Who Perform Valsalva Voiding

Han JS, Brucker BM, Demirtas A, et al (New York Univ School of Medicine)
J Urol 186:1370-1375, 2011

Purpose.—Male slings have emerged as a popular and efficacious treatment for men with post-prostatectomy stress urinary incontinence. Traditionally slings have been used with caution or avoided in men with impaired detrusor contractility or Valsalva voiding because of concern that patients will not be able to overcome the fixed resistance of a sling during micturition. We propose that men with post-prostatectomy urinary incontinence who have impaired contractility and/or void with abdominal straining for urodynamics can be safely treated with slings.

Materials and Methods.—A retrospective review of patients with post-prostatectomy urinary incontinence who underwent an initial sling procedure between January 2004 and January 2010 was conducted at a single institution. Preoperative urodynamic characteristics, and postoperative Patient Global Impression of Improvement, post-void residual and noninvasive uroflow data were examined. Patients were grouped by poor bladder contractility or Valsalva voiding status. Exclusion criteria were lack of preoperative urodynamics and/or postoperative post-void residual. A total of 92 patients were analyzed. The variables were compared using the Student t test and the chi-square test.

Results.—No statistically significant difference was shown in postoperative post-void residual (mean 4 months postoperatively) or urinary retention when comparing by bladder contractility or Valsalva voiding. In the subset of patients with available postoperative uroflow data, there were no differences in postoperative maximum flow rate or voided volume.

Conclusions.—Men with post-prostatectomy urinary incontinence with urodynamic findings suggesting impaired contractility or Valsalva voiding can be safely treated with sling surgery if they have normal preoperative emptying.

▶ There are a number of treatment options for postprostatectomy urinary incontinence. The optimal patient population for male slings or artificial urinary sphincter has yet to be defined. Some surgeons are reluctant to place male slings in patients with impaired contractility (detrusor underactivity) because of the risk of urinary retention. This study suggests that this patient population with impaired contractility is not at significant risk for postoperative urinary retention or elevated postvoid residuals. They are as likely to void successfully postoperatively as those with normal contractility. The patient population in this study was highly selected in that they all had satisfactorily low postvoid residuals preoperatively, and none of the patients had failed prior surgical treatment for their post-prostatectomy incontinence. Furthermore, it is unclear whether these authors included patients who had preoperative urinary retention prior to their prostatectomy, as they excluded "neurogenic" patients. Ultimately, when considering patients at risk for urinary retention following a fixed outlet procedure, such as a male sling, the patients who would likely be at highest risk would be those who had urinary retention prior to their prostatectomy, with preoperatively proven poor contractility, or those for whom urodynamics prior to their sling reproduced their Valsalva voiding pattern. This population is a very different patient population from the individuals studied in this analysis. Finally, it is interesting that none of the 92 patients included in this analysis required any surgical intervention or catheterization postoperatively following sling placement. This in itself would suggest some selection bias in the patients included in this study.

E. S. Rovner, MD

A New Quadratic Sling for Male Stress Incontinence: Retrograde Leak Point Pressure as a Measure of Urethral Resistance
Comiter CV, Nitti V, Elliot C, et al (Stanford Univ School of Medicine, CA; New York Univ School of Medicine; et al)
J Urol 187:563-568, 2012

Purpose.—Objective methods are essential for evaluating post-prostatectomy incontinence. While symptom score and pad weight may be the most useful methods to evaluate preoperative vs postoperative continence, neither is useful for guiding intraoperative sling tension. The Virtue quadratic sling (Coloplast, Humlebaek, Denmark) is a new device for treating post-prostatectomy incontinence that combines a transobturator and prepubic surgical approach. We examined urethral resistance by measuring retrograde leak point pressure during key portions of the surgery.

Materials and Methods.—A total of 22 consecutive men who elected to undergo Virtue sling surgery were evaluated with retrograde leak point pressure before and during the surgery. Retrograde leak point pressure was measured via perfusion sphincterometry at baseline, after transobturator tensioning, after prepubic tensioning, and after transobturator and prepubic arms were secured in place.

Results.—Mean patient age was 70 years. Mean baseline retrograde leak point pressure was 33.4 ± 8.8 cm water. After transobturator tensioning, mean retrograde leak point pressure increased to 43.3 ± 6.8 cm water. After prepubic tensioning mean retrograde leak point pressure was 55.8 ± 8.7, and final retrograde leak point pressure after transobturator and prepubic fixation increased to 68.8 ± 6.0 cm water. Each mean retrograde leak point pressure value was significantly higher than the preceding value.

Conclusions.—The Virtue sling provides ventral urethral elevation using a transobturator approach, and a long segment of urethral compression against the genitourinary diaphragm via a straightforward prepubic technique without the risks of bone screws or retropubic needle passage. Transobturator and prepubic components of the quadratic fixation contributed to increasing urethral resistance as measured by intraoperative retrograde leak point pressure. This quadratic technique has a potentially greater ability to provide urethral compression than does a purely perineal or transobturator sling.

▶ A variety of treatments exist for the therapy of postprostatectomy urinary incontinence, including a number of different types of male slings. This article describes urodynamic changes following placement of a new type of male sling. Clinical outcomes are not presented in this article beyond intraoperative urodynamic findings. The idea that a longer area of urethral compression, such as that seen with this new technique, would be beneficial for the therapy of male stress urinary incontinence is intriguing. However, whether such a rise in retrograde leak point pressure as seen in this study, and as a surrogate, urethral resistance, leads to improved clinical outcomes is, as of yet, unknown. It is anticipated that clinical outcomes with this new sling will be forthcoming shortly.

Results with currently used male slings, including the Schaefer perineal sling, the bone-anchored perineal sling, and the transobturator sling, are largely imperfect and probably somewhat inferior to the results with artificial urinary sphincter, especially in severely incontinent individuals. However, there has not been a randomized controlled trial between these two types of interventions.

E. S. Rovner, MD

17 Benign Prostatic Hyperplasia

Medical Treatment

The Effects of Chronic 5-Alpha-Reductase Inhibitor (Dutasteride) Treatment on Rat Erectile Function

Pinsky MR, Gur S, Tracey AJ, et al (Tulane Health Sciences Ctr, New Orleans, LA)
J Sex Med 2011 [Epub ahead of print]

Introduction.—Numerous clinical series have reported an association between 5-alpha-reductase inhibitors (5ARIs) and sexual dysfunction, but there are limited preclinical data available.

Aim.—To further investigate the mechanisms of erectile dysfunction (ED) related to 5ARI therapy using a rat model.

Main Outcome Measures.—Outcome measures include serum dihydro-testosterone (DHT), relaxant and contractile properties of cavernosal muscle, and nitric oxide synthase expression.

Methods.—Twenty adult male Sprague-Dawley rats were randomized into control (N = 10) and dutasteride (0.5 mg/rat/day, in drinking water, N = 10) groups. Serum samples were obtained at baseline, from which DHT was measured after 30 days of treatment via radioimmunoassay (Beckman Coulter, Fullerton, CA, USA). Before the terminal blood draw, erectile response was measured using cavernosal nerve stimulation. The relaxant and contractile properties of cavernosal muscle strips were evaluated in tissue baths, and immunohistochemical (IHC) staining for nitric oxide synthase (NOS) and collagen deposition was performed.

Results.—Mean serum DHT was suppressed by 86.5% (range 64.2–94.8%) after 30 days of 5ARI treatment and was statistically significant ($P = 0.0024$). In vivo erectile response in the dutasteride treated group decreased significantly compared with control ($P < 0.001$). While electrical field stimulation (EFS)-induced and acetylcholine-induced relaxation was decreased, EFS-induced and phenlyephrine-induced adrenergic contraction was significantly enhanced in the dutasteride group ($P < 0.01$). IHC studies demonstrated increased collagen deposition in the treatment arm as well as altered expression of neuronal NOS (nNOS) and inducible NOS (iNOS).

Conclusions.—The 5ARIs, as demonstrated in these rat cavernosal smooth muscle studies, have a detrimental effect on erectile function. Enhanced iNOS expression may protect penile smooth muscle from fibrosis. The effect of 5ARIs on human sexual function warrants further investigation.

▶ This small but potentially important study investigates histologic, molecular, and functional changes in rats treated with daily dutasteride versus placebo in drinking water. Five alpha reductase inhibitors (5ARI) have been associated with erectile dysfunction in randomized studies, and some experts have vociferously criticized these medications as high risks for development of sexual problems.[1] The dutasteride-treated group in this study evidenced poorer erectile function as well as fibrotic changes of the corporal tissues, increased response to adrenergic stimulation, and changes in nitric oxide synthase expression. Whether these effects were permanent or would have reversed with cessation of the drug is a topic worthy of consideration and further study.

The potential role for 5ARI in erectile dysfunction in older men is difficult to clearly ascertain, as many older men have numerous potential causes for sexual difficulties, including lower urinary tract symptoms, for which 5ARIs are typically prescribed. The potential for interference is perhaps greater in younger men who may take 5ARI for alopecia, an indication not currently present for dutasteride. Further studies and careful patient counseling are required when considering 5ARI therapy in men.

A. W. Shindel, MD

Reference

1. Traish AM, Hassani J, Guay AT, Ziltzmann M, Hansen ML. Adverse side effects of 5α-reductase inhibitors therapy: persistent diminished libido and erectile dysfunction and depression in a subset of patients. *J Sex Med.* 2011;8:872-884.

Efficacy and Safety of Tadalafil Once Daily in the Treatment of Men With Lower Urinary Tract Symptoms Suggestive of Benign Prostatic Hyperplasia: Results of an International Randomized, Double-Blind, Placebo-Controlled Trial
Porst H, for the LVHJ study team (Private Practice of Urology and Andrology, Hamburg, Germany; et al)
Eur Urol 60:1105-1113, 2011

Background.—Tadalafil is being investigated for the treatment of lower urinary tract symptoms (LUTS) suggestive of benign prostatic hyperplasia (BPH-LUTS).

Objective.—To assess efficacy, including onset, and safety of tadalafil on BPH-LUTS and the subject's and clinician's perception of changes in urinary symptoms.

Design, Setting, and Participants.—This randomized, double-blind, placebo-controlled, 12-week trial enrolled men ≥45 yr of age with

BPH-LUTS for > 6 mo, International Prostate Symptom Score (IPSS) ≥13, and maximum urine flow rate (Q_{max}) ≥ 4 to ≤15 ml/s.

Intervention.—Tadalafil 5 mg ($n = 161$) or placebo ($n = 164$), once daily.

Measurements.—Analysis of covariance (ANCOVA) modeling evaluated change from baseline in continuous efficacy variables. Categoric efficacy variables were analyzed with the Cochran-Mantel-Haenszel test, and between-group differences in treatment-emergent adverse events (TEAEs) were assessed using the Fisher exact test.

Results and limitation.—Tadalafil significantly improved IPSS results, from baseline to endpoint, compared to placebo (-5.6 vs -3.6; $p = 0.004$). Reduction in IPSS results was apparent after 1 wk and significant after 4 wk (tadalafil -5.3 vs placebo -3.5; $p = 0.003$). The BPH Impact Index (BII) was not assessed at week 1; however, BII improvement was apparent at 4 wk (tadalafil -1.8 vs placebo -1.2; $p = 0.029$) and continued at 12 wk (tadalafil -1.8 vs placebo -1.3; $p = 0.057$). Tadalafil significantly improved the International Index of Erectile Function—Erectile Function score in sexually active men with erectile dysfunction (ED; 6.7 vs 2.0; $p < 0.001$) at 12 wk (not assessed at week 1). Few subjects reported one TEAE or more ($p = 0.44$). For tadalafil, the most common TEAEs were headache (3.7%) and back pain (3.1%). Tadalafil did not significantly improve Q_{max} or reduce postvoid residual volume.

Conclusions.—Tadalafil 5 mg once daily for 12 wk resulted in a clinically meaningful reduction in total IPSS results as early as 1 wk and achieved statistical significance at 4 wk in men with BPH-LUTS. The adverse event profile was consistent with that previously reported in men with ED.

Trial registration.—This clinical trial is registered on the clinicaltrials. gov website (http://www.clinicaltrials.gov). The registration number is NCT00827242.

▶ PDE5 inhibitors have been promulgated for years as potential treatments for lower urinary tract symptoms (LUTS) in men. There is a physiological rationale for this because PDE5 expression has been detected in the prostate and other organs of the lower urinary tract in men. Although symptomatic benefit has also been demonstrated in small series, the lack of objective changes in parameters such as flow rate and post-void residual has cast something of a shadow on how these pills might improve voiding function. Is subjective improvement a factor of better erections, or are these medications exerting a genuine effect on urinary function in men with benign prostatic hyperplasia (BPH)?

This randomized controlled trial enrolled men older than 45 years of age with bothersome LUTS. Significant improvements were noted by week 4 in men taking the treatment as opposed to placebo. Also noted were substantial improvements in erectile function in those men with both ED and LUTS. Overall, there was no statistically significant difference in voiding symptoms response based on baseline ED severity; men with mild or moderate ED experienced an improvement in International Prostate Symptom Score (IPSS) scores with a confidence interval (CI) well within the 95% range considered statistically significant. However, men with severe ED at baseline experienced a more muted increase in IPSS improvement that did not attain statistical significance with 95% confidence bounds (mean difference in change between control and tadalafil group of 11.8 points on IPSS, 95% CI −4.8 to 1.3). This analysis included only 56 men, so the statistical power is somewhat limited; however, one might hypothesize that the men with the worst ED, least likely to respond to PDE5I, did not realize as much benefit on their voiding symptoms because their blunted response to the erectogenic drug led to subjectively worse assessment of the treatment as a whole.

In the end, the efficacy of these drugs for the management of LUTS appears clear-cut, and this newly approved indication for tadalafil is a welcome addition; a single daily dose medication that helps with both erectile problems and voiding problems is a welcome addition to our armamentarium.

A. W. Shindel, MD

Surgical Treatment

TURP and sex: patient and partner prospective 12 years follow-up study
Mishriki SF, Grimsley SJS, Lam T, et al (Grampian NHS Trust, Aberdeen, UK; Ninewells Hosp and Med School, Dundee, UK)
BJU Int 2011 [Epub ahead of print]

Objective.—• To evaluate the effect of transurethral resection of the prostate (TURP) on sexual function in the short (6 months), medium (6 years) and long (12 years) term and assess the conformity between patient and partner regarding sexual function.

Patients and Methods.—• A prospective cohort study set at the Aberdeen Royal Infirmary University Hospital.

• A total of 280 men referred with lower urinary tract symptoms (LUTS) to a university hospital underwent TURP between January 1993 and September 1994; 145 of their partners (partner or spouse) participated.

• Assessment included American Urological Association symptom score, flow rates and validated self-reported sexual questionnaires (SQ).

• Data were collected at baseline, 3 months, 6 months, 6 years and 12 years of follow-up.

Results.—• In all, 120 (43%) men were sexually active preoperatively. At 6 months, 73 (61%) of these 120 men completed the SQ and all were sexually active.

• No sexually active patient became impotent after the procedure. Moreover, 27 (15%) with pre-existing erectile dysfunction reported improved sexual activity and erection quality.

• At 6 years 101 men completed the SQ and 31 (30.7%) were sexually active. At 12 years, 36 (31.9%) of 113 who completed the SQ were sexually active.

• Partners agreed with the men's self assessment at all visits.

• Limitations include possible attrition bias and lack of information from non-responders.

Conclusions.—• Erectile dysfunction associated with LUTS frequently precedes TURP.

• The TURP did not adversely affect sexual function.

• Pre-operative erectile dysfunction can be improved by TURP and long-term sexual function is maintained after TURP. These findings, corroborated by the partners, were statistically significant.

▶ This very interesting prospective study examines sexual function outcomes of men undergoing transurethral resection of the prostate (TURP) and their partners in 1993 and 1994. Fewer than half of patients were sexually active at baseline; interestingly, just 82% of 66 partners who gave baseline sexual activity data agreed. No patients appeared to experience a worsening of erectile dysfunction after the procedure, and a small percentage endorsed improvement in erectile function and sexual activity after the procedure at up to 12-year follow-up time points.

Studies such as this are plagued by the inevitable attrition involved with studying an older population as well as frequent missing data points. Data on erectile function were not collected using validated instruments, a forgivable situation given that the initiation of this study was years before development of the International Index of Erectile Function. The authors state in the discussion that this study is evidence that TURP is more likely to improve than harm sexual function; this is a rather bold assertion but one that may be warranted in certain select men who have severe sexual bother related to lower urinary tract symptoms. Be that as it may, it cannot be denied that TURP (or any other genital surgery) has the capacity to exert a negative effect on erectile capacity for both physiologic and organic factors. Attention to technique and patient counseling are key to optimize satisfaction with this gold standard procedure.

A. W. Shindel, MD

18 Bladder Cancer

Half of Visible and Half of Recurrent Visible Hematuria Cases Have Underlying Pathology: Prospective Large Cohort Study With Long-Term Followup

Mishriki SF, Vint R, Somani BK (Grampian NHS Trust, Aberdeen, Scotland, UK)

J Urol 187:1561-1565, 2012

Purpose.—Visible hematuria has a cancer yield of up to 24.2%. A large proportion of cases will have no etiology. In this study we determined the incidence of pathology (benign and malignant) in patients with visible hematuria and those with persistent and recurrent visible hematuria, and evaluated the policy for investigations.

Materials and Methods.—Data were prospectively collected for 1,804 patients with visible hematuria at a United Kingdom teaching hospital from January 1999 to September 2007. In October 2010 the comprehensive hospital electronic database was checked for every individual patient to ensure no urological pathology was missed. All patients underwent standard hematuria investigations, including renal tract ultrasound and excretory urography or contrast enhanced computer tomography urogram, flexible cystoscopy and urine cytology.

Results.—The male-to-female ratio was 4.8:1. Median age ± SD was 67 ± 17.0 years (range 21 to 109). Median followup was 6.6 ± 2.5 years (range 1.5 to 11.6). No urological pathology was found in 965 (53.5%) patients. Malignant urological disease was found in 386 (21.4%) patients, of whom 329 had bladder tumors. There were 32 patients with persistent visible hematuria and no malignancy. Repeat investigation was performed in 69 patients reporting recurrence. Of these patients 35 received a significant urological diagnosis, including 12 (17.4%) urological malignancies, while 34 (49.3%) still had no diagnosis. Limitations include the possibility of missing pathology.

Conclusions.—Almost 50% of patients presenting with visible hematuria will have a diagnosis. Therefore, all cases of visible hematuria require full standard investigations. Patients with no diagnosis can be discharged from followup. Recurrent visible hematuria after full initial negative findings requires repeat full standard investigations because 11.6% will have malignant pathology.

▶ Gross hematuria is associated with identifiable malignant and benign etiologies. Despite the fact that in the majority of cases no definite etiology is identified, all cases of gross hematuria should be evaluated with urine cytology, computed tomography urography, and cystourethroscopy. Bladder cancer was the most common diagnosis (18%), and benign prostatic enlargement was second (13%). This study addresses which patients with a negative evaluation need a second evaluation. A patient with a normal initial evaluation for gross hematuria can be discharged from follow-up because no malignancy was identified in this subset with median 6.6 years of follow-up. Because malignancy was identified in 11.6% of patients, recurrent gross hematuria requires a repeat comprehensive evaluation. Patients and practitioners need to understand even with a subsequent evaluation, no etiology is identified 50% of the time. In this prospective study, not every patient with an initial negative evaluation had a comprehensive repeat evaluation at the end of the study. There is the theoretical possibility that some malignancies were missed, but the comprehensive EMR was queried 3 years after study completion, so the number would be very small.

D. E. Coplen, MD

Radiotherapy with or Without Chemotherapy in Muscle-Invasive Bladder Cancer

James ND, for the BC2001 Investigators (Univ of Birmingham, UK; et al)
N Engl J Med 366:1477-1488, 2012

Background.—Radiotherapy is an alternative to cystectomy in patients with muscle-invasive bladder cancer. In other disease sites, synchronous chemoradiotherapy has been associated with increased local control and improved survival, as compared with radiotherapy alone.

Methods.—In this multicenter, phase 3 trial, we randomly assigned 360 patients with muscle-invasive bladder cancer to undergo radiotherapy with or without synchronous chemotherapy. The regimen consisted of fluorouracil (500 mg per square meter of body-surface area per day) during fractions 1 to 5 and 16 to 20 of radiotherapy and mitomycin C (12 mg per square meter) on day 1. Patients were also randomly assigned to undergo either whole-bladder radiotherapy or modified-volume radiotherapy (in which the volume of bladder receiving full-dose radiotherapy was reduced) in a partial 2-by-2 factorial design (results not reported here). The primary end point was survival free of locoregional disease. Secondary end points included overall survival and toxic effects.

Results.—At 2 years, rates of locoregional disease-free survival were 67% (95% confidence interval [CI], 59 to 74) in the chemoradiotherapy group and 54% (95% CI, 46 to 62) in the radiotherapy group. With a median follow-up of 69.9 months, the hazard ratio in the chemoradiotherapy group was 0.68 (95% CI, 0.48 to 0.96; $P = 0.03$). Five-year rates of overall survival were 48% (95% CI, 40 to 55) in the chemoradiotherapy group and 35% (95% CI, 28 to 43) in the radiotherapy group (hazard ratio, 0.82; 95% CI, 0.63 to 1.09; $P = 0.16$). Grade 3 or 4 adverse events were slightly more common in the chemoradiotherapy group than in the radiotherapy group during treatment (36.0% vs. 27.5%, $P = 0.07$) but not during follow-up (8.3% vs. 15.7%, $P = 0.07$).

Conclusions.—Synchronous chemotherapy with fluorouracil and mitomycin C combined with radiotherapy significantly improved locoregional control of bladder cancer, as compared with radiotherapy alone, with no significant increase in adverse events. (Funded by Cancer Research U.K.; BC2001 Current Controlled Trials number, ISRCTN68324339.)

▶ The bottom line is that chemotherapy works. This randomized trial from the United Kingdom demonstrates that addition of relatively well-tolerated chemotherapy improves radiation therapy (Fig 2 in the original article). Is this treatment ready to replace radical cystectomy? No. The cure rate is just not good enough. Is it ready to replace cisplatin-based chemotherapy? Probably not, but I'm not as sure. However, a common problem is the patient who is too ill for either radical cystectomy or cisplatin. We now have level 1 data that this regimen will provide not only local control but will prolong life.

A. S. Kibel, MD

19 Urethral Strictures

Repeat Transurethral Manipulation of Bulbar Urethral Strictures is Associated With Increased Stricture Complexity and Prolonged Disease Duration
Hudak SJ, Atkinson TH, Morey AF (Univ of Texas Southwestern Med Ctr, Dallas)
J Urol 187:1691-1695, 2012

Purpose.—We examined the association of previous transurethral manipulation with stricture complexity and disease duration among men referred for bulbar urethral reconstruction.

Materials and Methods.—We retrospectively reviewed the records of 340 consecutive urethroplasties performed by a single surgeon between July 2007 and October 2010. Only men treated with initial open surgery for bulbar strictures were included in analysis, thus excluding those with hypospadias, lichen sclerosus, pelvic radiation, prior urethroplasty, incomplete data, or pure penile or posterior urethral stenosis. Cases were divided into 2 groups based on the history of transurethral treatment for urethral stricture before urethroplasty, including group 1—0 or 1 and group 2—2 or greater treatments.

Results.—Of 101 patients with bulbar urethral stricture and all data available 50 and 51 underwent 0 to 1 and 2 or greater previous transurethral treatments, respectively. Repeat transurethral manipulation was strongly associated with longer strictures and the need for complex reconstruction. Repeat transurethral manipulation of bulbar urethral strictures was also associated with an eightfold increase in disease duration between stricture diagnosis and curative urethroplasty.

Conclusions.—Repeat transurethral manipulation of bulbar strictures is associated with increased stricture complexity and a marked delay to curative urethroplasty.

▶ Direct vision internal urethrotomy is the most commonly performed procedure for urethral strictures. This is likely because urologists feel very comfortable with transurethral procedures, the procedure has minimal morbidity, and there is rapid convalescence. Since the long-term success rate for short bulbar strictures is 60%, endoscopic incision is a reasonable first approach. Historically, repeat urethrotomy unsuccessfully relieves obstruction. There is some evidence that urethroplasty is underutilized.[1] This is likely related to the complexity of urethroplasty. Since only a small number of men need urethroplasty, most urologists are not comfortable with either primary or augmented urethroplasty. The

Table in the original article shows increased stricture complexity in men presenting after more than 1 prior treatment. This may be related to the prior procedure but could also be related to practice patterns, because the authors treat many strictures primarily with open surgery. Regardless, the men in group 2 lived with stricture disease for a mean of 15 years. Given the morbidity of symptoms and the cost associated with repeated surgeries, urethroplasty is clearly the treatment of choice after a single failed urethrotomy.

D. E. Coplen, MD

Reference

1. Anger JT, Buckley JC, Santucci RA, et al. Trends in stricture management among male Medicare beneficiaries: underuse of urethoplasty? *Urology.* 2011;77:481.

Distal urethroplasty for isolated fossa navicularis and meatal strictures
Meeks JJ, Barbagli G, Mehdiratta N, et al (Northwestern Univ, Chicago, IL)
BJU Int 109:616-619, 2012

Objective.—• Urethral strictures located in the fossa navicularis are common and are often managed with meatotomy or meatoplasty.
• Few data have described the outcomes for men after urethroplasty or patient satisfaction following these procedures.
Methods.—• In all, 93 men at two different institutions underwent surgical repair of distal urethral stricture disease using meatotomy (73) or meatoplasty (20), with 13/20 (65%) of the latter group undergoing substitution urethroplasty.
• In patients with lichen sclerosus (LS), all involved tissue was excised prior to reconstruction.
• In a subset of men undergoing meatotomy, patient satisfaction was evaluated by questionnaire.
Results.—• Average clinical follow-up for men undergoing distal urethroplasty was 61 months.
• Successful reconstruction requiring no further intervention occurred in 84% of men overall. Subgroup analysis revealed success in 87% of men with meatotomy, 75% with meatoplasty and 66% with substitution urethroplasty.
• Men with LS had a significantly greater rate of stricture recurrence (20.5% vs 7.5%, $P = 0.04$).
• Of the subset of men who completed a patient-based questionnaire 84% reported they were either satisfied or very satisfied with the results of their meatotomy.
Conclusions.—• We report the success of distal urethral stricture management.
• Meatal strictures may be approached successfully in a stepwise manner progressing from meatotomy to meatoplasty for longer recurrent strictures, with a high overall success rate for meatotomy.

• Although substitution grafts may be useful for men with longer distal strictures and those with LS, the risk of recurrence was significantly higher in this cohort.

▶ The management of distal urethral (glandular) urethral strictures is very challenging. These are typically posttraumatic or may occur after prior hypospadias repair. As a result, ischemia and poor wound healing are etiologic and affect the healing of subsequent reconstructions. The ventral glans (spongiosum) is thin and gives minimal support for neovascularization of grafts. Lichen sclerosus is a chronic inflammatory condition that was present in 42% of the men in this series. Surprisingly, a substitution urethroplasty was performed in only half of these men. A meatotomy was successful in 16 of 19 (85%) men with lichen sclerosus and a meatoplasty was successful in 15 of 20 (75%). Patient selection and surgeon experience are the keys to long-term success. Urethral dilation is ill advised. The authors show that an aggressive ventral meatotomy is successful in the majority of men. Recurrence after meatotomy requires a more aggressive approach. Since local skin is often affected by lichen sclerosus, a vascularized flap is ill advised. In these cases the use of an oral mucosal graft should be considered since recurrence of lichen sclerosus has not been reported in this graft material.

D. E. Coplen, MD

Long-term Results of Small Intestinal Submucosa Graft in Bulbar Urethral Reconstruction
Palminteri E, Berdondini E, Fusco F, et al (Ctr for Urethral and Genitalia Reconstructive Surgery, Arezzo, Italy; Univ Federico II, Naples, Italy; "La Sapienza" Univ, Rome, Italy; et al)
Urology 79:695-701, 2012

Objective.—To retrospectively report the long-term results of the use of a small intestinal submucosa (SIS) graft in bulbar urethral repair.

Methods.—From 2003 to 2007, 25 men (mean age 40.5 years) with bulbar strictures underwent patch graft urethroplasty using SIS placed on the dorsal or ventral or dorsal plus ventral surface of the urethra. The mean follow-up period was 71 months (range 52-100). The clinical outcome was considered a failure when any postoperative instrumentation, including dilation, was needed.

Results.—Of the 25 cases, 19 (76%) were successful and 6 (24%) were failures. No postoperative complications were related to the use of heterologous graft material, such as infection or rejection. The failure rate was 14% for strictures < 4 cm and 100% for strictures > 4 cm.

Conclusion.—At long-term follow-up, in bulbar stricture repair, SIS grafts showed similar results to penile skin grafts but were less effective than buccal mucosa grafts. The use of SIS as graft material should not be the first choice but represents an alternative option for patients with bulbar strictures that are not long and who refuse the harvesting or are not ideal candidates for buccal mucosa or penile skin grafts. Larger series of patients with longer follow-up are needed before widespread use can be advocated.

▶ The authors use commercially available small intestinal submucosal (SIS) in augmented bulbar urethroplasty. This collagen matrix is a scaffold that promotes tissue regeneration. The authors state that they offered SIS as opposed to buccal mucosa to avoid the "eventual donor site discomfort." In my experience there is very little short- or long-term oral donor site morbidity regardless of whether or not the mucosal defect is closed. The excellent results in short (< 4 cm) strictures are somewhat surprising given the poor results in other studies using SIS in urethroplasty. All but 1 failure occurred when the SIS graft was placed ventrally. In 3 failures the entire urethroplasty was fibrotic. Despite reapproximation of the spongiosum over the graft this likely has poorer blood supply than when sutured dorsally to the corporal body. Follow-up length is reasonable. However, in the author's own series, there has been deterioration of success over time although all failures did occur by 18 months. The results are not as good as can be obtained using buccal mucosa. SIS can be considered when buccal mucosa is not available (a rare situation).

D. E. Coplen, MD

20 Cryptorchidism

Age at Cryptorchidism Diagnosis and Orchiopexy in Denmark: A Population Based Study of 508,964 Boys Born From 1995 to 2009
Jensen MS, Olsen LH, Thulstrup AM, et al (Aarhus Univ Hosp Skejby, Denmark; Aarhus Univ Hosp, Denmark; et al)
J Urol 186:1595-1600, 2011

Purpose.—Early treatment for cryptorchidism may be necessary to preserve fertility. International guidelines now recommend that congenital cryptorchidism be treated with orchiopexy before age 1 year. Acquired cryptorchidism should be treated at presentation. To our knowledge the rate of adherence to these guidelines in recent years is unknown. Thus, we present data on age at cryptorchidism diagnosis and orchiopexy in recent Danish birth cohorts.

Materials and Methods.—A population of 508,964 Danish boys born alive from January 1, 1995 to December 31, 2009 was identified using the Danish Civil Registration System. Five birth cohorts were defined, including 1995 to 1997, 1998 to 2000, 2001 to 2003, 2004 to 2006 and 2007 to 2009. The boys were followed in the Danish National Patient Registry for a diagnosis of cryptorchidism and for an orchiopexy procedure. Data were analyzed using the Kaplan-Meier estimator and Cox regression models.

Results.—During followup 10,094 boys were diagnosed with cryptorchidism, of whom 5,473 underwent orchiopexy. Mean age at diagnosis in boys followed at least 6 years was 3.3 years (95% CI 3.3–3.4) in the 1995 to 1997 cohort, 3.1 (95% CI 3.1–3.2) in the 1998 to 2000 cohort and 2.9 (95% CI 2.8–2.9) in the 2001 to 2003 cohort while mean age at orchiopexy was 3.8 (3.7–3.9), 3.6 (3.5–3.7) and 3.3 years (3.2–3.4), respectively.

Conclusions.—In the more recent birth cohorts of 1995 to 2009 we observed a shift toward younger age at cryptorchidism diagnosis and orchiopexy.

▶ Undescended testes are identified in 3% of full-term infants. Spontaneous descent will occur by 6 months of age in two-thirds of these boys. The figure in the article shows a shift toward younger age at referral and surgery, but this still lags far behind the international guidelines for evaluation and management of acquired cryptorchidism. The exact reason for delay in identification and referral for management is unclear. A small percentage of testes preferentially lie in the superficial ectopic pouch, and differentiation between retractility and true maldescent can be difficult. However, in many cases, these boys have maldescent that is simply not identified at birth. There is evidence that early orchiopexy protects spermatogenic function and may decrease the chance of malignancy. Anesthesia is very safe at 6 months of age, so there is little reason to delay surgery. Continued education of primary caregivers is required.

D. E. Coplen, MD

Long-term testicular position and growth of acquired undescended testis after prepubertal orchidopexy

Meij-de Vries A, Goede J, van der Voort L, et al (Med Centre Alkmaar, The Netherlands; et al)
J Pediatr Surg 47:727-735, 2012

Purpose.—The aim of the study was to determine long-term testicular position and growth of acquired undescended testis (UDT) after prepubertal orchidopexy.

Methods.—Patients who had undergone prepubertal orchidopexy for acquired UDT at our hospital between 1986 and 1999 were recruited to assess long-term testicular position and volume. Testis position was assessed by physical examination. Testis volume was measured with Prader orchidometry and ultrasound and was compared with normative values reported in the literature.

Results.—A total of 105 patients (aged 14.0-31.6 years) were included with 137 acquired UDT (32 bilateral, 33 left sided, and 40 right sided). All but 1 of the orchidopexied testes (99.3%) were in low scrotal position. The mean volume of the orchidopexied testes in unilateral UDT (n = 73, 10.57 ± 3.74 mL) differed significantly from the size of the testes at the contralateral side (14.11 ± 4.23 mL) (P = .000). The operated testes (10.28 ± 3.45 mL) were smaller than the mean adult testis volume reported in the literature (13.4-13.6 mL; cutoff, 13.2 mL).

Conclusion.—Testis position after prepubertal orchidopexy for acquired UDT was nearly always low scrotal. The volume of the orchidopexied testes was smaller than both the volume of the contralateral testes and the normative values reported in the literature.

▶ The differentiation between retractile testes and truly undescended testes can be very challenging on physical examination. A subclinical hernia or preferential ectopic testicular position can be hard to identify. Testes that ascend are retractile testes that subsequently lie outside the scrotum and cannot be brought into a dependent scrotal position. At the time of surgery, either a patent processus vaginalis or an ectopic gubernaculum is typically identified. The total number of orchiopexies performed at this institution during the study period is unknown, but the number of orchiopexies performed for testicular ascent does seem to be large. Some of these testes may have been undescended since birth (same physician did not examine the patients longitudinally from birth) and were always asymmetric related to testicular dysgenesis. Since testicular ascent does occur, the finding that previously descended testes were smaller after delayed orchiopexy reinforces the importance of serial examination of boys with retractile testes.

I typically encourage parents to return in 12 to 18 months for a repeat examination. In the absence of a clinical hernia, I quote a 1% incidence of testicular ascent that should be treated with orchiopexy.

D. E. Coplen, MD

Bilateral vanished testes diagnosed with a single blood sample showing very high gonadotropins (follicle-stimulating hormone and luteinizing hormone) and very low inhibin B

Thorup J, Petersen BL, Kvist K, et al (Rigshospitalet, Copenhagen, Denmark; Univ of Copenhagen, Denmark)

Scand J Urol Nephrol 45:425-431, 2011

Objective.—In boys with cryptorchidism median serum values of follicle-stimulating hormone (FSH) and luteinizing hormone (LH) are higher and median serum values of inhibin B lower than in normal controls. Serum values of inhibin B reflect the state of germinative epithelium in cryptorchid testes. The aim of the study was to evaluate whether a simple blood sample of gonadotropins and inhibin B could diagnose bilateral vanished testes.

Material and Methods.—Group I included five boys (4 months to 6 years and 3 months old) with bilateral vanished testes at laparoscopy. Group II included 82 boys with bilateral cryptorchidism younger than 7 years of age at surgery for bilateral cryptorchidism (median age 1 year and 9 months).

Results.—The serum levels of hormones for the patients with vanished testes were: inhibin B 5—18 pg/ml, FSH 41—191 IU/l and LH 3.9—56 IU/l. The patients all had karyotype 46,xy. The serum levels of hormones from group II were: inhibin B median 122 (range 20—404) pg/ml, FSH median 0.8 (range 0.2—3.5) IU/l and LH median 0.2 (range 0.1—3.2) IU/l. The serum levels of inhibin B, FSH and LH from the boys with vanished testes were significantly different from the serum levels of the boys with bilateral cryptorchidism ($p = 0.0026$, $p < 0.0001$ and $p < 0.0001$, respectively).

Conclusions.—The serum values of gonadotropins and inhibin B from boys with bilateral vanished testes were significantly different from those of bilateral cryptorchid boys, indicating no germinative epithelium, no Sertoli cells and compensatory high gonadotropins. If such abnormal serum values are obtained from boys with bilateral non-palpable testes, tubular tissue is not present and surgery can be avoided.

▶ Undescended testes are identified in 3% of full-term infants. Physical examination by an experienced pediatric urologist directs management. If a testicle is non-palpable, it is absent 10% to 30% of the time. If there is a unilateral undescended testicle, serologic tests have no utility in the evaluation. Ultrasound, CT, and MRI are not sensitive or specific for absence of a testis, and exploration (laparoscopic, inguinal, or scrotal approach) is required.

Bilateral intra-abdominal testes are much more common than bilateral vanishing testes. Human chorionic gonadotropin stimulation evaluates for the presence of functioning Leydig cells. A negative testosterone response does not exclude the presence of dysplastic gonads. Follicle-stimulating hormone (FSH) is routinely elevated in postpubertal males with abnormal spermatogenesis and is typically elevated in infants with anorchia. Twenty percent of males with bilateral cryptorchidism and impaired fertility do not have marked elevations of gonadotropins.

Müllerian-inhibiting substance and inhibin-B are produced by Sertoli cells. If levels are at or below the lower limit of detection, then Sertoli cells and germ cells are absent. In theory there is no risk of cancer development.

If FSH and luteinizing hormone are elevated and inhibin-B levels are low in an infant with nonpalpable gonads, it is exceedingly unlikely that viable testes are present. In these rare cases, surgical exploration may be excluded.

A. Makhlouf, MD, MD

The Volume of Retractile Testes
Goede J, van der Voort-Doedens LM, Sijstermans K, et al (Med Centre Alkmaar, The Netherlands)
J Urol 186:2050-2055, 2011

Purpose.—We used ultrasound to determine the volume of retractile testes in boys and compared these volumes with normative testicular volume values.

Materials and Methods.—A total of 171 boys were enrolled in the study, of whom 14 were excluded from analysis. The 157 boys included (age 0.8 to 11.5 years) were recruited from 2 different populations. The first subgroup comprised 92 boys previously excluded from a study aimed at obtaining normative values of ultrasonographically scanned testes. The second group included 65 boys who had been referred to our outpatient clinic for nonscrotal testis and who were diagnosed with retractile testis. Testicular volume was measured by ultrasound in a scrotal position or in an inguinal position. Three separate transverse and longitudinal images of each testis were recorded. Length, width and height were measured, and the volume was calculated with the formula for an ellipsoid, $\pi/6 \times$ length $\times$ width $\times$ height. The highest value of the 3 testicular volumes was determined and taken as the volume measurement.

Results.—The volumes measured by ultrasound for the 157 boys with 276 retractile testes ranged from 0.18 to 1.49 ml (mean 0.50). The volumes of the retractile testes were significantly smaller than normative values ($p < 0.001$). Furthermore, the testicular volumes of retractile testes measured in an inguinal position were significantly smaller than those measured in a scrotal position ($p < 0.001$).

Conclusions.—The volumes of retractile testes are significantly smaller than recently determined normative values.

▶ A retractile testicle is considered to be a normal variant. As the cremasteric reflex blunts, the testicle remains in the scrotum at all times. Differentiation between retractile and undescended testes can be difficult, and ascent can occur (often ectopia that becomes apparent at an older age). The authors evaluated ultrasound-determined testicular volume in 2 discrete populations with retractile testes. The figures show that testicular size is smaller in boys with retractile testes than in age-related reference values in boys with descended testes. This is of some concern because we have been taught that retractile testes are normal. Does the smaller size mean that at puberty these testes will not have normal function? There is no study evaluating postpubertal function in boys with histories of retractility. Would surgery in these testicles be associated with catch-up growth? Careful evaluation of boys referred for undescended testes is required, and follow-up of boys with retractile testes is warranted.

D. E. Coplen, MD

Histological Examination of Solitary Contralateral Descended Testis in Congenital Absence of Testis

Kraft KH, Bhargava N, Schast AW, et al (Univ of Pennsylvania School of Medicine, Philadelphia)
J Urol 187:676-681, 2012

Purpose.—Congenital absence of the testis is believed to be secondary to prenatal torsion, differing from the isolated undescended testis. We determined whether congenital absence of the testis is associated with abnormal histology in the solitary contralateral descended testis.

Materials and Methods.—A total of 239 boys with a primary diagnosis of unilateral absent testis underwent orchiectomy and testis biopsy. Germ cell counts were compared between solitary contralateral descended testes and contralateral descended testes in a randomly selected, age matched cohort of patients with unilateral undescended testes. Subanalyses evaluating hypertrophic testes and hypertrophic prepubertal testes between the study groups were performed.

Results.—The solitary contralateral descended testis group exhibited a significantly greater volume ($p < 0.001$) and a significantly greater germ cell count ($p = 0.001$). In the hypertrophied testes there was a greater gonocyte count ($p = 0.02$), greater percentage of gonocytes ($p = 0.02$), greater primary spermatocyte count ($p = 0.04$) and greater percentage of primary spermatocytes ($p = 0.03$). No significant differences in adult dark spermatogonia or Leydig cells were detected. Primary spermatocytes did not differ significantly in prepubertal patients.

Conclusions.—The solitary contralateral descended testis exhibits increased volume, increased germ cell proliferation and dissimilar maturation patterns compared to the contralateral descended testis in unilateral cryptorchidism. These findings support prenatal torsion rather than endocrinopathy as the etiology for the congenitally absent testis. In the postpubertal solitary contralateral descended testis more germ cell maturation is seen and primary spermatocytes account for the increased total germ cell count. Patients with a solitary testis are likely not at additional risk for infertility.

▶ Evaluation of the contralateral descended testicle in boys with an absent testicle shows compensatory enlargement and an increased number of germ cells in the descended gonad when compared with the findings in boys with a unilateral undescended testicle. This clearly supports the concept that torsion is a mechanical event, whereas maldescent is the result of an endocrinopathy. Contralateral hypertrophy is commonly observed in infancy (when the boys present for evaluation of a nonpalpable testicle), but at times it is not apparent until progression through puberty. There is a gonadotropin surge between 60 and 90 days of life (important for the maturation of germ cells), and I have always thought that this may result in the compensatory enlargement. Because not all testes demonstrate hypertrophy, perhaps there are other factors that are important in the expansion of the germ cell population. Based on the histology, the authors conclude that normal fertility is anticipated in a male who has a solitary testicle secondary to prenatal torsion. Even though pregnancy was not a study end point, this is a reasonable supposition.

D. E. Coplen, MD

21 Hypospadias

Analysis of Risk Factors for Glans Dehiscence After Tubularized Incised Plate Hypospadias Repair
Snodgrass W, Cost N, Nakonezny PA, et al (Univ of Texas Southwestern Med Ctr and Children's Med Ctr, Dallas)
J Urol 185:1845-1851, 2011

Purpose.—We determined the incidence of glans dehiscence and the associated risk factors after tubularized incised plate hypospadias repair.

Materials and Methods.—All data for patients undergoing tubularized incised plate hypospadias repair, surgical details and postoperative outcomes were prospectively maintained in databases. Data were analyzed with simple and multiple logistic regression to determine if patient age, preoperative testosterone use, meatal location (distal, mid shaft or proximal), glansplasty sutures (chromic catgut vs polyglactin) or primary vs revision tubularized incised plate procedure was associated with an increased risk of glans dehiscence.

Results.—Glans dehiscence occurred in 32 of 641 patients (5%). Age at surgery, preoperative testosterone use and glansplasty suture did not impact the risk of glans dehiscence. Glans dehiscence occurred in 20 of 520 distal (4%), 1 of 47 mid shaft (2%) and 11 of 74 proximal (15%) tubularized incised plate repairs, with the odds of glans dehiscence being 3.6 times higher in patients with proximal vs distal meatal location. Patients undergoing reoperative (9 of 64, 14%) vs primary tubularized incised plate (23 of 577, 4%) had a 4.7-fold increased risk of glans dehiscence.

Conclusions.—Proximal meatal location and revision surgery, most commonly for prior glans dehiscence, increase the odds of glans dehiscence by 3.6 and 4.7-fold, respectively, suggesting anatomical and/or host factors (wound healing) are more important than age, type of suture or preoperative testosterone use in the development of this postoperative complication (Table 1).

▶ The glansplasty is the key to a normal-appearing hypospadias repair. To the parents, the flattened glans that is present after dehiscence looks unchanged when compared with their preoperative recollections. A percentage of children with glans dehiscence will have an abnormal urinary stream. The authors evaluate potential relationships between 6 variables and glans dehiscence in primary and reoperative hypospadias. The patient characteristics and outcomes are shown in Table 1. Proximal hypospadias and prior failure are risk factors for

TABLE 1.—Patient Demographics and Clinical Characteristics of Glans Dehiscence after TIP Urethroplasty

	GD Present	GD Absent	p Value*
Mean ± SD age (mos)	16.8 ± 26.9	19.5 ± 33.6	0.65 (unpaired 2-sample t test)
Mean ± SD followup (mos)	7.1 ± 5.3	9.2 ± 12.3	0.05 (unpaired 2-sample t test)[†]
No. chromic glansplasty suture (%)	7 (21.9)	106 (17.4)	0.52 (chi-square)
No. TIP revision (%)	9 (28.1)	55 (9.0)	0.003 (chi-square)
No. preop testosterone (%)	4 (12.5)	30 (4.9)	0.10 (chi-square)
No. meatal location at primary surgery (%):			0.002 (chi-square)
Distal	20 (62.5)	500 (82.1)	
Mid shaft	1 (3.1)	46 (7.6)	
Proximal	11 (34.4)	63 (10.3)	

*Tested for differences between presence and absence of GD on each demographic/clinical characteristic in separate model with p values left unadjusted for multiple testing.
[†]Satterthwaite method for unequal variances.

deshiscence. Prior failure may be the result of surgical technique or an inherent disorder of wound healing related to the diagnosis of hypospadias. Because suture material, age at surgery, and preoperative testosterone were not related to deshiscence, it is less likely that technical factors play an important role. The authors suggest that a small glans impacts healing and propose the use of preoperative testosterone to decrease dehiscence. This needs to be further evaluated in a prospective fashion (Table 1).

D. E. Coplen, MD

Androgen receptor is overexpressed in boys with severe hypospadias, and *ZEB1* regulates androgen receptor expression in human foreskin cells
Qiao L, Tasian GE, Zhang H, et al (Weifang Med College, Shandong, China; The Children's Hosp of Philadelphia, PA; Univ of California, San Francisco)
Pediatr Res 71:393-398, 2012

Introduction.—*ZEB1* is overexpressed in patients with severe hypospadias. We examined the interaction between ZEB1 and the androgen receptor (AR) *in vitro* and the expression of AR in boys with hypospadias.

Results.—ZEB1 and AR colocalize to the nucleus. Estrogen upregulated ZEB1 and AR expression. Chromatin immunoprecipitation (ChIP) demonstrated that ZEB1 binds to an E-box sequence in the AR gene promoter. AR expression is higher in subjects with severe hypospadias than those with mild hypospadias and control subjects ($P < 0.05$). ZEB1 physically interacts with AR in human foreskin cells.

Discussion.—AR is overexpressed in patients with severe hypospadias. Environmental estrogenic compounds may increase the risk of hypospadias by facilitating the interaction between ZEB1 and AR.

Methods.—Hs68 cells, a fibroblast cell line derived from neonatal human foreskin, were exposed to 0, 10, and 100 nmol/l of estrogen, after which the cellular localization of ZEB1 and AR was assessed using immunocytochemistry. To determine if ZEB1 interacted with the AR gene, ChIP was performed using ZEB1 antibody and polymerase chain reaction (PCR) for AR. Second, AR expression was quantified using real-time PCR and western blot in normal subjects ($n = 32$), and subjects with mild ($n = 16$) and severe hypospadia ($n = 16$).

▶ Diminished androgen signaling results in a spectrum of incompletely virilized external genitalia (complete insensitivity gives a normal female external phenotype). Estrogen is a potential disrupter of normal androgen signaling. The authors evaluate the molecular mechanisms underlying the association between estrogen exposure, androgen signaling, and the development of hypospadias. It seems counterintuitive that the androgen receptor is upregulated in severe hypospadias. It is conceivable that this is a feedback phenomenon related to abnormal androgen receptor function. The authors show in vitro upregulation of androgen receptor by estrogen. Estrogen also upregulates ZEB1 (a transcription regulator). This may be 1 mechanistic pathway for altered androgen signaling, but there are likely other pathways that need to be explored.

D. E. Coplen, MD

22 Infertility

Analysis of the outcome of intracytoplasmic sperm injection using fresh or frozen sperm
Kalsi J, Thum MY, Muneer A, et al (Univ College London Hosps NHS Foundation Trust, UK; The Lister Hosp, London, UK)
BJU Int 107:1124-1128, 2011

Objectives.—• To compare the outcome of first-attempt intracytoplasmic sperm injection (ICSI) ICSI–embryo transfer (ET) cycles using frozen-thawed testicular sperm (FTTS), fresh testicular sperm (FTS), frozen-thawed epididymal sperm (FTES) and fresh epididymal sperm (FES) so as to determine which of these has the most successful ICSI outcome with respect to fertilization rate (FR), pregnancy rate (PR) and birth rate.
• To assess the outcomes according to the underlying aetiology of azoospermia.
Patients and Methods.—• The records of 493 patients undergoing first-attempt ICSI between 1993 and 2008 were reviewed retrospectively. FTS was used in 112 cycles, FTTS in 43 cycles, FES in 279 cycles, and FTES in 59 cycles.
• Within each group, the aetiology of the azoospermia was recorded according to history, clinical examination and histological analysis ($n = 316$).
• The FR, clinical PR and delivery rate were calculated for each group with respect to the type of sperm retrieval used.
Results.—• Analysis of the data showed no significant differences between any of the four groups in the FR, PR or delivery rate ($P > 0.05$).
• There were no significant differences seen between fresh sperm (FTS and FES) and frozen sperm (FTTS and FTES) or between epididymal sperm (FES and FTES) and testicular sperm (FTS and FTTS) in any of the outcomes measured ($P > 0.05$). However, subset analysis showed a statistically higher FR and PR for FTTS over fresh sperm.
• When comparing aetiologies, there was no significant difference in the FR, clinical PR and delivery rate between obstructive azoospermia (OA) and non-obstructive azoospermia (NOA) groups. However, sub-set analysis showed a higher PR and birth rate for FTTS over fresh sperm in both OA and NOA groups.
Conclusions.—• The results of the present study suggest that using frozen sperm in ICSI cycles is a reliable and favourable method with the same outcome as fresh sperm.
• Testicular and epididymal sperm have similar ICSI outcomes for both fresh and frozen samples. However, results suggest a tendency for higher

PRs and birth rates for frozen than for fresh testicular sperm in both OA and NOA aetiologies.

• The aetiology of azoospermia does not significantly affect the outcome of first-attempt ICSI. The higher rates in the frozen groups suggest that these patients have had better quality semen when they were initially harvested and frozen.

▶ There is concern that freezing and thawing of sperm may have a detrimental effect on the morphology of sperm. These morphologic changes may disrupt cellular and nuclear membranes and affect DNA integrity. This is a retrospective review evaluating fertility rates using fresh and frozen sperm either from the epididymis or testicle. The unique component of this study is that couples had cycles of intracytoplasmic sperm injection (ICSI) with both fresh and frozen-thawed spermatozoa in their first cycle and not in consecutive cycles. Frozen sperm was as good as fresh sperm in all domains evaluated. The results of this study showed no difference in outcome using ICSI either with respect to the site of retrieval or whether the sperm used was fresh or frozen (Table 1 in the original article). The study also shows that the outcome of ICSI is not related to the underlying cause of the azoospermia (Table 2 in the original article). Elective verification of the presence of sperm and storage (freezing) prior to egg harvest makes good sense. Frozen sperm eliminates the need for repeat sperm harvesting if a second ICSI cycle is required.

D. E. Coplen, MD

Physical activity and semen quality among men attending an infertility clinic
Wise LA, Cramer DW, Hornstein MD, et al (Boston Univ, MA; Brigham and Women's Hosp and Harvard Med School, Boston, MA)
Fertil Steril 95:1025-1030, 2011

Objective.—To examine the association between regular physical activity and semen quality.

Design.—Prospective cohort study.

Setting.—Couples attending one of three IVF clinics in the greater Boston area during 1993–2003. At study entry, male participants completed a questionnaire about their general health, medical history, and physical activity. Odds ratios (ORs) and 95% confidence intervals (CIs) were derived using generalized estimating equations models, accounting for potential confounders and multiple samples per man.

Patient(s).—A total of 2,261 men contributing 4,565 fresh semen samples were enrolled before undergoing their first IVF cycles.

Intervention(s).—None.

Main Outcome Measure(s).—Semen volume, sperm concentration, sperm motility, sperm morphology, and total motile sperm (TMS).

Result(s).—Overall, none of the semen parameters were materially associated with regular exercise. Compared with no regular exercise, bicycling ≥5 h/wk was associated with low sperm concentration (OR 1.92, 95% CI

1.03—3.56) and low TMS (OR 2.05, 95% CI 1.19—3.56). These associations did not vary appreciably by age, body mass index, or history of male factor infertility.

Conclusion(s).—Although the present study suggests no overall association between regular physical activity and semen quality, bicycling ≥5 h/wk was associated with lower sperm concentration and TMS.

▶ There is concern that bicycling might be a risk factor for erectile dysfunction. It is unknown if this or other physical activity adversely affects semen quality/ fertility. The authors used reported physical activity (running, bicycling, and weightlifting) on an entry questionnaire completed at fertility clinics. They correlated these findings with seminal parameters. Self-report of cycling greater than 5 hours per week was associated with diminished sperm count and motility (odds ratio of only 2). Whether this is a real association needs to be determined prospectively.

D. E. Coplen, MD

Anabolic steroids and male infertility: a comprehensive review
de Souza GL, Hallak J (Sao Paulo State Military Police Hosp, Brazil; Univ of Sao Paulo Med School, Brazil)
BJU Int 108:1860-1865, 2011

What's known on the subject? and What does the study add?
The negative impact of AAS abuse on male fertility is well known by urologists. The secondary hypogonadotropic hypogonadism is often highlighted when AAS and fertility are being discussed. On the other hand, the patterns of use, mechanisms of action and direct effects over the testicle are usually overseen. The present study reviews the vast formal and "underground" culture of AAS, as well as their overall implications. Specific considerations about their impact on the male reproductive system are made, with special attention to the recent data on direct damage to the testicle. To our knowledge this kind of overview is absolutely unique, offering a distinguished set of information to the day-by-day urologists.

For several decades, testosterone and its synthetic derivatives have been used with anabolic and androgenic purposes. Initially, these substances were restricted to professional bodybuilders, becoming gradually more popular among recreational power athletes. Currently, as many as 3 million anabolic-androgenic steroids (AAS) users have been reported in the United States, and considering its increasing prevalence, it has become an issue of major concern. Infertility is defined as the failure to achieve a successful pregnancy after 12 months or more of regular unprotected intercourse, with male factor being present in up to 50% of all infertile couples. Several conditions may be related to male infertility. Substance abuse, including AAS, is commonly associated to transient or persistent impairment on male reproductive function, through different pathways. Herein, a brief overview on

AAS, specially oriented to urologists, is offered. Steroids biochemistry, patterns of use, physiological and clinical issues are enlightened. A further review about fertility outcomes among male AAS abusers is also presented, including the classic reports on transient axial inhibition, and the more recent experimental reports on structural and genetic sperm damage.

▶ Infertility commonly occurs after anabolic steroid abuse. Typically this presents with oligospermia or azoospermia in association with abnormal motility and morphology. These results are related to negative feedback of androgens on the hypothalamic—pituitary axis. Although serum testosterone levels may be high, the decreased follicle-stimulating hormone and luteinizing hormone lower the intratesticular testosterone concentration that is necessary for normal spermatogenesis. Typically the sperm quality will recover within 6 months of cessation of exogenous androgens, but treatment with gonadotropin analogs may be required if azoospermia persists. Given the prevalence of steroid use, this should be considered during infertility evaluation.

A. Makhlouf, MD, MD

Low-Dose Lisinopril in Normotensive Men With Idiopathic Oligospermia and Infertility: A 5-Year Randomized, Controlled, Crossover Pilot Study

Mbah AU, Ndukwu GO, Ghasi SI, et al (Univ of Nigeria, Enugu; et al)
Clin Pharmacol Ther 91:582-589, 2012

The outcomes of drug treatment for male infertility remain conjectural, with controversial study results. Our pilot study employed a randomized, placebo-controlled, crossover methodology with intention-to-treat analysis. Thirty-three men with idiopathic oligospermia were randomized to start either daily oral lisinopril 2.5 mg ($n = 17$) or daily oral placebo ($n = 16$). Lisinopril was found to cause a normalization of seminal parameters in 53.6% of the participants. Although the mean ejaculate volume was unchanged ($P \geq 0.093$), the total sperm cell count and the percentage of motile sperm cells increased ($P \leq 0.03$ and $P < 0.001$, respectively), whereas the percentage of sperm cells with abnormal morphology decreased ($P \leq 0.04$). The pregnancy rate was 48.5%, and there was no serious adverse drug event. It is concluded, albeit cautiously, that prolonged treatment with 2.5 mg/day of oral lisinopril may be well tolerated in normotensive men with idiopathic oligospermia, may improve sperm quantity and quality, and may enhance fertility in approximately half of those treated.

▶ This National Institutes of Health—supported clinical trial showed that total sperm cell count increased in men while they were taking lisinopril and decreased when the medication was substituted by a placebo. This shows that lisinopril is linked to the observed changes in sperm cell count. The medication also improved total sperm motility and morphology. There were wide individual variations, and in some men the parameters actually worsened when compared with baseline. This supports the concept that oligospermia has multiple etiologies. The spontaneous pregnancy rate was high, although 5 of the pregnancies occurred in the placebo group after crossover from medication. The exact mechanism of action of the angiotensin-converting enzyme inhibitor that improved seminal parameters is not known. The sample size is very small, and interactions with other medications or substances cannot be excluded. These results require confirmation in a larger multicenter trial.

D. E. Coplen, MD

Use of laptop computers connected to internet through Wi-Fi decreases human sperm motility and increases sperm DNA fragmentation
Avendaño C, Mata A, Sanchez Sarmiento CA, et al (Nascentis Medicina Reproductiva, Córdoba, Argentina; et al)
Fertil Steril 97:39-45, 2012

Objective.—To evaluate the effects of laptop computers connected to local area networks wirelessly (Wi-Fi) on human spermatozoa.

Design.—Prospective in vitro study.

Setting.—Center for reproductive medicine.

Patient(s).—Semen samples from 29 healthy donors.

Intervention(s).—Motile sperm were selected by swim up. Each sperm suspension was divided into two aliquots. One sperm aliquot (experimental) from each patient was exposed to an internet-connected laptop by Wi-Fi for 4 hours, whereas the second aliquot (unexposed) was used as control, incubated under identical conditions without being exposed to the laptop.

Main Outcome Measure(s).—Evaluation of sperm motility, viability, and DNA fragmentation.

Result(s).—Donor sperm samples, mostly normozoospermic, exposed ex vivo during 4 hours to a wireless internet-connected laptop showed a significant decrease in progressive sperm motility and an increase in sperm DNA fragmentation. Levels of dead sperm showed no significant differences between the two groups.

Conclusion(s).—To our knowledge, this is the first study to evaluate the direct impact of laptop use on human spermatozoa. Ex vivo exposure of human spermatozoa to a wireless internet-connected laptop decreased motility and induced DNA fragmentation by a nonthermal effect. We speculate that keeping a laptop connected wirelessly to the internet on the lap near the testes may result in decreased male fertility. Further in vitro and in vivo studies are needed to prove this contention.

▶ The use of laptop computers that wirelessly (Wi-Fi) communicate with the Internet is commonplace. Some of the transmitted energy from the radio signals may be absorbed into the body. With laptop use, the testicles (and spermatozoa) may be exposed to electromagnetic waves. The authors evaluated the effect of electromagnetic radiation on sperm motility and viability. Temperature was controlled and the same in both groups. A third study arm using exposure to a laptop without a Wi-Fi connection would have been ideal. The authors demonstrate decreased sperm quality secondary to a nonthermal effect. Similar findings have been observed when spermatozoa are exposed to mobile phone radiation. The mechanisms involved in altering sperm motility and DNA integrity require additional study.

D. E. Coplen, MD

23 Urinary Tract Infection

Antibiotic Prophylaxis for Urinary Tract Infections in Children With Spina Bifida on Intermittent Catheterization
Zegers B, Uiterwaal C, Kimpen J, et al (Wilhelmina Children's Hosp, Utrecht, The Netherlands; Julius Ctr for Health Sciences and Primary Care, Utrecht, The Netherlands; Univ Med Ctr, Utrecht, The Netherlands; et al)
J Urol 186:2365-2371, 2011

Purpose.—Antibiotic prophylaxis (low dose chemoprophylaxis) has been prescribed since the introduction of clean intermittent catheterization in children with spina bifida. We hypothesized that stopping low dose chemoprophylaxis does not increase the number of urinary tract infections in these patients.

Materials and Methods.—A total of 176 patients with spina bifida participated in a randomized controlled trial (ISRCTN trial number 56278131) of either continuation or discontinuation of low dose chemoprophylaxis. During the 18-month study period biweekly urine samples were evaluated for leukocyturia and bacteriuria with dipsticks and cultures. Asymptomatic significant bacteriuria (positive culture results without clinical symptoms) and urinary tract infections (significant bacteriuria with clinical symptoms and leukocyturia) were analyzed.

Results.—Discontinuation of low dose chemoprophylaxis resulted in higher rates of asymptomatic significant bacteriuria (incidence rate ratio 1.23, 95% CI 1.08–1.40, $p = 0.002$) and urinary tract infection (IRR 1.44, 95% CI 1.13–1.83, $p = 0.003$). For urinary tract infection the number needed to harm was 2.2, that is if 2 patients discontinued low dose chemoprophylaxis for a year, 1 extra urinary tract infection would result. Febrile urinary tract infection occurred once in every 30 patient-years and slightly more often in the discontinuation group (relative risk 2.0, 95% CI 0.38–10.6, $p = 0.4$). Of 88 patients allocated to discontinuation of low dose chemoprophylaxis 38 (43%) switched back to chemoprophylaxis. The urinary tract infection rate was nonsignificantly higher in the presence of vesicoureteral reflux. Male gender and a low prestudy rate of urinary tract infection predicted successful discontinuation.

Conclusions.—Patients with spina bifida on clean intermittent catheterization and antibiotic prophylaxis for urinary tract infections can safely discontinue this prophylaxis, in particular males, patients with low urinary tract infection rates and patients without vesicoureteral reflux.

▶ I was somewhat surprised that the standard of care for children on clean intermittent catheterization (CIC) in Belgium included daily prophylactic antibiotics. As long as the bladder is low pressure, most children are colonized with bacteria but do not develop symptomatic urinary tract infections. In this study, there was a clinically insignificant increase in urinary tract infections once prophylaxis was stopped. It is unclear from the data why 43% of children randomized to prophylaxis restarted the medication. Presumably this is because a subset of children have symptomatic infections (incontinence, pain, fevers) and are more comfortable on antibiotics. Significant antibiotic resistance can develop while on prophylaxis, so it should not routinely be utilized in patients on CIC.

D. E. Coplen, MD

Lactobacilli vs Antibiotics to Prevent Urinary Tract Infections: A Randomized, Double-blind, Noninferiority Trial in Postmenopausal Women

Beerepoot MAJ, ter Riet G, Nys S, et al (Academic Med Ctr, Amsterdam, the Netherlands; Maastricht Univ Med Ctr, the Netherlands; et al)
Arch Intern Med 172:704-712, 2012

Background.—Growing antibiotic resistance warrants studying nonantibiotic prophylaxis for recurrent urinary tract infections (UTIs). Use of lactobacilli appears to be promising.

Methods.—Between January 2005 and August 2007, we randomized 252 postmenopausal women with recurrent UTIs taking part in a double-blind noninferiority trial to receive 12 months of prophylaxis with trimethoprim-sulfamethoxazole, 480 mg, once daily or oral capsules containing 10^9 colony-forming units of *Lactobacillus rhamnosus* GR-1 and *Lactobacillus reuteri* RC-14 twice daily. Primary end points were the mean number of symptomatic UTIs, proportion of participants with at least 1 UTI during 12 months, time to first UTI, and development of antibiotic resistance by *Escherichia coli.*

Results.—The mean number of symptomatic UTIs in the year preceding randomization was 7.0 in the trimethoprim-sulfamethoxazole group and 6.8 in the lactobacilli group. In the intention-to-treat analysis, after 12 months of prophylaxis, these numbers were 2.9 and 3.3, respectively. The between-treatment difference of 0.4 UTIs per year (95% CI, −0.4 to 1.5) was outside our noninferiority margin. At least 1 symptomatic UTI occurred in 69.3% and 79.1% of the trimethoprim-sulfamethoxazole and lactobacilli participants, respectively; median times to the first UTI were 6 and 3 months, respectively. After 1 month of trimethoprim-sulfamethoxazole prophylaxis, resistance to trimethoprim-sulfamethoxazole, trimethoprim, and amoxicillin had increased from approximately 20% to 40% to approximately 80% to 95% in *E coli* from the feces and urine of asymptomatic women and among *E coli* causing a UTI. During the 3 months after trimethoprim-sulfamethoxazole discontinuation, resistance levels gradually decreased. Resistance did not increase during lactobacilli prophylaxis.

Conclusions.—In postmenopausal women with recurrent UTIs, *L rhamnosus* GR-1 and *L reuteri* RC-14 do not meet the noninferiority criteria in the prevention of UTIs when compared with trimethoprim-sulfamethoxazole. However, unlike trimethoprim-sulfamethoxazole, lactobacilli do not increase antibiotic resistance.

Trial Registration.—isrctn.org Identifier: ISRCTN50717094.

▶ Antibiotics do not prevent urinary tract infections (UTI) in 100% of cases, and use of them may cause bacterial resistance. The authors evaluate the ability of daily trimethoprim-sulfa (TMP-SMX) and lactobacilli to prevent UTI in women with chronic cystitis (average 7 UTIs per year prior to study initiation). There was no difference in the clinical recurrence rate between the 2 groups (2.9 vs 3.3), although women in both groups had fewer symptoms than at baseline. There were fewer microbiological recurrences in the TMP-SMX group (culture positive 33% to 60% of the time in the 2 groups when symptomatic). Recurrences occurred earlier in the lactobacilli group (3 months vs 6 months). Lactobacilli therapy was clearly second best to TMP-SMX for the prevention of UTI. As might be anticipated, patients on TMP-SMX did develop antibiotic resistance when compared to the lactobacilli group. Even after being off of the antibiotic for 3 months, antibiotic resistance was higher than at study entry. The authors do not show that orally administered lactobacilli actually reach the vagina. There seem to be few adverse effects of lactobacillus administration, and it is clear that this group was exposed to fewer antibiotics during the study time period and that this may be a reasonable alternative to prophylactic antibiotics in the treatment of chronic cystitis.

D. E. Coplen, MD

Overtreatment of Enterococcal Bacteriuria

Lin E, Bhusal Y, Horwitz D, et al (Baylor College of Medicine, Houston, TX; et al)
Arch Intern Med 172:33-38, 2012

Background.—The purposes of this study were to investigate the clinical outcomes of enterococcal bacteriuria and to determine whether current management is adherent to Infectious Diseases Society of America guidelines.

Methods.—We conducted a retrospective medical record review of patients from 2 academic teaching hospitals for 3 months (September 1 through November 30, 2009). Patients were classified as having urinary tract infection (UTI) or asymptomatic bacteriuria (ABU) by applying the guidelines. Antibiotic use was deemed appropriate in patients with UTI and inappropriate in ABU. Medical records were reviewed for *Enterococcus* cultured from another sterile site within 30 days.

Results.—A total of 375 urine cultures growing *Enterococcus* were reviewed, with 339 cultures meeting inclusion criteria. Of these 339 episodes, 183 (54.0%) were classified as ABU and 156 (46.0%) as UTI. In 289 episodes accompanied by urinalysis, pyuria was associated with UTI in 98 of 140 episodes (70.0%) compared with 63 of 149 episodes of ABU (42.3%) (odds ratio, 3.19; 95% CI, 1.96-5.18). Providers inappropriately treated 60 of 183 episodes of ABU (32.8%) with antibiotics. In multivariate analysis, only pyuria was associated with the inappropriate use of antibiotics (odds ratio, 3.27; 95% CI, 1.49-7.18). Only 7 subsequent infections with *Enterococcus* occurred in the 339 episodes of bacteriuria overall (2.1%), with 2 of the 183 cases of ABU (1.1%) having distant infection.

Conclusions.—Providers often overtreat enterococcal ABU with antibiotics, particularly in patients with pyuria. Given the low incidence of infectious complications, efforts should be made to optimize the use of antibiotics in enterococcal bacteriuria.

▶ Asymptomatic bacteriuria is commonly identified in hospitalized patients. Treatment risks increased antimicrobial resistance and *Clostridium difficile* colitis. The positive urine culture may not be the clinical explanation in an ill patient with complex multisystem concerns. The authors retrospectively evaluate antibiotic utilization in patients with enterococcal bacteriuria. They assumed that the absence of symptoms recorded in the medical records meant that symptoms were absent, so there is a chance of misclassification. Clinically, there is always some concern that asymptomatic bacteria will become symptomatic and, in the worst case scenario, cause sepsis. This may explain some of the inappropriate treatment of the positive urine cultures. The natural reflex to treat a positive urine culture needs to be addressed. Care pathways and management by hospitalists may be one way to achieve appropriate hospital-based antibiotic use.

D. E. Coplen, MD

Long-term Fluoroquinolone Use Before the Prostate Biopsy May Increase the Risk of Sepsis Caused by Resistant Microorganisms
Akduman B, Akduman D, Tokgöz H, et al (Zonguldak Karaelmas Univ School of Medicine, Turkey)
Urology 78:250-256, 2011

Objectives.—To evaluate the effect of long-term fluoroquinolone treatment before the biopsy in terms of post procedure sepsis. Three-week fluoroquinolone management before the biopsy may lower serum prostate specific antigen (PSA) levels and prevent unnecessary biopsies.

Methods.—A total of 558 patients were referred to our clinic for transrectal ultrasound (TRUS)—guided prostate biopsy. Of the patients, 205 had received levofloxacin 500 mg once a day for 3 weeks before the biopsy to lower the serum PSA levels (group 1). A total of 353 patients had not received any antibiotics before the procedure (group 2). In terms of the postbiopsy sepsis rate, group 1 and group 2 as well as patients who underwent biopsies in the early period and the latter period of the study were compared.

Results.—Sepsis was diagnosed in 17 patients (3.0%) after biopsy. Of these patients, 11 (5.4%) and 6 (1.7%) were in group 1 and group 2, respectively ($P = .0297$, OR: 3.28, 95% CI: 1.10-10.13). Sepsis was diagnosed in 7 patients (1.9%) and 10 patients (5.0%) in the early and the latter period of the study, respectively ($P = .0771$, OR: 0.38, 95% CI: .13-1.09). *Escherichia coli* was the causative agent in all patients with a positive culture. In addition, 1 patient also had meticillin resistant *Staphylococcus epidermidis* (MRSE). All of the *E. coli* isolates were resistant to fluoroquinolones, and 55.6% were positive for extended spectrum β-lactamases (ESBL).

Conclusions.—Long-term fluoroquinolone use to prevent unnecessary prostate biopsy may result in postbiopsy sepsis caused by fluoroquinolone resistant microorganisms.

▶ The rate of sepsis following prostate biopsy appears to be increasing, and the primary etiology is the increased prevalence of quinolone-resistant organisms in the fecal flora. This article adds to the evidence that prior fluoroquinolone (FQ) use increases the risk of sepsis following a prostate needle biopsy. FQ antibiotics may be administered to treat a clinical infection or to potentially reduce prostate-specific antigen values in asymptomatic patients with suspected or documented prostatic inflammation. The use of antibiotics for the latter indication does not appear to be efficacious[1] and should be discouraged. We currently do not know how long it takes the fecal flora to return to normal after FQ administration, but FQ treatment within the preceding 3 months appears to be a reasonable reason to either defer prostate biopsy or to broaden the empiric antimicrobial coverage if a biopsy is performed. Furthermore, sepsis after a prostate biopsy should be assumed to be a result of quinolone-resistant organisms and should be managed as such until culture data become available.

J. Q. Clemens, MD

Reference

1. Stopiglia RM, Ferreira U, Silva MM Jr, Matheus WE, Denardi F, Reis LO. Prostate specific antigen decrease and prostate cancer diagnosis: antibiotic versus placebo prospective randomized clinical trial. *J Urol.* 2010;183:940-945.

Prostate Specific Antigen Decrease and Prostate Cancer Diagnosis: Antibiotic Versus Placebo Prospective Randomized Clinical Trial
Stopiglia RM, Ferreira U, Silva MM Jr, et al (State Univ of Campinas — UNICAMP, Brazil)
J Urol 183:940-945, 2010

Purpose.—Prostate inflammation can lead to an increase in serum prostate specific antigen concentration and confound the use of prostate specific antigen kinetics. Repeat prostate specific antigen measurements after a period of observation or a course of empirical antibiotics are controversial in terms of the optimal approach to reduce the confounding impact on prostate cancer screening. This issue was analyzed in patients with a diagnosis of type IV or asymptomatic prostatitis (National Institutes of Health classification) and high prostate specific antigen.

Materials and Methods.—We studied 200 men between 50 and 75 years old with a high prostate specific antigen (between 2.5 and 10 ng/dl). Of these patients 98 (49%) had a diagnosis of type IV prostatitis. In a prospective, double-blind trial they were randomized to receive placebo (49 patients, group 1) or 500 mg ciprofloxacin (49 patients, group 2) twice a day for 4 weeks. Prostate specific antigen was determined after treatment and all patients underwent transrectal ultrasound guided biopsy of the prostate.

Results.—In group 1, 29 (59.18%) patients presented with a decrease in prostate specific antigen and 9 (31%) had cancer on biopsy, while in group 2 there were 26 (53.06%) patients with a decrease in prostate specific antigen and 7 (26.9%) with prostate cancer. There was no statistical difference in either group in relation to prostate specific antigen decrease after treatment or the presence of tumor.

Conclusions.—A considerable number of patients (49%) were diagnosed with type IV prostatitis and high prostate specific antigen in agreement with the current literature. Of the patients 26.9% to 31% presented with a decrease in prostate specific antigen after the use of antibiotic or placebo and harbor cancer as demonstrated on prostate biopsy. Prostate specific antigen decreases do not indicate the absence of prostate cancer.

▶ It is well documented that prostate-specific antigen (PSA) is an imperfect test due to its lack of specificity for the detection of prostate cancer. One reason for this is that prostatic inflammation (type IV prostatitis) may cause PSA values to be elevated. In men with documented type IV prostatitis, it has been a common practice to administer antimicrobials to treat the prostatic inflammation/infection, with the expectation that this may reduce PSA levels and prevent unnecessary prostate biopsies. This study calls that practice into question. Other investigations of asymptomatic men have found that PSA levels decrease slightly and to a similar degree with either antimicrobial administration or with observation.[1] These findings suggest that a prudent approach may be to obtain a repeat PSA measurement after at least a 4-week interval in patients suspected of having prostatic inflammation as the cause of a PSA elevation. Treatment with a nonsteroidal anti-inflammatory agent might also make intuitive sense, although I am not aware of evidence regarding the efficacy of these agents in reducing PSA levels.

J. Q. Clemens, MD

Reference

1. Heldwein FL, Teloken PE, Hartmann AA, Rhoden EL, Teloken C. Antibiotics and observation have a similar impact on asymptomatic patients with a raised PSA. *BJU Int.* 2011;107:1576-1581.

24 Hypogonadism

Changes in Prostate Specific Antigen in Hypogonadal Men After 12 Months of Testosterone Replacement Therapy: Support for the Prostate Saturation Theory
Khera M, Bhattacharya RK, Blick G, et al (Baylor College of Medicine, Houston, TX; Univ of Kansas Med Ctr; Circle Med LLC, Norwalk, CT; et al)
J Urol 186:1005-1011, 2011

Purpose.—We measured prostate specific antigen after 12 months of testosterone replacement therapy in hypogonadal men.

Materials and Methods.—Data were collected from the TRiUS (Testim® Registry in the United States), an observational registry of hypogonadal men on testosterone replacement therapy (849). Participants were Testim naïve, had no prostate cancer and received 5 to 10 gm Testim 1% (testosterone gel) daily.

Results.—A total of 451 patients with prostate specific antigen and total testosterone values were divided into group A (197 with total testosterone less than 250 ng/dl) and group B (254 with total testosterone 250 ng/dl or greater). The groups differed significantly in free testosterone and sex hormone-binding globulin, but not in age or prostate specific antigen. In group A but not group B prostate specific antigen correlated significantly with total testosterone ($r = 0.20$, $p = 0.005$), free testosterone ($r = 0.22$, $p = 0.03$) and sex hormone-binding globulin ($r = 0.59$, $p = 0.002$) at baseline. After 12 months of testosterone replacement therapy, increase in total testosterone (mean ± SD) was statistically significant in group A ($+326 \pm 295$ ng/dl, $p < 0.001$; final total testosterone 516 ± 28 ng/dl) and group B ($+154 \pm 217$ ng/dl, $p < 0.001$; final total testosterone 513 ± 20 ng/dl). After 12 months of testosterone replacement therapy, increase in prostate specific antigen was statistically significant in group A ($+0.19 \pm 0.61$ ng/ml, $p = 0.02$; final prostate specific antigen 1.26 ± 0.96 ng/ml) but not in group B ($+0.28 \pm 1.18$ ng/ml, $p = 0.06$; final prostate specific antigen 1.55 ± 1.72 ng/ml). The average percent prostate specific antigen increase from baseline was higher in group A (21.9%) than in group B (14.1%). Overall the greatest prostate specific antigen was observed after 1 month of treatment and decreased thereafter.

Conclusions.—Patients with baseline total testosterone less than 250 ng/dl were more likely to have an increased prostate specific antigen after testosterone replacement therapy than those with baseline total testosterone

250 ng/dl or greater, supporting the prostate saturation hypothesis. Clinicians should be aware that severely hypogonadal patients may experience increased prostate specific antigen after testosterone replacement therapy.

▶ Optimal use of testosterone replacement therapy requires close attention to the risk for prostate cancer development/progression and changes in prostate-specific antigen (PSA). The traditional dogma that testosterone causes prostate cancer has not been well supported, but concern for patient well-being and defensive medical practice warrant close attention to prostate issues in men receiving supplemental androgen therapy for hypogonadism. The "saturation hypothesis" of Morgentaler suggests that supplementation of testosterone beyond a very low baseline level does not meaningfully alter prostate cancer/PSA growth.

This retrospective review of men taking supplemental testosterone by Khera et al attempts to provide further evidence for the saturation hypothesis. Men with baseline total testosterone less than 250 ng/dL were more likely to have significant changes in serum PSA 12 months after beginning testosterone therapy. Men with baseline testosterone did not have a statistically significant change in PSA at 12-month follow-up; however, the change in PSA approached significance with a P value of 0.06 for change; it seems likely that inclusion of a few more data points might have shifted this group into the "strictly" significant category.

Whether 250 ng/dL represents an optimal cutpoint is not at this time clear, but this is an important step toward intelligent risk stratification and patient notification when beginning testosterone therapy.

A. W. Shindel, MD

25 Voiding Dysfunction/ Enuresis

Doxazosin Versus Tizanidine for Treatment of Dysfunctional Voiding in Children: A Prospective Randomized Open-Labeled Trial
El-Hefnawy AS, Helmy T, El-Assmy MM, et al (Mansoura Univ, Egypt)
Urology 79:428-433, 2012

Objective.—To examine the efficacy and tolerability of tizanidine for the treatment of dysfunctional voiding in children compared with those of doxazosin.

Methods.—A total of 40 children with dysfunctional voiding were enrolled in a prospective, randomized, 2-parallel group, flexible-dose study. The evaluations were performed in accordance with the International Children's Continence Society guidelines. The children were followed up after 1 week and then monthly for 6 months for the clinical, urine culture, and urodynamic parameters. The degree of improvement was assessed using a satisfaction scale that ranged from 0 (no improvement at all) to 10 (total improvement).

Results.—A total of 40 patients with a mean ± SD age of 7 ± 2.6 years were enrolled. The clinical and urodynamic parameters were comparable between both groups. At the last follow-up visit, both groups had had similar improvement in the severity of symptoms, satisfaction scale, and noninvasive flowmetry parameters. In the doxazosin group, urge episodes was the only symptom that showed a significant reduction compared with the baseline values ($P = .028$). However, the incidence of nocturnal enuresis, urgency attacks, and daytime incontinence were significantly reduced compared with baseline in the tizanidine group ($P = .003$, $P = .008$, and $P = .017$, respectively). Adverse effects were recorded in 6 patients (15%). Epigasteric pain was reported in 2 children (10%) who received doxazosin. In the tizanidine group, a loss of appetite was noted in 2 children (10%), epigastric pain in 1 (5%), and headache in 1 (5%).

Conclusion.—Tizanidine could be a safe and effective treatment of children with dysfunctional voiding due to pelvic floor/skeletal sphincter dysfunction. More placebo-controlled trails with larger sample sizes are needed.

▶ The authors compare a muscle relaxant (imidazoline) with an alpha-adrenergic blocker (doxazosin) in the management of detrusor sphincter dyssynergia (DSD) and incomplete bladder emptying. Alpha-blockers are used in the treatment of bladder outlet obstruction in adult males. DSD in children most commonly involves the external sphincter and less commonly the bladder neck. Doxazosin (the control) has been previously evaluated in the treatment of DSD, and no definite benefit has been shown in randomized trials. The 0.5 mg dose of doxazosin used in this trial is likely too low to evaluate efficacy. The skeletal muscle relaxant seems to have an effect when compared to the α-blocker, but the improvement in voiding symptoms may have been impacted by the use of oxybutynin in two-thirds of patients.

D. E. Coplen, MD

Animated Biofeedback: An Ideal Treatment for Children With Dysfunctional Elimination Syndrome
Kajbafzadeh AM, Sharifi-Rad L, Ghahestani SM, et al (Children's Hosp Med Ctr, Tehran, Iran; Univ of Med Sciences, Tehran, Iran)
J Urol 186:2379-2385, 2011

Purpose.—Animated biofeedback is an established treatment for pediatric dysfunctional voiding. Bowel dysfunction is closely associated with dysfunctional voiding. We evaluated the efficacy of animated biofeedback urotherapy in bowel and voiding dysfunction in children with dysfunctional elimination syndrome.

Materials and Methods.—A total of 80 children with dysfunctional elimination syndrome were randomly assigned to undergo animated biofeedback (group A, 40 patients) or conservative therapy (group B, 40 patients). Group A underwent animated biofeedback along with pelvic floor muscle exercises and behavioral modification (hydration, high fiber diet, scheduled voiding). Group B underwent behavioral modification only. Dysfunctional voiding symptom score, constipation and fecal soiling episodes per week (according to Paris Consensus on Childhood Constipation Terminology criteria), and uroflowmetry parameters were evaluated before and 6 and 12 months after treatment in both groups.

Results.—Subjective and objective voiding problems were significantly improved. Vesicoureteral reflux resolved in 7 of 9 children (78%) and urinary tract infection did not recur in 10 of 14 children (71%) within 1 year. Bladder capacity and voided volume did not significantly improve. Post-void residual and voiding time decreased considerably, while maximum and average urine flow increased significantly. All children with fecal soiling and 17 of 25 with constipation (68%) in group A were symptom-free within 1 year after treatment. Animated biofeedback therapy was more efficient than nonbiofeedback management regarding objective and subjective voiding problems and bowel dysfunction ($p < 0.05$).

Conclusions.—Animated biofeedback effectively treats bowel and voiding dysfunction in children with dysfunctional voiding. Pelvic floor muscle exercises coordinate breathing and pelvic floor muscle contractions, and are beneficial in improving bowel dysfunction.

▶ The authors compare animated biofeedback and standard behavioral therapy in the management of voiding dysfunction. These approaches should give a more durable response than urethral dilation (mostly historical), botulinum toxin (some utility in neurogenic with sphincter dyssynergia), and smooth (alpha blocker) or skeletal (baclofen) muscle relaxants. Patients were maintained on antibiotics for reflux but were not started on anticholinergics because of potential exacerbation of constipation that might alter response. The figure in the original article shows the marked improvement (decrease) in pelvic floor electromyogram activity that can be observed after successful treatment. There was improvement in voiding parameters in both treatment arms (up to 50% of patients in the control arm), although animation resulted in a larger improvement in all parameters measured. There was not continued improvement after active therapy stopped, but the improvements were durable. Since animated biofeedback is more time intensive and expensive, identification of parameters predictive of a poor response to behavioral modification is important in directing therapy.

D. E. Coplen, MD

Is the Screening Method of Sacral Neuromodulation a Prognostic Factor for Long-Term Success?

Marcelissen T, Leong R, Serroyen J, et al (Maastricht Univ Med Centre, The Netherlands; Univ of Maastricht, The Netherlands)
J Urol 185:583-587, 2011

Purpose.—We evaluated whether there is a difference in long-term outcomes between patients screened with percutaneous nerve evaluation and a first stage tined lead procedure. We also evaluated the outcome in patients who only responded to screening with the tined lead procedure after failed initial percutaneous nerve evaluation.

Materials and Methods.—We evaluated all patients screened for eligibility to receive sacral neuromodulation treatment since the introduction of the tined lead technique in our center in 2002. In May 2009 all implanted patients were asked to maintain a voiding diary to record the effect of sacral neuromodulation on urinary symptoms. Chi-square analysis was used to evaluate differences in the long-term outcomes of the separate screening methods.

Results.—A total of 92 patients were screened for sacral neuromodulation. Of the 76 patients screened with percutaneous nerve evaluation 35 (46%) met the criteria for permanent implantation. In 11 of the 16 patients (69%) who underwent direct screening with the tined lead procedure permanent stimulators were placed. Of the 41 patients in whom percutaneous nerve evaluation failed and who subsequently underwent screening with tined lead procedure 18 (44%) were implanted with a neurostimulator after a successful response. Statistical analysis showed no difference between screening type and long-term success ($p = 0.94$).

Conclusions.—The first stage tined lead procedure is a more sensitive screening tool than percutaneous nerve evaluation but long-term success seems to be independent of the screening method. Patients in whom percutaneous nerve evaluation initially failed but who responded to prolonged screening the with tined lead procedure appeared to be as successful as those who directly responded to percutaneous nerve evaluation or the tined lead procedure.

▶ Patients who are candidates for a sacral neuromodulation tril can undergo test stimulation either using the percutaneous nerve evaluation (PNE) technique or with a so-called staged technique. The PNE test is typically performed in the office setting, with or without fluoroscopic guidance. After a needle is placed through the S3 sacral foramen, the tiny PNE electrode is then passed through the needle and is taped to the skin. Given the size and the limited tissue attachments provided by the PNE electrode, it is typically only tested for a period of 3 to 5 days. If PNE testing is successful, a permanent lead and battery are subsequently placed surgically for long-term stimulation. The staged test involves fluoroscopic placement of the permanent tined lead in the operating room as the first step, with attachment of a percutaneous extension wire for external test stimulation (stage I). Given the more robust attachments of the tined lead, staged test stimulation can be performed for up to 4 weeks. If the stage I test is successful, the tined lead is kept in place and attached to an implanted subcutaneous battery (stage II). Of note, if a patient has an unsuccessful PNE test, he or she may proceed to a staged test.

Although the PNE test is convenient for many patients, it has demonstrated a lower test response rate than staged testing. Furthermore, it is possible that the PNE test stimulation and the subsequent permanent stimulation may yield different results, as the PNE lead is removed after the testing and is replaced with a different, permanent lead during the implantation surgery. In this retrospective study, the authors found that the outcomes were similar regardless of the initial testing strategy. In other words, some patients responded to initial PNE testing and underwent implantation, while others did not respond to PNE testing and went on to a staged test. The eventual outcomes (number of implants, symptoms response) in the patients who were initially tested using the PNE approach were equivalent to those who had an initial staged test performed. This is reassuring and suggests that the initial sacral neuromodulation testing approach can be guided by patient and clinician preferences rather than variability in outcomes.

J. Q. Clemens, MD

Behavioral Versus Drug Treatment for Overactive Bladder in Men: The Male Overactive Bladder Treatment in Veterans (MOTIVE) Trial

Burgio KL, Goode PS, Johnson TM II, et al (Education and Clinical Ctr, Birmingham, AL; et al)
J Am Geriatr Soc 59:2209-2216, 2011

Objectives.—To compare the effectiveness of behavioral treatment with that of antimuscarinic therapy in men without bladder outlet obstruction who continue to have overactive bladder (OAB) symptoms with alpha-blocker therapy.

Design.—The Male Overactive Bladder Treatment in Veterans (MOTIVE) Trial was a two-site randomized, controlled, equivalence trial with 4-week alpha-blocker run-in.

Setting.—Veterans Affairs Medical Center outpatient clinics.

Participants.—Volunteer sample of 143 men aged 42 to 88 who continued to have urgency and more than eight voids per day, with or without incontinence, after run-in.

Interventions.—Participants were randomized to 8 weeks of behavioral treatment (pelvic floor muscle exercises, urge suppression techniques, delayed voiding) or drug therapy (individually titrated, extended-release oxybutynin, 5–30 mg/d).

Measurements.—Seven-day bladder diaries and a validated urgency scale were used to calculate changes in 24-hour voiding frequency, nocturia, urgency, and incontinence. Secondary outcomes were global patient ratings and American Urological Association Symptom Index.

Results.—Mean voids per day decreased from 11.3 to 9.1 (−18.8%) with behavioral treatment and 11.5 to 9.5 (−16.9%) with drug therapy. Equivalence analysis indicated that posttreatment means were equivalent ($P < .01$). After treatment, 85% of participants rated themselves as much better or better; more than 90% were completely or somewhat satisfied, with no between group differences. The behavioral group showed greater reductions in nocturia (mean $= -0.70$ vs -0.32 episodes/night; $P = .05$). The drug group showed greater reductions in maximum urgency scores (mean $= -0.44$ vs -0.12; $P = .02$). Other between-group differences were nonsignificant.

Conclusion.—Behavioral and antimuscarinic therapy are effective when added to alpha-blocker therapy for OAB in men without outlet obstruction. Behavioral treatment is at least as effective as antimuscarinic therapy.

▶ It is still surprising how few studies have looked at behavioral therapy for the treatment of lower urinary tract symptoms in men. In this well-done randomized trial, drug therapy was as effective as behavioral therapy, which included pelvic floor muscle training, delayed voiding, and urge suppression techniques as well as fluid moderation for the treatment of nocturia. The results were not surprising in that several trials have demonstrated that behavioral therapy can be as effective as drug therapy in women. There is a modest increment of improvement when these 2 therapies are combined, which was not looked at in this particular study. It is notable that all the men in this trial were on α-blocker therapy at entry, so it is unclear whether the results would be applicable to men not already on such therapy. Finally, the authors attempted to exclude men with bladder outlet obstruction using uroflowmetry and postvoid residuals. However, such testing cannot definitively exclude bladder outlet obstruction, because the only test that allows for such a diagnosis is a simultaneous pressure-flow urodynamics study. Thus, such an exclusion is a limitation of this study, because we do not know whether these individuals were actually obstructed.

E. S. Rovner, MD

Efficacy and Safety of Low Doses of OnabotulinumtoxinA for the Treatment of Refractory Idiopathic Overactive Bladder: A Multicentre, Double-Blind, Randomised, Placebo-Controlled Dose-Ranging Study
Denys P, for the VESITOX study group in France (Univ of Versailles Saint Quentin, France; et al)
Eur Urol 61:520-529, 2012

Background.—In the treatment of patients with idiopathic overactive bladder (iOAB), high doses of botulinum toxin type A (BoNTA) were often associated with complications resulting from high postvoid residuals (PVR), leading to clean intermittent catheterisation (CIC) and urinary tract infections (UTI).

Objective.—Evaluate the efficacy and tolerability of low doses of onabotulinumtoxinA compared to placebo in patients with iOAB.

Design, Setting, and Participants.—Between 2005 and 2009, adults with persistent iOAB were included in a prospective, randomised, double-blind, placebo-controlled comparative trial.

Intervention.—Patients were randomised to undergo a single intradetrusor injection procedure of either placebo or onabotulinumtoxinA (50 U, 100 U or 150 U).

Measurements.—The initial evaluations (ie, clinical and urodynamic variables as well as quality of life [QoL]) were repeated at day 8 and months 1, 3, 5, and 6.

Results and Limitations.—Ninety-nine patients were included in the efficacy analysis. Three months after the procedure, we observed >50% improvement versus baseline in urgency and urge urinary incontinence (UUI) in 65% and 56% of patients who respectively received 100 U ($p = 0.086$) and 150 U ($p = 0.261$) BoNTA injections and >75% improvement in 40% of patients of both groups (100 U [$p = 0.058$] and 150 U [$p = 0.022$]). Complete continence was observed in 55% and 50% patients after 100 U and 150 U BoNTA treatment, respectively, at month 3. Frequency symptoms and QoL improved up to the 6-mo visit. We observed only three patients with a PVR >200 ml in the 150 U group and a few UTIs.

Conclusions.—100 U and 150 U BoNTA injections were well tolerated and have both shown to improve symptoms and QoL in patients with iOAB. Nevertheless, 100 U injections showed a reasonable efficacy, with a lower risk of high PVR.

Trial Registration.—ClinicalTrials.gov NCT00231491.

▶ This is a well-done randomized controlled trial examining onabotulinumtoxinA in idiopathic overactive bladder in patients who have failed prior therapy. This dose-ranging study suggests that 50 U is an inadequate dose in this patient population, whereas the 2 higher doses (100 or 150 U) are both efficacious. The intervention was well tolerated, with a total of 9 patients requiring intermittent catheterization at some point in this study, and 1 of these was in the placebo group. These data strongly suggest that onabotulinumtoxinA at a dose of 100 or 150 U is a reasonable treatment for refractory idiopathic overactive bladder. Several other large-scale multicenter trials examining this agent in the treatment of idiopathic overactive bladder are ongoing. If similar results are seen in these studies, then regulatory approval for this agent in idiopathic overactive bladder should be forthcoming as this agent is already approved for neurogenic detrusor overactivity-related incontinence.

E. S. Rovner, MD

26 Imaging

Diagnostic Yield of CT Urography in the Evaluation of Young Adults With Hematuria
Lokken RP, Sadow CA, Silverman SG (Brigham and Women's Hosp, Boston, MA)
AJR Am J Roentgenol 198:609-615, 2012

Objective.—CT urography is increasingly used as the initial imaging test in patients with hematuria. The aim of our study was to determine the yield of CT urography in young adults with hematuria to see whether single phase unenhanced CT would have been sufficient.

Materials and Methods.—We reviewed medical records of consecutive patients undergoing CT urography between March 2000 and July 2009 at our tertiary medical center. Of 5400 CT urograms performed, 375 (6.9%) in 359 patients aged 40 years or younger with hematuria were included in the study. Urographic findings were tabulated according to their clinical significance. CT images were reviewed to see whether contrast-enhanced images were necessary for diagnosis.

Results.—A clinically significant source was found in 83 of 375 examinations (22.1%), including 42 of 142 (29.6%) for gross hematuria, 29 of 181 (16.0%) for microscopic hematuria, and 12 of 52 (23.1%) for hematuria of unspecified subtype. The most common clinically significant findings were renal or ureteral calculi ($n = 73$ [75.3%]); four malignancies were also detected. Ninety-two (94.8%) of 97 clinically significant findings were evident on unenhanced images. All significant findings that required contrast-enhanced images for diagnosis occurred in patients with predisposing medical conditions.

Conclusion.—A clinically significant source of hematuria was detected in 22.1% of CT urograms of young adults. However, an unenhanced CT alone may be sufficient in patients without additional predisposing medical conditions, thereby reducing radiation dose in this radiosensitive population.

▶ The American Urological Association and American College of Radiology recommend upper tract imaging in adults with hematuria. Patients with gross hematuria are more likely to have malignancy than those with microscopic hematuria. The vast majority of "clinically significant" lesions were stones (57/83-69%) that would clearly not require intravenous contrast for diagnosis and likely not contribute to formulation of a treatment plan. Only 1 renal cancer and no urothelial malignancies were identified in this young population. Three other nonurothelial or renal cancers were identified. Many of the insignificant findings could likely have been identified using the medical history in conjunction with ultrasound. There were 12 false positives on the contrast images that led to cystoscopic evaluation or additional imaging exposure and expense. It is true that CT urography is more sensitive than excretory urography in detection of renal masses and urothelial cancer, but it is clear that intravenous contrast is not required for a younger population with a known lower prevalence of abnormalities.

D. E. Coplen, MD

Prospective Measurement of Patient Exposure to Radiation During Pediatric Ureteroscopy
Kokorowski PJ, Chow JS, Strauss K, et al (Harvard Med School, Boston, MA)
J Urol 187:1408-1415, 2012

Purpose.—Few data have been reported regarding radiation exposure during pediatric endourological procedures, including ureteroscopy. We measured radiation exposure during pediatric ureteroscopy and identify opportunities for exposure reduction.

Materials and Methods.—We prospectively observed ureteroscopy procedures as part of a quality improvement initiative. Preoperative patient characteristics, operative factors, fluoroscopy settings and radiation exposure were recorded. Our outcomes were entrance skin dose and midline dose (both mGy). Specific modifiable factors were identified as targets for potential quality improvement.

Results.—Direct observation was performed in 54 consecutive ureteroscopy procedures. Mean ± SD patient age was 14.8 ± 3.8 years (range 7.4 to 19.2), with 9 children being younger than 12 years. Mean ± SD entrance skin dose was 46.4 ± 48 mGy. Mean ± SD midline dose was 6.2 ± 5.0 mGy. The most important major determinant of radiation dose was total fluoroscopy time (mean ± SD 2.68 ± 1.8 minutes) followed by dose rate setting, child anteroposterior diameter and source to skin distance (all $p < 0.01$). Analysis of factors affecting exposure levels revealed that use of ureteral access sheaths ($p = 0.01$) and retrograde pyelography ($p = 0.04$) were significantly associated with fluoroscopy time. We also found that dose rate settings were higher than recommended in up to 43% of cases and ideal C-arm positioning could have reduced exposure by 14% (up to 49% in some cases).

Conclusions.—Children receive biologically significant radiation doses during ureteroscopy procedures. Several modifiable factors contribute to dose and could be targeted in efforts to implement dose reduction strategies.

▶ Children are particularly vulnerable to ionizing radiation. There is significant emphasis on decreasing the use of computerized tomography (CT) in the evaluation of children with symptoms suspicious for urolithiasis. Ureteroscopic stone management is increasingly popular, and reduction of fluoroscopic radiation exposure is another potential quality improvement. In this study, the average radiation exposure (46.4 mGy) exceeds that of 2 stone protocol CTs.

The author's data suggest several potential ways to reduce radiation exposure. Fluoroscopy time is clearly a key component of exposure. Setting an alarm to prompt the surgeon regarding exposure time (20-second increments) and reporting the total exposure to the surgeon at the end of the procedure will increase awareness and may change practice patterns. The image intensifier (not the source) should be as close to the patient as possible. The machine dose rate settings should be matched to the patient size. Additionally, high-definition images are not required for most of the manipulations performed during ureteroscopy (eg, guide wire passage, flexible scope placement, stent placement). Systematic investigation of current practices is important not only in the pediatric population.[1] Patient outcomes can be preserved while minimizing radiation exposure.

D. E. Coplen, MD

Reference

1. Lipkin ME, Wang AJ, Toncheva G, Ferrandino MN, Yoshizumi TT, Preminger GM. Determination of patient radiation dose during ureteroscopic treatment of urolithiasis using a validated model. *J Urol.* 2012;187:920-924.

27 Pediatric Imaging

The Efficacy of Oral Midazolam for Decreasing Anxiety in Children Undergoing Voiding Cystourethrogram: A Randomized, Double-Blind, Placebo Controlled Study
Ferguson GG, Chen C, Yan Y, et al (Washington Univ School of Medicine, St Louis, MO)
J Urol 185:2542-2546, 2011

Purpose.—Voiding cystourethrogram is an invasive test that evokes anxiety. Our primary aim was to determine whether midazolam is beneficial in decreasing anxiety in children who undergo voiding cystourethrogram. Secondary aims were an examination of parent anxiety, health care professional perceptions and post-procedure behavioral outcomes in children after voiding cystourethrogram.

Materials and Methods. A total of 44 children were randomized to placebo or oral midazolam before voiding cystourethrogram in double-blind fashion. The Modified Yale Preoperative Anxiety Scale was used to evaluate child behavior before and during voiding cystourethrogram, and the Post Hospitalization Behavior Questionnaire was used to investigate any short-term and intermediate-term behavioral outcomes. The State-Trait Anxiety Inventory was used to evaluate parent personal anxiety during voiding cystourethrogram. A separate questionnaire was administered to radiology staff. Statistical analysis included the 2-sample t and Fisher exact tests.

Results.—There was no difference in Modified Yale Preoperative Anxiety Scale scores in children randomized to midazolam or placebo. There was also no significant difference in parent anxiety. Radiology care providers identified no reliable benefit when blinded to sedation vs placebo. We did not note any post-procedural behavior issues after voiding cystourethrogram at up to 6 months of followup.

Conclusions.—Midazolam may not significantly help with child or parent anxiety during voiding cystourethrogram. No reliable benefit was noted according to radiology health care provider perception and there was no significant post-procedural behavior benefit. Midazolam may not provide a significant benefit in decreasing anxiety during voiding cystourethrogram.

▶ Detection of reflux currently requires urethral catheterization for a voiding cystourethrogram. Families prefer either a noninvasive test (thermography is being studied) or no testing at all. For the pediatric urologist, informed and selective testing for detection of reflux is required because of changing concepts regarding the indications for testing (pediatric reference) after UTI and parental reluctance to proceed with a voiding cystourethrogram. Hypnosis, topical anesthetics, oral sedatives, and inhalational anesthetics have been utilized to decrease the discomfort and stress associated with the test. Midazolam is the drug most commonly used for sedation during medical procedures. Because of the difficulty in recruiting patients, this study is underpowered to show a difference between treatment arms. Based on this and other studies, sedation should be selectively used in children undergoing cystogram (prior exposure or experience with testing, complex anatomy with anticipated difficult catheterization, significant behavioral issues, etc).

D. E. Coplen, MD

28 Pediatric Laparoscopy/ Reconstruction

Endoscopic Management and the Role of Double Stenting for Primary Obstructive Megaureters
Christman MS, Kasturi S, Lambert SM, et al (Children's Hosp of Philadelphia, PA; Perelman School of Medicine at the Univ of Pennsylvania, Philadelphia)
J Urol 187:1018-1023, 2012

Purpose.—We determined the efficacy and potential complications of endoscopic incision and balloon dilation with double stenting for the treatment of primary obstructive megaureter in children.

Materials and Methods.—We prospectively reviewed cases of primary obstructive megaureter requiring repair due to pyelonephritis, renal calculi and/or loss of renal function. A total of 17 patients were identified as candidates for endoscopy. Infants were excluded from study. All patients underwent cystoscopy and retrograde ureteropyelography to start the procedure. In segments less than 2 cm balloon dilation was performed, and for those 2 to 3 cm laser incision was added. Two ureteral stents were placed within the ureter simultaneously and left indwelling for 8 weeks. Imaging was performed 3 months after stent removal and repeated 2 years following intervention.

Results.—Mean patient age was 7.0 years (range 3 to 12). Of the patients 12 had marked improvement of hydroureteronephrosis on renal and bladder ultrasound. The remaining 5 patients had some improvement on renal and bladder ultrasound, and underwent magnetic resonance urography revealing no evidence of obstruction. All patients were followed for at least 2 years postoperatively and were noted to be symptom-free with stable imaging during the observation period.

Conclusions.—Endoscopic management appears to be an alternative to reimplantation for primary obstructive megaureter with a narrowed segment shorter than 3 cm. Double stenting seems to be effective in maintaining patency of the neo-orifice. Followup into adolescence is needed.

▶ Ureterovesical (UVJ) obstruction secondary to a distal aperistaltic segment is the second most common site of congenital upper tract obstruction. Ipsilateral renal function is usually reasonably normal. This is likely secondary to capacitance from the markedly dilated ureter. Over 90% of prenatally identified UVJ obstructions (megaureters) spontaneously improve. Endoscopic management of neonates or infants has not been successful, likely related to technical issues with instrumentation and stent size. The authors report on endoscopic management for older children with UVJ obstruction. There is no mention as to whether the children had been followed expectantly or if they presented symptomatically at an older age. As such it is unknown if there was loss of function or if these patients (15 of 17) had stable diminished function since birth.

An endoscopic approach was technically feasible in all patients. It is unknown if a failure would increase the complexity of tapered reimplantation either acutely or after healing and development of some periureteral scarring. The prompt improvement in dilation is a bit surprising, given the chronicity (mean age 7 years). Dilation did not significantly improve in 5 patients, although drainage was improved on MR urogram. In older children with megaureter, an endoscopic approach is a reasonable alternative that is less morbid and likely does not preclude subsequent successful reimplantation.

D. E. Coplen, MD

Prospective Long-term Analysis of Nerve-sparing Extravesical Robotic-assisted Laparoscopic Ureteral Reimplantation
Kasturi S, Sehgal SS, Christman MS, et al (Hosp of the Univ of Pennsylvania, Philadelphia; Children's Hosp of Philadelphia, PA)
Urology 79:680-683, 2012

Objective.—To prospectively review our experience with extravesical robotic-assisted laparoscopic ureteral reimplantation to determine whether postoperative voiding dysfunction can be avoided with pelvic plexus visualization and to assess the efficacy of this approach for the treatment of vesicoureteral reflux (VUR).

Methods.—We prospectively followed 150 patients who underwent bilateral extravesical robotic-assisted laparoscopic ureteral reimplantation by a single surgeon at an academic institution. Each patient was followed for a 2-year period. All 150 patients had primary VUR of grade 3 or greater bilaterally, with 127 having parenchymal defects found on renal scans. All patients were toilet trained before surgical intervention. The operation was performed with an extravesical transperitoneal approach with robotic assistance using the daVinci Surgical System. All patients underwent voiding cystourethrography at 3 months postoperatively to document the resolution of VUR. Voiding dysfunction was assessed in each patient by uroflow, postvoid residual urine volume, and a validated questionnaire.

Results.—The operative success rate was 99.3% for VUR resolution on voiding cystourethrography. One patient with bilateral grade 5 VUR that was downgraded to unilateral grade 2 VUR was considered to have treatment failure. This patient ultimately underwent subsequent subureteral injection therapy after an episode of pyelonephritis. No patient experienced de novo voiding dysfunction.

Conclusion.—Bilateral nerve-sparing robotic-assisted extravesical reimplantation has the same success rate as the traditional open approaches, with minimal morbidity and no voiding complications in our series.

▶ This is a large case series of bilateral extravesical ureteral reimplantation. Notably, there was no postoperative voiding dysfunction that can rarely occur after bilateral detrusorrhaphy. The authors claim that the visualization of the pelvic plexus is the key to elimination of postoperative voiding dysfunction. Similar success can be obtained with open surgery and similar overnight or short-stay hospitalization. Whether robotic reimplantation is cost effective cannot be determined from this study.

D. E. Coplen, MD

29 Pediatric Urinary Tract Infection

Acute Tc-99m DMSA Scan for Identifying Dilating Vesicoureteral Reflux in Children: A Meta-analysis
Mantadakis E, Vouloumanou EK, Georgantzi GG, et al (Democritus Univ of Thrace and Univ General Hosp of Alexandroupolis, Thrace, Greece; Alfa Inst of Biomedical Sciences (AIBS), Athens, Greece)
Pediatrics 128:e169-e179, 2011

Controversy exists regarding the type and/or sequence of imaging studies needed during the first febrile urinary tract infection (UTI) in young children. Several investigators have claimed that because acute-phase Tc-99m dimercaptosuccinic acid (DMSA) renal-scan results are abnormal in the presence of dilating vesicoureteral reflux, a normal DMSA-scan result makes voiding cystourethrography (VCUG) unnecessary in the primary examination of infants with UTI. To evaluate the accuracy of acute-phase DMSA scanning in identifying dilating (grades III through V) vesicoureteral reflux documented by VCUG in children with a first febrile UTI, we performed a meta-analysis of the accuracy of diagnostic tests as reported from relevant studies identified through the PubMed and Scopus databases. Patient-based and renal unit–based analyses were performed. Overall, 13 cohort studies were identified. Nine studies involved patients younger than 2 years, 3 involved children aged 16 years or younger, and 1 involved exclusively neonates. Girls constituted 22% to 85% of the involved children. Pooled (95% confidence intervals) sensitivity and specificity rates of DMSA scanning were 79% and 53%, respectively, for the patient-based analysis (8 studies) and 60% and 65% for the renal unit–based analysis (5 studies). The respective areas under the hierarchical summary receiver operating curves were 0.71 and 0.67. Marked statistical heterogeneity was observed in both analyses, as indicated by I^2 test values of 91% and 87%, respectively. Acute-phase DMSA renal scanning cannot be recommended as replacement for VCUG in the evaluation of young children with a first febrile UTI.

▶ Historically, children with a febrile urinary tract infection (UTI) are evaluated with an ultrasound scan (US) and voiding cystourethrography (VCUG). The new AAP UTI guidelines recommend a VCUG only if a renal US is abnormal. Because US is not a sensitive predictor of reflux, this approach will not identify all high-grade reflux. In the alternative top-down approach, a dimercaptosuccinic acid (DMSA) scan is obtained in all children with a febrile UTI. A VCUG is obtained in children with a positive scan. This approach is not necessarily trying to identify patients with high-grade reflux but only those with clinically significant reflux. This meta-analysis shows that a positive DMSA scan has poor sensitivity for detection of grade III-V reflux. If one accepts the premise of the top-down approach, then the sensitivity and specificity for reflux detection are not important. The goal is to prevent renal scarring. The imaging of children with urinary tract infections is the subject of much debate. There is a subpopulation of children with reflux who have a normal US and normal DMSA scan and will have recurrent infections. Delay in diagnosis may not result in renal scarring but may subject the child and family to the morbidity of recurrent infections.

D. E. Coplen, MD

Randomized Trial of Oral Versus Sequential IV/Oral Antibiotic for Acute Pyelonephritis in Children

Bocquet N, Sergent Alaoui A, Jais J-P, et al (Hôpital Necker Enfants Malades, Paris, France; Hôpital Armand Trousseau, Paris, France; et al)
Pediatrics 129:e269-e275, 2012

Objective.—To confirm whether oral antibiotic treatment is as efficacious as sequential intravenous/oral antibiotic treatment in the prevention of renal scarring in children with acute pyelonephritis and scintigraphy-documented acute lesions.

Methods.—In a prospective multicenter trial, children aged 1 to 36 months with their first case of acute pyelonephritis, a serum procalcitonin concentration ≥ 0.5 ng/mL, no known uropathy, and a normal ultrasound exam were randomized into 2 treatment groups. They received either oral cefixime for 10 days or intravenous ceftriaxone for 4 days followed by oral cefixime for 6 days. Patients with acute renal lesions detected on early dimercaptosuccinic acid scintigraphy underwent a follow-up scintigraphy 6 to 8 months later.

Results.—The study included 171 infants and children. There were no significant differences between the 2 groups in any clinical characteristic. Initial scintigraphy results were abnormal for 119 children. Ninety-six children were measured for renal scarring at the follow-up scintigraphy (per protocol analysis population). The incidence of renal scarring was 30.8% in the oral treatment group and 27.3% for children who received the sequential treatment.

Conclusions.—Although this trial does not statistically demonstrate the noninferiority of oral treatment compared with the sequential treatment, our study confirmed the results of previously published reports and therefore supports the use of an oral antibiotic treatment of primary episodes of acute pyelonephritis in infants and young children (Fig 1).

▶ Hospital admissions are expensive and can be a major social issue for working parents. The authors compare oral and sequential antibiotic regimens

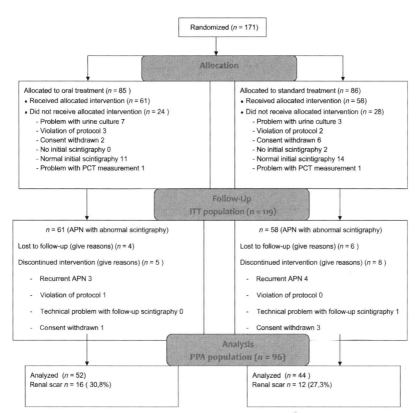

FIGURE 1.—Randomization and children flow chart. (Reprinted from Bocquet N, Sergent Alaoui A, Jais J-P, et al. Randomized Trial of Oral Versus Sequential IV/Oral Antibiotic for Acute Pyelonephritis in Children. *Pediatrics*. 2012;129:e269-e275, Copyright 2012, with permission from the American Academy of Pediatrics.)

in the treatment of acute pyelonephritis (confirmed by a positive DMSA [^{99m}Tc dimercaptosuccinic acid] scan). Children with abnormal sonography were excluded. A voiding cystourethrogram was eventually obtained, but reflux was not an inclusion or exclusion criteria. Fig 1 shows the randomization, flow, and outcomes of the children enrolled in the study. Only patients with elevated procalcitonin levels (>0.5 ng/mL) were included in the initial enrollment. Eighty-five percent of children had a positive DMSA. The study is not sufficiently powered to show that oral therapy is better, but there is little difference in the incidence of renal scarring at 8 months. In selected patients, oral antibiotic treatment of acute pyelonephritis is appropriate.

D. E. Coplen, MD

Urinary Tract Infection: Clinical Practice Guideline for the Diagnosis and Management of the Initial UTI in Febrile Infants and Children 2 to 24 months
Subcommittee on Urinary Tract Infection, Steering Committee on Quality Improvement and Management
Pediatrics 128:595-610, 2011

Objective.—To revise the American Academy of Pediatrics practice parameter regarding the diagnosis and management of initial urinary tract infections (UTIs) in febrile infants and young children.

Methods.—Analysis of the medical literature published since the last version of the guideline was supplemented by analysis of data provided by authors of recent publications. The strength of evidence supporting each recommendation and the strength of the recommendation were assessed and graded.

Results.—Diagnosis is made on the basis of the presence of both pyuria and at least 50 000 colonies per mL of a single uropathogenic organism in an appropriately collected specimen of urine. After 7 to 14 days of antimicrobial treatment, close clinical follow-up monitoring should be maintained to permit prompt diagnosis and treatment of recurrent infections. Ultrasonography of the kidneys and bladder should be performed to detect anatomic abnormalities. Data from the most recent 6 studies do not support the use of antimicrobial prophylaxis to prevent febrile recurrent UTI in infants without vesicoureteral reflux (VUR) or with grade I to IV VUR. Therefore, a voiding cystourethrography (VCUG) is not recommended routinely after the first UTI; VCUG is indicated if renal and bladder ultrasonography reveals hydronephrosis, scarring, or other findings that would suggest either high-grade VUR or obstructive uropathy and in other atypical or complex clinical circumstances. VCUG should also be performed if there is a recurrence of a febrile UTI. The recommendations in this guideline do not indicate an exclusive course of treatment or serve as a standard of care; variations may be appropriate. Recommendations about antimicrobial prophylaxis and implications for performance of VCUG are based on currently available evidence. As with all American Academy of Pediatrics clinical guidelines, the recommendations will be reviewed routinely and incorporate new evidence, such as data from the Randomized Intervention for Children With Vesicoureteral Reflux (RIVUR) study.

Conclusions.—Changes in this revision include criteria for the diagnosis of UTI and recommendations for imaging.

▶ The new American Academy of Pediatrics (AAP) urinary tract infections guidelines update guidelines previously issued in 1999. This guideline recommends selective testing for UTI in febrile children. Table 1 in the guideline delineates the probability of UTI. The AAP recommends a high index of suspicion and recognizes that urine samples should be obtained in many more children than will actually have a UTI (33/1). The rationale for this recommendation is prevention of scarring and other sequelae of UTI. There is no cookbook approach to evaluation, and there is a need to factor the severity of illness and the reliability of the care-givers to follow up.

The guidelines cite the good evidence that in most instances, oral antibiotics are as effective as parenteral therapy. Oral therapy should be utilized in the absence of clinical contraindications.

While the majority of renal anomalies are now detected with prenatal imaging, an ultrasound scan is still recommended after the first febrile UTI in all children. However, the current guideline states that if a renal ultrasound scan is normal, a VCUG should not be routinely obtained after a febrile UTI. However, most chil-dren with reflux have normal renal ultrasound scans. Additionally, a normal renal ultrasound scan does not exclude the presence of renal inflammation that poten-tially results in renal scarring.

There are 2 downsides to a VCUG. One is the discomfort associated with the test. The second is the identification and overtreatment of reflux. The guidelines committee concludes that detection is of little benefit. This is largely based on recent trials that show little to no benefit of antibiotic prophylaxis in low-grade reflux. However, children with high-grade reflux are at risk for recurrent infec-tions and, based on trials, are most likely to develop renal scarring and benefit from prophylaxis. The International Reflux Study found a similar incidence of scarring in the surgical and antibiotic arms, but surgery clearly decreased the incidence of febrile UTI.

It is clear that it is very unlikely that a 5-year-old with a first febrile urinary tract infection and a normal renal ultrasound scan has significant reflux. The natural history in this child reveals a low risk for UTI. A 3-month-old with bacteremia secondary to UTI should have a cystogram regardless of the ultrasound scan findings. If the VCUG is normal, the family is reassured. If reflux is identified, then the physician and family can ascertain risk and determine if antibiotic prophylaxis or observation is the best course of action.

D. E. Coplen, MD

Prediction of Moderate and High Grade Vesicoureteral Reflux After a First Febrile Urinary Tract Infection in Children: Construction and Internal Validation of a Clinical Decision Rule

Leroy S, Romanello C, Smolkin V, et al (Univ of Oxford, UK; Univ of Udine, Italy; Ha'Emek Med Ctr, Afula, Israel; et al)
J Urol 187:265-271, 2012

Purpose.—Urinary tract infection leads to a diagnosis of moderate or high grade (III or higher) vesicoureteral reflux in approximately 15% of children. Predicting reflux grade III or higher would make it possible to restrict cystog-raphy to high risk cases. We aimed to derive a clinical decision rule to predict vesicoureteral reflux grade III or higher in children with a first febrile urinary tract infection.

Materials and Methods.—We conducted a secondary analysis of prospec-tive series including all children with a first febrile urinary tract infection from the 8 European participating university hospitals.

Results.—A total of 494 patients (197 boys, reflux grade III or higher in 11%) were included. Procalcitonin and ureteral dilatation on ultrasound were significantly associated with reflux grade III or higher and then combined into a prediction model with an ROC AUC of 0.75 (95% CI 0.69—0.81). Given the prespecified constraint of achieving at least 85% sensitivity, our model led to the clinical decision rule, for children with a first febrile urinary tract infection cystography should be performed in cases with ureteral dilatation and serum procalcitonin level 0.17 ng/ml or higher, or without ureteral dilatation (ie ureter not visible) when serum procalcitonin level is 0.63 ng/ml or higher. The rule had 86% sensitivity (95% CI 74—93) with 47% specificity (95% CI 42—51). Internal cross-validation produced 86% sensitivity (95% CI 79—93) and 43% specificity (95% CI 39—47).

Conclusions.—A clinical decision rule was derived to enable a selective approach to cystography in children with urinary tract infection. The rule predicts high grade vesicoureteral reflux with approximately 85% sensitivity and avoids half of the cystograms that do not find reflux grade III or higher. Further validation is needed before its widespread use.

▶ In the past, a voiding cystourethrogram (VCUG) was recommended in all children with urinary tract infections (UTI). Using this approach, there was over-diagnosis and almost certainly overtreatment of reflux. The goal is to identify patients who will benefit from early diagnosis and treatment. Recent American Academy of Pediatrics recommendations recommend limiting VCUG in infants older than 2 months to those with an abnormal renal ultrasound scan. This approach does not necessarily focus on the clinical characteristics of the individual patient. For example, to better define risk for subsequent UTI, I think a VCUG should be obtained in a 3-month-old with a UTI and bacteremia even if the renal ultrasound scan is normal.

Procalcitonin (PCT) is a sensitive and specific marker for bacterial infections. Elevation is consistent with renal parenchymal involvement (pyelonephritis) at the time of UTI. The role of PCT may be as a surrogate for a positive dimercapto-succinic acid scan (blood test obviously much easier to obtain than the nuclear medicine scan). The authors describe a rule combining ureteral dilation and PCT dilation to predict high-grade reflux. Ureteral dilation was utilized because it is less subjective than the magnitude of renal dilation. Table 3 in the original article shows the performance of the rules. There does not seem to be an advantage when compared with PCT alone. PCT may be a useful adjunct in counseling parents in evaluation after febrile UTI.

D. E. Coplen, MD

Childhood Urinary Tract Infections as a Cause of Chronic Kidney Disease

Salo J, Ikäheimo R, Tapiainen T, et al (Univ of Oulu, Finland; Oulu Univ Hosp, Finland)

Pediatrics 128:840-847, 2011

Objective.—Urinary tract infections (UTIs) in childhood are considered a risk for chronic kidney disease (CKD), but this association is poorly verified. We wanted to determine the etiologic fraction of UTIs in childhood as a cause of CKD.

Methods.—A systematic literature search on the association between childhood UTIs and CKD was conducted, and data for patients with CKD in the area of 1 tertiary care hospital were reviewed.

Results.—In our literature search, we found no patients among the 1576 reviewed cases for whom childhood UTIs were the main cause of subsequent CKD. However, there were 3 patients with childhood UTIs for whom the results of kidney imaging studies were not reported. Of the 366 patients with CKD who were monitored in the Oulu University Hospital, 308 had a specific noninfectious cause of CKD. Of the remaining 58 patients, 13 had a history of UTIs in childhood. In their first imaging studies, all of those 13 patients demonstrated kidney tissue abnormalities, which could have been observed through ultrasonography. Recurrent UTIs in childhood were possibly the cause of CKD in 1 case; therefore, the etiologic fraction of recurrent childhood UTIs as a main cause of CKD was, at most, 0.3%.

Conclusions.—In the absence of structural kidney abnormalities evident in imaging studies after the first childhood UTI, the etiologic fraction of recurrent childhood UTIs as a main cause of CKD seems to be small. A child with normal kidneys is not at significant risk of developing CKD because of UTIs.

► Childhood urinary tract infections (UTIs) can cause renal scarring. It is unclear if these infections and scarring are a significant etiology of chronic kidney disease. An evaluation of the etiology of chronic kidney disease (CKD) in Australia found that routine imaging after UTI and proactive treatment of reflux did not decrease CKD related to renal scarring.[1] There is some thought that some CKD previously ascribed to reflux may actually be congenital dysplasia identified later in life.

The authors use 2 methodologies to evaluate the fraction of CKD with UTI as a major etiologic factor. First, literature review allowed evaluation of 1576 patients with CKD in 10 articles. Table 2 in the original article summarizes the findings, and there were 12 patients of 1576 with symptomatic UTIs in childhood and CKD without a definite noninfectious cause. Second, the authors reviewed data at a single tertiary care center and found that patients with a history of UTI and CKD all had structural abnormalities on their initial renal imaging studies.

These data do not mean that the evaluation and treatment of UTIs are not important. Even if UTIs are a rare cause of CKD, there is morbidity related to the UTIs and prevention is important. Upper tract evaluation with an ultrasound scan and/or DMSA should be obtained in infants with a febrile UTI and perhaps those with multiple UTIs without systemic symptoms. A VCUG should be obtained in children with an abnormal ultrasound scan and those with recurrent febrile UTIs because there is evidence that treatment of high-grade reflux can decrease the frequency of infections.

D. E. Coplen, MD

Reference

1. Craig JC, Irwig LM, Knight JF, Roy LP. Does treatment of vesicoureteric reflux in childhood prevent end-stage renal disease attributable to reflux nephropathy? *Pediatrics.* 2000;105:1236-1241.

The Role of Procalcitonin for Acute Pyelonephritis and Subsequent Renal Scarring in Infants and Young Children

Sheu J-N, Chang H-M, Chen S-M, et al (Chung Shan Med Univ Hosp, Taichung, Taiwan; Chung Shan Med Univ, Taichung, Taiwan)
J Urol 186:2002-2008, 2011

Purpose.—We assessed the usefulness of procalcitonin as a biological marker in diagnosing acute pyelonephritis and for predicting subsequent renal scarring in young children with a first febrile urinary tract infection.

Materials and Methods.—Children 2 years old or younger with a first febrile urinary tract infection were prospectively studied. Renal parenchymal involvement was assessed by ^{99m}Tc-dimercaptosuccinic acid scan within 5 days of admission and after 6 months. Serum samples from all patients were tested for procalcitonin, C-reactive protein and white blood cell count measurements.

Results.—The 112 enrolled patients (age range 24 days to 24 months old) were divided into acute pyelonephritis (76) and lower urinary tract infection (36) groups according to the results of ^{99m}Tc-dimercaptosuccinic acid scans. Median values of procalcitonin, C-reactive protein and white blood cell count at hospitalization were significantly higher in patients with acute pyelonephritis than in those with lower urinary tract infection. The area under receiver operating characteristic curves showed that procalcitonin was superior to C-reactive protein and white blood cell count as a marker for diagnosing acute pyelonephritis. Initial and post-antibiotic treatment procalcitonin values were significantly higher in children with renal scarring than in those without scarring ($p < 0.001$). Procalcitonin values at hospitalization and after treatment were independent predictors of later renal scarring on logistic regression analysis.

Conclusions.—Our results indicate the superior diagnostic accuracy of procalcitonin for predicting acute pyelonephritis in children 2 years old or younger. Higher initial and posttreatment procalcitonin values are independent risk factors for later renal scarring.

▶ Accurate identification of pyelonephritis in children with urinary trackt infection (UTI) guides therapy and subsequent evaluation. Those with renal involvement are at risk for renal injury. The gold standard for acute pyelone-phritis (^{99m}Tc dimercaptosuccinic acid [DMSA] scan) is not uniformly available in all centers. It is expensive and exposes infants to radiation. Biomarkers could effectively assess renal risk. The authors obtained DMSA scans in infants with UTI. The procalcitonin (PCT) level was correlated with the severity of the renal lesion on DMSA (Fig 1 in the original article). Receiver operating characteristic analysis shows that PCT distinguishes acute pyelonephritis from cystitis much better that white cell count and C-reactive protein. Additionally, higher PCT levels correlated with a higher risk of renal scarring 6 months after UTI. As with any biomarker, the cutoff levels may not apply in a given patient. The clin-ical course, presence of renal structural anomalies on ultrasound, and patient age may impact decision making for additional testing.

D. E. Coplen, MD

Utility of Post–Urinary Tract Infection Imaging in Patients With Normal Prenatal Renal Ultrasound
Sasaki J, Parajuli N, Sharma P, et al (Elmhurst Hosp Ctr, NY; et al)
Clin Pediatr 51:244-246, 2012

The American Academy of Pediatrics recommends renal ultrasound (RUS) and voiding cystourethrography (VCUG) for all infants after a first urinary tract infection (UTI). However, many congenital renal anomalies are identified by a prenatal US. At the present time, there are no data regarding the yield of post-UTI imaging among infants who have a docu-mented normal prenatal US. We retrospectively reviewed the charts of all patients <1 year of age with a first UTI who had normal kidneys noted on prenatal US to determine the frequency of abnormal findings. Abnormal RUS and VCUG results were noted in 5.1% (24 of 471) and 20.4% (75 of 368) of infants, respectively. While the abnormal US rate is significantly less than what has been previously reported, the frequency of abnormal VCUGs is similar. These results suggest that a post-UTI RUS may not be needed if the prenatal US was normal. However, a VCUG continues to be indicated.

▶ The authors show that a standard prenatal screening ultrasound scan (US) (obtained at 17 to 22 weeks in obstetric office) reliably excludes most renal-level anomalies in infants with a febrile urinary tract infection (UTI). Obstruc-tion was identified in 1 infant, and a small atrophic kidney was found in another. Nonobstructive dilation was seen in 17 infants. The authors studied only infants that had prenatal imaging/care and hospitalization in the same institution. In most cases, prenatal care is not in the same institution, and the ability to review images and confirm normalcy is difficult. Because US is very easily obtained and obstruction is potentially more devastating than reflux, it is hard to argue against obtaining US, especially in cases in which the infant's fever persists or clinical course is otherwise abnormal.

As expected, the authors identify reflux in 20% of infants with a febrile UTI. The authors conclude that a cystogram is indicated in all infants with a febrile

UTI regardless of the US findings. However, reflux was grade IV (2) and V (5) in only 7 of 76 infants. Based on recent studies, it is unknown if there is a benefit to detecting all infants with reflux, as many will never have another UTI and will outgrow the reflux. Selective utilization of a voiding cystourethrography based on US findings and clinical scenario is a reasonable approach.

D. E. Coplen, MD

30 Quality Improvement

Targeted Antimicrobial Prophylaxis Using Rectal Swab Cultures in Men Undergoing Transrectal Ultrasound Guided Prostate Biopsy is Associated With Reduced Incidence of Postoperative Infectious Complications and Cost of Care

Taylor AK, Zembower TR, Nadler RB, et al (Northwestern Univ Feinberg School of Medicine, Chicago, IL; et al)

J Urol 187:1275-1279, 2012

Purpose.—We evaluated targeted antimicrobial prophylaxis in men undergoing transrectal ultrasound guided prostate biopsy based on rectal swab culture results.

Materials and Methods.—From July 2010 to March 2011 we studied differences in infectious complications in men who received targeted vs standard empirical ciprofloxacin prophylaxis before transrectal ultrasound guided prostate biopsy. Targeted prophylaxis used rectal swab cultures plated on selective media containing ciprofloxacin to identify fluoroquinolone resistant bacteria. Patients with fluoroquinolone susceptible organisms received ciprofloxacin while those with fluoroquinolone resistant organisms received directed antimicrobial prophylaxis. We identified men with infectious complications within 30 days after transrectal ultrasound guided prostate biopsy using the electronic medical record.

Results.—A total of 457 men underwent transrectal ultrasound guided prostate biopsy, and of these men 112 (24.5%) had rectal swab obtained while 345 (75.5%) did not. Among those who received targeted prophylaxis 22 (19.6%) men had fluoroquinolone resistant organisms. There were no infectious complications in the 112 men who received targeted antimicrobial prophylaxis, while there were 9 cases (including 1 of sepsis) among the 345 on empirical therapy ($p = 0.12$). Fluoroquinolone resistant organisms caused 7 of these infections. The total cost of managing infectious complications in patients in the empirical group was $13,219. The calculated cost of targeted vs empirical prophylaxis per 100 men undergoing transrectal ultrasound guided prostate biopsy was $1,346 vs $5,598, respectively. Cost-effectiveness analysis revealed that targeted prophylaxis yielded a cost savings of $4,499 per post-transrectal ultrasound guided prostate biopsy infectious complication averted. Per estimation, 38 men would need to undergo rectal swab before transrectal ultrasound guided prostate biopsy to prevent 1 infectious complication.

Conclusions.—Targeted antimicrobial prophylaxis was associated with a notable decrease in the incidence of infectious complications after transrectal ultrasound guided prostate biopsy caused by fluoroquinolone resistant organisms as well as a decrease in the overall cost of care.

▶ According to the AUA Best Practice Statement, the recommended antimicrobial prophylaxis prior to transrectal prostate needle biopsy (PNB) includes (1) oral fluoroquinolones, (2) intramuscular (IM)/intravenous (IV) first-/second-/third-generation cephalosporins, (3) IM/IV aminoglycoside + (IV metronidazole or IV clindamycin) or (4) IV aztreonam + (IV metronidazole or IV clindamycin). Oral fluoroquinolones are by far the most common agent used, as they are the only option that can be administered orally, and they have been shown to be effective in reducing the incidence of infectious complications following PNB. However, several recent studies have found an increased trend of infectious complications following the procedure, typically due to the presence of fluoroquinolone-resistant organisms. Health care workers and men with previous exposure to fluoroquinolone antibiotics appear to be at increased risk for harboring fluoroquinolone resistance. In men who present with a fever or other signs of infection after PNB, it is very likely that the infection is due to quinolone resistance, and empiric antimicrobial therapy should be chosen accordingly.

The authors of this study found that they were able to reduce the risk of postoperative infectious complications by screening for the presence of fluoroquinolone-resistant organisms using rectal swab cultures. This is a promising preventive measure that deserves additional study.

J. Q. Clemens, MD

31 Training

High Fidelity Simulation Based Team Training in Urology: A Preliminary Interdisciplinary Study of Technical and Nontechnical Skills in Laparoscopic Complications Management
Lee JY, Mucksavage P, Canales C, et al (St Michael's Hosp, Toronto, Ontario, Canada; Univ of California Irvine Med Ctr, Orange)
J Urol 187:1385-1391, 2012

Purpose.—Simulation based team training provides an opportunity to develop interdisciplinary communication skills and address potential medical errors in a high fidelity, low stakes environment. We evaluated the implementation of a novel simulation based team training scenario and assessed the technical and nontechnical performance of urology and anesthesiology residents.

Materials and Methods.—Urology residents were randomly paired with anesthesiology residents to participate in a simulation based team training scenario involving the management of 2 scripted critical events during laparoscopic radical nephrectomy, including the vasovagal response to pneumoperitoneum and renal vein injury during hilar dissection. A novel kidney surgical model and a high fidelity mannequin simulator were used for the simulation. A debriefing session followed each simulation based team training scenario. Assessments of technical and nontechnical performance were made using task specific checklists and global rating scales.

Results.—A total of 16 residents participated, of whom 94% rated the simulation based team training scenario as useful for communication skill training. Also, 88% of urology residents believed that the kidney surgical model was useful for technical skill training. Urology resident training level correlated with technical performance ($p = 0.004$) and blood loss during renal vein injury management ($p = 0.022$) but not with nontechnical performance. Anesthesia resident training level correlated with nontechnical performance ($p = 0.036$). Urology residents consistently rated themselves higher on nontechnical performance than did faculty ($p = 0.033$). Anesthesia residents did not differ in the self-assessment of nontechnical performance compared to faculty assessments.

Conclusions.—Residents rated the simulation based team training scenario as useful for interdisciplinary communication skill training. Urology resident training level correlated with technical performance but not with nontechnical performance. Urology residents consistently overestimated their nontechnical performance.

▶ Changes in medical education (eg, decreased resident work hours, decreased hands-on [console] time, new technologies requiring postgraduate training) and a push by regulatory agencies to validate competence will almost certainly increase the use of simulators in medical education. The authors evaluate not only surgical skills but interdisciplinary communication skills in this simulation model. A nonvalidated checklist was utilized to assess technical skills (Fig 4 in the original article), while validated scales (nonoperative surgeon technical skills) were used to assess interaction with the team. The task-specific checklist was reliable but will need to be validated in further studies. This is a small group of 8 simulations evaluating urology and anesthesiology residents who were not paired based on level of training. The resident performance was evaluated by the institutional faculty members, so complete blinding was difficult. Video recordings were obtained and reviewed. The debriefing session may be the most educational component of the simulation. Further study is required but with appropriately developed models, simulation-based team training will be important in training and assessment.

D. E. Coplen, MD

32 Trauma

Conservative Management vs Early Surgery for High Grade Pediatric Renal Trauma—Do Nephrectomy Rates Differ?
Jacobs MA, Hotaling JM, Mueller BA, et al (Univ of Texas, Southwestern, Dallas; Univ of Washington School of Medicine, Seattle; et al)
J Urol 187:1817-1822, 2012

Purpose.—Guidelines for management of pediatric high grade renal injuries are currently based on limited pediatric data and algorithms from adults, for whom initial nonoperative management is associated with decreased nephrectomy risk. Using a national database, we compared nephrectomy rates between children with high grade renal injury managed conservatively and those undergoing early surgical intervention.

Materials and Methods.—All children with high grade renal injuries were identified in the National Trauma Data Bank®. High grade renal injuries were defined as American Association for the Surgery of Trauma grade IV or V renal injuries. After excluding fatalities within 24 hours of hospitalization, 419 pediatric patients comprised our study cohort. A total of 81 patients underwent early (within 24 hours of hospitalization) surgical intervention, while 338 were initially treated conservatively. Using stratified analysis with adjustment for relevant covariates, we compared nephrectomy rates between these groups.

Results.—Nephrectomy was performed less often in patients treated conservatively (RR 0.24, 95% CI 0.16 to 0.36, adjusted for age, renal injury grade and injury mechanism). The decreased risk of nephrectomy was more marked among children with grade IV vs grade V renal injuries (adjusted RR 0.16, 95% CI 0.08 to 0.23). Multiple procedures were more common in patients initially observed. Of pediatric patients with grade IV and V renal injuries 11% still underwent nephrectomy.

Conclusions.—Conservative management of high grade renal injuries is common in children. Although mechanism of injury and renal injury grade impact initial clinical management decisions, the risk of nephrectomy was consistently decreased in children with high grade renal trauma managed conservatively regardless of injury characteristics.

▶ Regardless of the severity of renal injury, conservative management of renal trauma is recommended. Renal embolization, ureteral stenting, or delayed exploration and nephrectomy may be subsequently indicated. Rarely, marked hemodynamic instability and ureteropelvic junction disruption are indications for emergent exploration. In this series, children were more likely to undergo immediate exploration if they had grade V or penetrating injuries. The 6-fold higher nephrectomy rate in this group may be in part related to the severity of the injury. Unfortunately, the retrospective database analysis does not allow an assessment of the indications for nephrectomy (bleeding, shattered kidney not amenable to reconstruction, or intraoperative instability requiring aggressive treatment). Although nephrectomy may be required in conservatively managed patients (11%), it is unlikely that nephrectomy would have been performed in the same number had all these children been initially managed conservatively. Observed patients may need additional intervention, but a conservative approach to renal trauma almost certainly decreases unnecessary nephrectomy.

D. E. Coplen, MD

A National Study of Trauma Level Designation and Renal Trauma Outcomes
Hotaling JM, Wang J, Sorensen MD, et al (Univ of Washington School of Medicine, Seattle)
J Urol 187:536-541, 2012

Purpose.—We examined the initial management of renal trauma and assessed patterns of management based on hospital trauma level designation.

Materials and Methods.—The National Trauma Data Bank is a comprehensive trauma registry with records from hospitals in the United States and Puerto Rico. Renal injuries treated at a member hospital from 2002 to 2007 were identified. We classified initial management as expectant, minimally invasive (angiography, embolization, ureteral stent or nephrostomy) or open surgical management based on ICD-9 procedure codes. The primary outcome was use of secondary therapies.

Results.—Of 3,247,955 trauma injuries in the National Trauma Data Bank 9,002 were renal injuries (0.3%). High grade injuries demonstrated significantly higher rates of definitive success with the first urological intervention at level I trauma centers vs other trauma centers (minimally invasive 52% vs 26%, p <0.001), and were more likely treated successfully with conservative management (89% vs 82%, p <0.001). When adjusting for other known indices of injury severity, and examining low and high grade injuries, level I trauma centers were 90% more likely to offer an initial trial of conservative management (OR 1.90; 95% CI 1.19, 3.05) and had a 30% lower chance of patients requiring multiple procedures (OR 0.70; 95% CI 0.52, 0.95).

Conclusion.—Following multivariate analysis conservative therapy was more common at level I trauma centers despite the patient population being more severely injured. Initial intervention strategies were also more definitive at level I trauma centers, providing additional support for tiered delivery of trauma care.

▶ Level 1 trauma centers treat more severely injured patients than do non—level 1 centers. Mortality rates, however, after renal trauma, are not significantly higher at these centers despite the higher injury severity score, longer intensive care unit (ICU) stays, and decreased Glasgow Coma scores. Despite the higher acuity level 1 trauma centers are more likely to observe renal injuries. After adjusting for more severe renal injuries, there is improved survival at level I trauma centers. This is likely secondary to better access to fully staffed trauma ICUs that are capable of providing acute trauma care. Studies have clearly found that nontrauma centers deliver less efficient trauma care and have increased mortality rates. Transfer of patients with grades IV and V renal injuries to level I trauma centers should be considered to decrease the number of interventions and likely improve patient survival. Despite the potential flaws of database analysis (eg, improper coding, exclusion of patients with incomplete data entry, overrepresentation of level I and II trauma centers) this article provides additional support for tiered delivery of trauma care.

D. E. Coplen, MD

33 Urethral Reconstruction

Changes in Uroflowmetry Maximum Flow Rates After Urethral Reconstructive Surgery as a Means to Predict for Stricture Recurrence
Erickson BA, Breyer BN, McAninch JW (Univ of California, San Francisco)
J Urol 186:1934-1937, 2011

Purpose.—A reliable, noninvasive screening method for urethral stricture recurrence after urethroplasty is needed. We hypothesized that changes in flow rates on uroflowmetry relative to preoperative values might help predict stricture recurrence.

Materials and Methods.—All men who underwent urethral reconstructive surgery from 2000 to 2009 with adequate preoperative and postoperative uroflowmetry studies were included in the study. Preoperative and postoperative maximum flow rates were compared. The absolute change in maximum flow rate was compared between patients with and those without recurrence as determined by retrograde urethrogram.

Results.—A total of 125 patients treated with urethroplasty were included in the study. Mean ± SD preoperative maximum flow rate was 11.8 ± 9.1 ml per second, which did not vary by stricture length ($p = 0.11$), patient age ($p = 0.46$) or stricture location ($p = 0.58$). The change in maximum flow rate in men without recurrence was 19.2 ± 11.7 vs 0.2 ± 6.4 ml per second ($p < 0.001$) in failed repairs. Setting a change in maximum flow rate of less than 10 ml per second as a screen for stricture recurrence would have resulted in a test sensitivity and specificity of 92% and 78%, respectively. There were 85 men without stricture recurrence who underwent more than 1 postoperative uroflowmetry study. Repeated maximum flow rate values achieved reasonable test reproducibility ($r = 0.52$), further supporting the use of uroflowmetry.

Conclusions.—Change in flow rate after urethral reconstruction represents a promising metric to screen for stricture recurrence that is noninvasive and has a high sensitivity (Fig).

▶ A prior study by these authors showed that uroflow did not accurately predict or indicate stricture recurrence after urethroplasty.[1] There are many factors that affect uroflow. For example, coexisting benign prostatic hyperplasia may result in a lower flow rate despite successful correction of a stricture. Similarly, a younger patient with a postoperative flow rate of 15 mL/sec may not

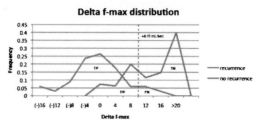

FIGURE.—Distribution of Δ*f*max (preoperative vs postoperative *f*max) in patients with and those without stricture recurrence. *TP*, true positives. *TN*, true negatives. *FP*, false-positives. *FN*, false-negatives. (Reprinted from Erickson BA, Breyer BN, McAninch JW. Changes in Uroflowmetry Maximum Flow Rates After Urethral Reconstructive Surgery as a Means to Predict for Stricture Recurrence. *J Urol.* 2011;186:1934-1937, Copyright 2011, with permission from American Urological Association.)

have a good result if preoperatively the flow was only 10 mL/sec. The authors use the change in postoperative flow rate as a surrogate for successful urethroplasty. The figure shows the findings in their patient population. A change from a flat to a bell-shaped curve postoperatively would likely increase the sensitivity of the flow rate. Because the study population was heavily weighted to patients with failure (26%), the positive predictive value of the test may be falsely increased.

D. E. Coplen, MD

Reference

1. Erickson BA, Breyer BN, McAninch JW. The use of uroflowmetry to diagnose recurrent stricture after urethral reconstructive surgery. *J Urol.* 2010;184:1386-1390.

34 Varicocele

Persistent or recurrent varicocoele after failed varicocoelectomy: Outcome in patients treated using percutaneous transcatheter embolization
Kim J, Shin JH, Yoon HK, et al (Hanyang Univ, Gyeonggi-do, Republic of Korea; Univ of Ulsan, Seoul, Republic of Korea)
Clin Radiol 67:359-365, 2012

Aim.—To determine the efficacy of percutaneous transcatheter embolization in the management of patients with spermatic varicocoeles persisting or recurring after surgery.

Materials and Methods.—Over a period of 10 years, 28 patients (age range 13—55 years) were referred for percutaneous transcatheter embolization of postsurgical, recurrent varicocoeles. Medical documents were retrospectively reviewed to evaluate past surgical history, subjective symptoms, and results of scrotal examination, ultrasound, and semen parameters. Pre-embolization venograms were analysed to assess the anatomy of the testicular vein. The technical and clinical outcomes of embolization were then determined.

Results.—The 28 patients included in the study had undergone laparoscopic varicocoelectomy (39.3%), high retroperitoneal ligation (25%), or inguinal ligation (25%). Subjective symptoms were scrotal pain (60.7%) and a palpable scrotal mass (50%) exclusively on the left side. Venograms revealed abnormalities of the left testicular vein in all cases. Embolization was technically successful in all but two cases, thus yielding an occlusion rate of 93%; a single case of suspected thrombophlebitis was the only complication. After excluding two, technically unsuccessful cases and one patient who was lost to follow-up, 25 patients underwent scrotal examination after embolization, which revealed complete resolution in 20 cases (80%), partial improvement in four cases (16%), and no improvement in a single case (4%). Among the follow-up group of patients, of the 12 who initially presented with scrotal pain, six (50%) were symptom-free and four (33.3%) had partial improvement.

Conclusion.—Percutaneous transcatheter embolization of the testicular vein is technically feasible and effective for managing postsurgical recurrent varicocoeles.

▶ Percutaneous transcatheter embolization can be performed as either a primary or salvage procedure in the management of spermatic varicocoeles. Primary embolization has equivalent efficacy when compared with open (subinguinal or retroperitoneal) or laparoscopic ligations. Embolization is historically associated with a lower incidence of postoperative hydrocele, likely because there is no disruption of the lymphatics in the spermatic cord. In secondary cases, embolization helps avoid scarring and the increased potential of arterial or lymphatic injury. The authors used embolization (coils or foam sclerosant) to treat recurrent (18) and persistent (10) varicoceles after prior surgery. Venography showed the presence of patent drainage pathway to the pampiniform plexus in all patients. Iliac venography was also performed to exclude aberrant collaterals. Embolization was not technically feasible when the testicular vein could not be directly catheterized in 2 patients. The procedure was associated with morbidity in only 1 patient felt to have thrombosis of the pampiniform plexus from reflux of the sclerosing agent. The procedure was successful in 80% of patients. The reported data do not allow insight into the cause of the failures. When experienced interventional radiologists are available, venography and embolization should be strongly considered in the management of recurrent varicoceles.

D. E. Coplen, MD

Article Index

Chapter 6: Renal Tumors

Chapter 7: Prostate Cancer

Chapter 8: Testicular Cancer

Chapter 9: Sexual Function

Chapter 14: Neurogenic Reconstruction

Chapter 15: Vesicoureteral Reflux

Chapter 16: Male Incontinence/Voiding Dysfunction

Chapter 17: Benign Prostatic Hyperplasia

Chapter 18: Bladder Cancer

Chapter 19: Urethral Strictures

Chapter 25: Voiding Dysfunction/Enuresis

Chapter 26: Imaging

Chapter 27: Pediatric Imaging

Chapter 28: Pediatric Laparoscopy/Reconstruction

Chapter 29: Pediatric Urinary Tract Infection

Chapter 30: Quality Improvement

Chapter 31: Training

Chapter 32: Trauma

Chapter 33: Urethral Reconstruction

Chapter 34: Varicocele

Author Index

Printed and bound by CPI Group (UK) Ltd, Croydon, CR0 4YY

14/05/2025

01870851-0001